DVD CONTENTS

1. ABC of Hysterectomy

2. Myomectomy

Videos by
Dr Resad Pasic
President
The American Association of
Gynecologic Laparoscopist (AAGL) 2009

A Manual of
Minimally Invasive
GYNECOLOGICAL SURGERY

Editor

Meenu Agarwal
MBBS DGO DNB (Diplomate of National Board)
Dip in Gynecological Endoscopy (Germany)
Fellow Advanced Endometriosis and Laser Surgeries (Austria)
Training in IVF (Germany)
Bachelor in Endoscopy, Gynecological Endoscopic Surgeon
(Certified by European Academy of Gynaecological Surgery)
Endoscopic Surgeon and Infertility Specialist
Morpheus Bliss Fertility Centre
Consultant Gynecologist
Ruby Hall Clinic and Grant Medical Foundation
Pune, Maharashtra, India

Co-editors

Liselotte Mettler MD PhD
Professor Emeritus
Department of Obstetrics and Gynecology
University Hospitals Schleswig-Holstein
Kiel, Germany

Ibrahim Alkatout MD PhD MA
Senior Consultant
Department of Obstetrics and Gynecology
University Hospitals Schleswig-Holstein
Kiel, Germany

Forewords

Liselotte Mettler

Ibrahim Alkatout

Prashant Mangeshikar

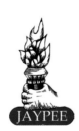

JAYPEE *The Health Sciences Publisher*

New Delhi | London | Philadelphia | Panama

Jaypee Brothers Medical Publishers (P) Ltd

Headquarters

Jaypee Brothers Medical Publishers (P) Ltd
4838/24, Ansari Road, Daryaganj
New Delhi 110 002, India
Phone: +91-11-43574357
Fax: +91-11-43574314
Email: jaypee@jaypeebrothers.com

Overseas Offices

J.P. Medical Ltd
83, Victoria Street, London
SW1H 0HW (UK)
Phone: +44 20 3170 8910
Fax: +44 (0)20 3008 6180
Email: info@jpmedpub.com

Jaypee-Highlights Medical Publishers Inc
City of Knowledge, Bld. 237, Clayton
Panama City, Panama
Phone: +1 507-301-0496
Fax: +1 507-301-0499
Email: cservice@jphmedical.com

Jaypee Medical Inc
The Bourse
111 South Independence Mall East
Suite 835, Philadelphia, PA 19106, USA
Phone: +1 267-519-9789
Email: jpmed.us@gmail.com

Jaypee Brothers Medical Publishers (P) Ltd
17/1-B Babar Road, Block-B, Shaymali
Mohammadpur, Dhaka-1207
Bangladesh
Mobile: +08801912003485
Email: jaypeedhaka@gmail.com

Jaypee Brothers Medical Publishers (P) Ltd
Bhotahity, Kathmandu
Nepal
Phone: +977-9741283608
Email: kathmandu@jaypeebrothers.com

Website: www.jaypeebrothers.com
Website: www.jaypeedigital.com

Inquiries for bulk sales may be solicited at: jaypee@jaypeebrothers.com

A Manual of Minimally Invasive Gynecological Surgery

First Edition: **2015**

ISBN 978-93-5152-766-4

Printed at Sanat Printers, Kundli

Dedicated to

My parents,
for giving me the education and freedom
to explore my dreams, and
my dear husband Dr Sanjay Agarwal,
for being my ultimate support

—Meenu Agarwal

All laparoscopic surgeons,
who in the face of criticism and skepticism
continued to pursue the development of
minimally invasive techniques

—Liselotte Mettler
—Ibrahim Alkatout

CONTRIBUTORS

Artin Ternamian MD FRCSC
Associate Professor
Department of Obstetrics and Gynecology
Faculty of Medicine
University of Toronto
Director of Gynecologic Endoscopy
St. Joseph's Health Centre
Toronto, Canada

Carlos Ferreira MD
Unidade Local de Saúde de Matosinhos

Dilip Walke MBBS MD
Founder Director and Consultant
Gynecology and Obstetrics
Aster Medipoint Hospital
Pune, Maharashtra, India

Geetanjali Joshi MS
Consultant Oncosurgeon and
Laparoscopic Oncosurgeon
Galaxy Care Laparoscopy Institute
Pune, Maharashtra, India

Gregoris Grimbizis
Aristotle University of Thessaloniki
First Department of Obstetrics and Gynecology
Papageorgiou Hospital
Thessaloniki, Greece

Guenter K Noé
Medical Director
Communal Hospital of the City of Dormagen
Head of Department Department OB/GYN
comunal Clinics Rhein-Kreis-Neuss
Witten/Herdecke, University
Witten, Germany

Helder Ferreira MD
Associate Professor
Head of Gynecology, Minimally Invasive
Surgery
Centro Hospitalar do Porto-Porto, Portugal
Life and Health Sciences Research Institute
(ICVS)
School of Health Sciences
University of Minho, Braga, Portugal
ICVS/3B's PT Government Associate
Laboratory
Braga/Guimarães, Portugal

Ibrahim Alkatout MD PhD MA
Senior Consultant
Head, Kiel School of Gynecological Endoscopy
Department of Obstetrics and Gynecology
University Hospitals Schleswig-Holstein
Campus Kiel, Kiel, Germany

JP Rath MD
Consultant, Critical Care Obstetrics
Nandadeep Critical Care Center
Pune, Maharashtra, India

Linda Shiber MD MSc
Instructor of OB/GYN and
Minimally Invasive Gynecology Surgery
Department of Obstetrics and Gynecology
University of Louisville School of Medicine
Louisville, Kentucky, US

Liselotte Mettler MD PhD
Professor Emeritus
Department of Obstetrics and Gynecology
University Hospitals Schleswig-Holstein
Kiel, Germany

Madhuri Kashyap MD (Ob and Gyn)
Diploma in Endoscopy (Germany)
Consultant Gynecologist and Endoscopic Surgeon
Director, Kashyap Nursing Home
Panel Consultant Ruby Hall Clinic
Pune, Maharashtra, India

Manisha Bijlani MD (Anesthesiology)
Associate Professor (Anesthesiology)
MA Rangoonwalla Dental College, Pune
Maharashtra University of Health Sciences (MUHS)
Nashik, Maharashtra, India

Meenu Agarwal MBBS DGO DNB
(Diplomat of national Board)
Dip in Gynecological Endoscopy (Germany)
Fellow Advanced Endometriosis and Laser
Surgeries (Austria)
Training in IVF (Germany)
Bachelor in Endoscopy, Gynecological
Endoscopic Surgeon (Certified by European
Academy of Gynaecological Surgery)
Endoscopic Surgeon and Fertility Specialist
Morpheus Bliss Fertility Centre
Consultant Gynecologist
Ruby Hall Clinic and Grant Medical Foundation
Pune, Maharashtra, India

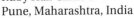

Nagendra Sardeshpande DNB FCPS DGO DFP
MBBS
Consultant Endoscopic Surgeon
Bombay Hospital Institute of Medical Sciences
Mumbai, Maharashtra, India

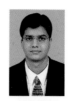

Nalini Bagul MD DGO Bachelor of Endoscopy
(Europe)
Director, Dr Bagul Hospital
Nashik, Maharashtra, India
Consultant, Wockhardt Hospital Nashik,
Maharashtra, India and Many Multispecialty
Hospitals (Laparoscopy)

Nandan Purandare MS (obgyn)
Fellow in Gynecology Laparoscopy
Galaxy Care Laparoscopy Institiute
Pune, Maharashtra, India

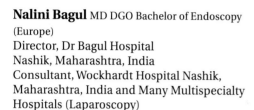

Namita Joshi DGO
Consultant
Morpheus Bliss Fertility Center
Pune, Maharashtra, India

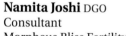

Pranay Shah MD DGO
Gynecologist and Endoscopic Surgeon
Bhatia, Jaslok, HN Reliance
Saifee Hospitals, Mumbai, Maharashtra, India

Resad Pasic MD PhD
Professor
Director of the Section of Advanced Gynecologic
Endoscopy
Fellowship Director of AAGL
Fellowship in Minimally Invasive Gynecologic
Surgery
Department of Obstetrics and Gynecology
University of Louisville School of Medicine
Louisville, Kentucky, USA

Seema Puntambekar MD DGO
Consultant Laparoscopic Gynecologist
Galaxy Care Laparoscopy Institute
Pune, Maharashtra, India

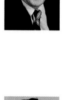

Shailesh Puntambekar MS
Medical Director
Consultant Laparoscopic and
Robotic Oncosurgeon
Galaxy Care Laparoscopy Institute
Pune, Maharashtra, India

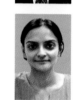

Shinjini Pande MS
Gynecology Laparoscopy Surgeon
Nalini Endoscopy Unit
Mumbai, Maharashtra, India

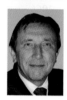

Stephan Gordts MD
Scientific Director Leuven Institute for Fertility
and Embryology (LIFE)
Leuven, Belgium

Themistoklis Mikos MSc MD PhD
First Department of Obstetrics and Gynecology
School of Medicine, Aristotle University of
Thessaloniki, Papageorgiou General Hospital,
Thessaloniki, Greece

Thomas Lang MD MSc
Clinical Affiliate Assistant Professor of
Biomedical Science Charles E Schmidt
College of Medicine
Florida Atlantic University, Boca Raton,
Florida, USA
Instructor of Obstetrics and Gynecology
and Minimally Invasive Gynecology Surgery
Department of Obstetrics and Gynecology
University of Louisville School of Medicine,
Louisville, Kentucky, USA

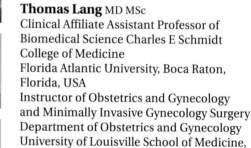

Ulrich Honemeyer MD
Professor
Dubrovnik International University, Croatia

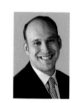

Vivek Salunke MD
Gynecology Endoscopy Surgeon
Nalini Endoscopy Unit
Mumbai, Maharashtra, India

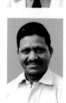

FOREWORD

The book *A Manual of Minimally Invasive Gynecological Surgery* is an example of global medical and, in particular, Indo-German cooperation. It gives us great pleasure to invite you to study this new landmark in gynecological endoscopy. This book further complements the *Practical Manual for Laparoscopic and Hysteroscopic Gynecological Surgery*, released in 2013 by the same publishing house.

For the last 30 years, the Kiel School of Gynecological Endoscopy has welcomed annually more than 50 Indian gynecologists for training. It is a special pleasure to see that a number of these colleagues have surpassed their teachers in their development. Two of our teachers, Kurt Semm (1927–2003) and Thoralf Schollmeyer (1962–2014), laid the foundation for gynecological endoscopy worldwide, and their spirit is to be found within all the chapters. The editors are proud to have been able to weave together a rich diversity of subjects and authors from different specialties. The content is current, concise, and well-presented. The scholarly contribution of basic endoscopic topics will help to generate a greater understanding of gynecological endoscopy. With the ever-accelerating progress of new technologies, this book elegantly demonstrates where we are in 2015. The publication of *A Manual of Minimally Invasive Gynecological Surgery* is timely and the book will serve as a valuable resource for all laparoendoscopic surgeons and their trainees.

Liselotte Mettler
Professor Emeritus
Department of Obstetrics and Gynecology
University Hospitals Schleswig-Holstein
Kiel, Germany

Ibrahim Alkatout
Senior Consultant
Department of Obstetrics and Gynecology
University Hospitals Schleswig-Holstein
Kiel, Germany

FOREWORD

It is an honor that I have been asked to write the Foreword to this interesting book: *A Manual of Minimally Invasive Gynecological Surgery.*

As newer technologies evolve, there is further update in publications with advances in instrumentation and technique. This book covers both laparoscopic as well as hysteroscopic surgery. Written by a mixed array of contributors ranging from youthful endoscopists with great enthusiasm to internationally known exponents known for their expertise in gynecological endoscopy, this book has great promise to the gynecologists in practice as well as in training.

The chapters give practical advice and focus on tips and tricks on various techniques in gynecological endoscopic surgery. The operative photographs and line drawings aid the understanding of the chapters. Almost all operations in gynecology can now be safely performed via endoscopy and the purpose of the book is to serve as a primer to the budding surgeons to be trained in the nuances of minimally invasive gynecological surgery.

This book, edited by Meenu Agarwal, Liselotte Mettler and Ibrahim Alkatout, should be a must-read book and housed in all postgraduate medical libraries that will help promote the practice of safe gynecological endoscopic surgery.

Prashant Mangeshikar
President
International Society for Gynecological Endoscopy (ISGE)

PREFACE

Laparoscopic surgery is an evolving science and it was my passion to place before the fraternity, innovations and advances in a concise and comprehensible manner. It has been my sincere effort to bring specifics about instrumentation and share our experience in both basics and advances of this growing branch. The pearls and pitfalls have been highlighted at every step so as to guide the practicing gynecologist.

The first section covers the basic OT armamentarium and safe access into peritoneal cavity for the residents and gynecologists to begin their journey of endoscopy. A very meticulous presentation of "port placement" will be highly appreciated. There is a lot to learn about newer energy sources and correct methodology of suturing, which has been covered in detail. The global understanding of various surgical procedures by the pioneers in the respective fields is the highlight of this book.

Pelvic floor repair, an upcoming surgical modality by laparoscopic route, has been included to add greater value to the content.

Every modality has its pitfalls. We have, in detail, covered the management of complications of laparoscopy and medicolegal aspects in the form of clinical cases.

The adage "old is gold" does not stand true for hysteroscopic surgery which has grown by leaps and bounds in the last few years. The instrumentation and the procedure of hysteroscopy have been discussed in detail. Again a very balanced description of complications along with fluid management during hysteroscopy has been incorporated in this section on hysteroscopy.

The journey to completion of this book has been both enlightening and rewarding. It is hoped that it will do the same for its readers.

Meenu Agarwal

In less than 30 years, so much has happened in the young field of microinvasive surgery. The major crossroad has already been passed—the transition from large incision surgery to microincision surgery. The upcoming questions are the feasibility and efficacy of advanced surgical techniques and the right selection of alternative methods. Furthermore, we should not forget manual tools that have been valuable for centuries.

Every gynecological specialty is seeing new and innovative methods using minimally invasive surgery. This is so important to our society not only because of the benefit to patients in the form of rapid recovery and minimal discomfort, but also because of the promise it holds in providing improved healthcare in a cost-effective, outcome-oriented way.

This landmark publication, encompassing hysteroscopy and laparoscopy, is a result of the collaboration of specialists from all over the world sharing their knowledge and experience. This book *A Manual of Minimally Invasive Gynecological Surgery,* reveals the multifaceted possibilities for the application of minimally invasive surgery and describes all currently available techniques.

It is an honor for us from the Kiel School of Gynecological Endoscopy to be the co-editors with our distinguished Indian colleague, Meenu Agarwal.

This book represents an important work and is an excellent addition to any reference library. It brings together ideas from the experts who are helping to forge our future practice and by its very nature helps us enhance the science and art of surgical practice. Our and your patients will be very grateful.

Liselotte Mettler
Ibrahim Alkatout

ACKNOWLEDGMENTS

Writing this book has been a great learning experience for me. Right from the inception to the completion with all the highs and lows, it has been a roller-coaster ride. It was a mammoth task to have the globally renowned endoscopic surgeons to contribute to this book, but each one came forward on this common platform with the only mission of propagating safe endoscopic surgery.

I express my heartfelt gratitude to all the contributing authors, pioneers in their respective fields, who in spite of their busy schedule took out time to write the chapters of immense scientific value.

I profusely thank the publishers M/s Jaypee Brothers Medical Publishers (P) Ltd, New Delhi, India and their entire team, especially Shri Jitendar P Vij (Group Chairman), Mr Sabarish Menon (Commissioning Editor) and Mr Tupe (Branch In-Charge, Pune, Maharashtra, India). It was a pleasant experience working with them.

My special thanks to Lilo, for her love and invaluable contribution toward this book. I feel privileged to have her as the co-author.

A heartfelt gratitude to Dr Ibrahim Alkatout for not only coauthoring this book, but also for making sure that the work is completed on time.

My sincere thanks to my support team of Dr Namita Joshi and Shanta Borkar who have always completed the work assigned, on time, and Dr Pramod Tejane for his contribution in sketching images for the book.

I am grateful to Dr Resad Pasic for contributing videos for the book for better understanding of the techniques.

My journey toward excellence in laparoscopic surgery would not have been easy without the unwavering support of my very dear friend Dr Madhuri Kashyap. I thank her from the bottom of my heart.

I thank Dr Shirin Venkat for her loving presence and guidance.

I greatly appreciate the wholehearted support of my family members, especially my dear husband Sanjay and my loving boys Varun and Aryan, who have been extremely caring and supportive of my work.

I take this opportunity to thank all my teachers who nurtured my skills, taught me and enabled my skills in laparoscopic surgery. The special mention here are: Col AK Srivastava, Dr Rakesh Sinha, Prof Lisolette Mettler, Prof Jeorge Keckstein and last but not the least, Dr Prashant Mangeshikar, for being my mentor in my endeavor toward excellence in endoscopic surgery.

CONTENTS

SECTION 2

The Learning Curve

SECTION 4

Special Situations for Minimally Invasive Approach

SECTION 5

Complications

SECTION 6

Hysteroscopy

Section 1

TO KNOW YOUR BASICS

- Equipment in Laparoscopic Surgery
- Peritoneal Access in Laparoscopy
- Port Placement in Laparoscopy

"Give me six hours to chop down a tree and I will spend the first four sharpening the axe."

Abraham Lincoln

CHAPTER 1

Equipment in Laparoscopic Surgery

Helder Ferreira

"Before a new instrument is used, the surgeon should know and test it. It is always better to test a device before a procedure than during it!"

▌ INTRODUCTION

Over the last 30 years, laparoscopic procedures have become standard in most surgical diseases. The rise of abdominal and pelvic laparoscopic surgery has been a true revolution in medical practice. The concept of minimally invasive approach, with all its advantages such as quicker recovery, shorter hospital stay and a far superior aesthetic results has been gaining more and more supporters among the international surgical community. The old paradigm that a big incision meant a big surgeon has dramatically changed.

The equipment and instruments for performing these minimally access procedures has, over the years, greatly improved. Following the surgeons' demands, the increasing investment and research on better tools have provided more sophisticated and efficient equipment that offers lower risk and thus higher safety to our patients.

An organized and well-equipped operating room is essential for successful laparoscopy. The surgical team and the operating room staff should be familiar with the instruments and their functions. If they are not aware of an instrument's mechanism of action, it can interfere with surgery progression, increasing not only risks for patients but also surgeon's anxiety and fatigue. Each instrument should be inspected periodically. Scissors, graspers, trocars, trocar sleeves are checked for loose or broken tips,

even if the same instruments were used during a previous procedure.

One of the most important benefits of laparoscopy is the magnified vision offered by the optics and high definition cameras and thus better identifies anatomical structures and dissection plans. This improved image often permits a more precise surgical gesture, better hemostasis and probably less postoperative adhesions.

Almost all instruments available for laparotomy are now available in a specialized form for laparoscopy. Instruments and devices that are used in laparoscopy include the laparoscope (camera), trocars and port devices, instruments for dissection, hemostasis and ultrasound. Laparoscopic instruments attempt to reproduce the effects of conventional laparotomic instruments: Grasping, dissecting, cutting and coagulation.

▌ LAPAROSCOPY VERSUS OPEN SURGERY

Operative laparoscopy requires an advanced degree of technical skills and training. The smaller size incisions and instruments implicate a huge degree of precision only dealt by imaging systems of high magnification.

In spite of the same final objective, we have to distinguish the laparoscopic field from the open surgery field. Contrary to open surgery where surgeons have a direct view and manually manipulate and palpate tissues during the operation, the challenge in laparoscopy is the absence of stereoscopic vision and the need of transpositioning the movement of surgeons' hand through a long small diameter trocar creating one or more output functions at the distal part of body cavity.

Some of the specificities of laparoscopic surgery are:

❑ *Limited field of vision controlled by an assistant*: Surgeons need an increased cognitive and physical load to perform the surgery (i.e. the instruments may intermittently disappear from the surgeon's vision while manipulating structures).

❑ *Reduced depth perception:* The monitors used in laparoscopic surgery filter three-dimensional cues from the operative field such as interposition or overlap, lighting, outline and texture.[1] The effect of reduction in depth cues can be inferred from performance differences under different viewing conditions, as 3D video systems that restore stereoscopic vision are currently available.

❑ *Impaired hand-eye coordination:* The main variables are the location of the monitor, degree of amplification, mirrored movement and misorientation.[2]

❑ *Motion limitation:* The trocar restricts movement by acting as invariant points.[3] The surgeon´s dexterity is affected because the range of motion is reduced to four degrees of freedom compared to six needed to perform free motion. This movement restriction leads to increased physical discomfort.

❑ *Reduction of haptic feedback:* The role of haptic feedback is of special interest because it is used in important decision-making scenarios such as the discrimination of healthy versus abnormal tissues, identification of organs and motor control. In laparoscopic surgery, it is reduced but not absent as in robotic surgery.[4-5]

❑ *Vision is dependent on the cleanliness of laparoscopic optic, intra-abdominal smoke and light absorption:* Irrigation, blood, organic fluids, intra-abdominal pressure and smoke can impair surgeon vision. The irrigation of the operative field should be minimal as the mixture of blood with serum alters light absorption creating difficulties to discriminate structures and surgical planes. Equilibrium is necessary between smoke evacuation and pneumoperitoneum preservation.

▮ IMAGING DEVICES

Minimally invasive surgery resulted from the introduction of new imaging devices to look at internal organs through pericentimetric or shorter incisions. Surgical scopes are recognized as very old medical instruments conceived many centuries ago when simple hollow tubes were used to observe intracorporeal cavities. Philip Bozzini in 1805 used the first illuminated scope consisted in a viewing tube with a series of mirrors which reflected light from a burning wax candle. However, only in the 20th century, a light scope was used to perform a diagnostic laparoscopy and only after the success obtained with laparoscopic cholecystectomies (1986), the medical industry started to develop better imaging and optical devices.[6]

Although the skepticism of some during the years, today we are facing a rapid advancement of minimally invasive surgery in different disciplines and pathologies, and in parallel, new imaging devices are appearing. The surgeon must be familiar with these developments.

Laparoscope: Traditionally, the laparoscope is a rigid endoscope which is made of an outer ring of optical fibers, used to transmit light into the abdominal and pelvic cavity and an inner core of rod lenses via which the illuminated operative field is captured by a camera. Digital imaging chips located within the camera allow the image from the scope to be transmitted to an external display.

Various different types of laparoscope are available, specified in terms of overall length, number of rods, diameter and angle of view. The diameter of laparoscopes varies from 3 mm to 12 mm and the objective located at the distal end offers an angle of view from 0 to 120 degrees. The brightness of the image is lower in thinner scopes, due to less light transmission through the central channel lenses. However, with the improvement in the optical fiber technology, even laparoscopes with 3 mm of diameter are able to produce brighter and clearer images. The "angle of view" enables the operator to see objects that might otherwise be out of camera view. A 30° telescope provides a total field of view of 152° enabling the visualization of the anterior abdominal wall and working around masses or within deeper spaces. A 0° telescope provides a field of view of 76°, but offers a panoramic view and more usual perspective (Fig. 1). There is a laparoscope model that has the possibility of changing the view angle from 0° to 120° (Fig. 2). Flexible tip laparoscopes are also available.

In gynecology, telescopes without instrument channels are used in the majority of cases, as they give a better overview and offer better image resolution. However, in some cases, it may be useful to use telescopes with an integrated instrument channel (Fig. 3). These laparoscopes are generally 0° straightforward scopes. The diameter of the instrument channel is 5–7 mm; thus, a correspondingly large instrument can be inserted. CO_2 laser can also be connected to this laparoscope.

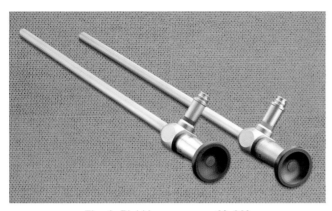

Fig. 1: Rigid laparoscopes 0°, 30°

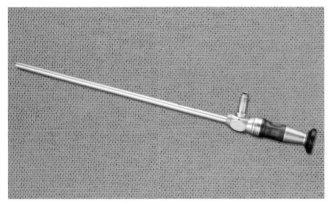

Fig. 2: EndoCameleon® by Karl Storz (direction of view can be adjusted ranging from 0°–120°)

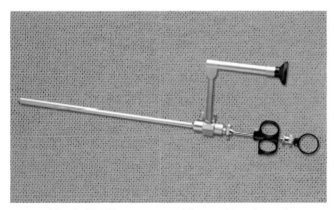

Fig. 3: Rigid laparoscope with a working channel

In gynecology, a good application for these instruments is in performing laparoscopic sterilization. In addition, tissue fragments or biopsy specimens can also be extracted with the aid of a grasping forceps introduced through the telescope's instrument channel. On other hand, a disadvantage of using telescopes with instrument channels is the deterioration in image quality. This is due to the lower light intensity that can be picked up by the video camera, when compared with telescopes that do not have an instrument channel.

The light sources and light cables: No light, no laparoscopy! The light is transmitted from a light source (located separately off the patient table) to the operative field through a light cable and the fiber bundle in the laparoscope. High-intensity light is created with bulbs of halogen gas, xenon gas or mercury vapor. The bulbs are available in different potencies (150 and 300 Watts) and should be chosen based on the type of procedure being performed.

Nowadays, there are two types of light cables available: fiberoptic or liquid crystal gel cables. Fiberoptic cables are made up of a bundle of optical fiber glass thread swaged at both ends. Light transmission occurs by total internal reflection and is improved with an increasing number of light fibers and increased diameter cable. These cables offer little light loss but are less durable than the liquid-filled light guide cables, because, some optical fibers break with continuous usage. However, the liquid crystal gel cables are made more rigid by a metal sheath, which makes them less flexible and more difficult to maintain and store.

Laparoscopic Camera

A high quality image is essential to perform the procedure safely. The laparoscopic camera has undergone some of the biggest changes in the last decade (Fig. 4). Most endoscopic surgery is being done now with high-definition technology. With this improved image quality cameras, the surgeon can more readily identify the relevant anatomy. Nowadays, systems that produce three-dimensional images are currently under development and seem to facilitate surgical performance.[7]

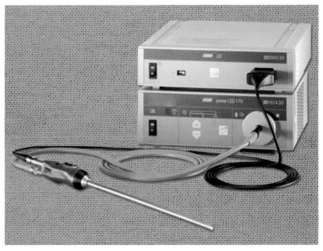

Fig. 4: 3D Laparoscopic camera by Karl Storz

Video Monitors

The sizes of the screen vary. To accommodate high-definition cameras, the medical industry has adopted the flat-panel monitors whose resolution determines a better image. Some monitors include sterile touchscreen functionality, offering the surgeon control over the entire imaging system via the monitor.

Video Recording Systems

The video recording systems document and record the performed procedures. They are of paramount importance for scientific and educational purposes.

▌CO_2 GAS INSUFFLATOR

The pneumoperitoneum offers the surgical field and the access for the procedure itself. Conventional gas insufflators are sufficient for a purely diagnostic laparoscopy. However, in surgical laparoscopies performed today, accurate pressure control insufflators are necessary to compensate considerable volume losses that occur, for example due to frequent suction of irrigation solutions using high-performance irrigation-aspiration units. High-flow CO_2 insufflators are a basic prerequisite for surgical laparoscopy, as they monitor intra-abdominal pressure constantly and halt the flow immediately when the set intra-abdominal pressure is reached. Electronically controlled insufflators have become the preferred choice in this respect. The insufflator's display indicates all the vital information that is needed for the surgeon (Fig. 5):

❑ Patient's intra-abdominal pressure (should not exceed a value of 15 mm Hg)

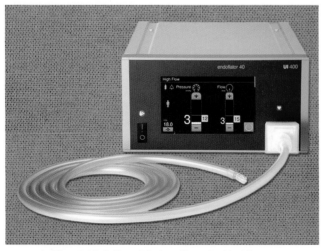

Fig. 5: High-flow CO_2 insufflator by Karl Storz

❑ Rate of inflow of the gas
❑ Volume of CO_2 insufflated
❑ Gas reserve.

When the pressurized CO_2 expands, it cools down and has the potential to reduce the body temperature of the patient. Some insufflators are equipped with facilities to heat the CO_2 before its passage into the abdomen. In order to avoid the disadvantages of CO_2 insufflation, gasless laparoscopy could be an alternative.

▌PORTS OF ENTRANCE IN ABDOMINAL CAVITY

Veress Needle

Disposable and reusable Veress needles for creating pneumoperitoneum are available. Veress needle is used to create the initial pneumoperitoneum. A trocar can be introduced safely because the distance from the abdominal wall to the organs is increased. The Veress needle technique is the most widely practiced method to access the peritoneal cavity. Veress needle compromises two components—an outer hollow needle with a sharp beveled edge, and an inner, spring-loaded, retractable blunt obturator with the stop position beyond the tip of the hollow needle. Once the peritoneal cavity is entered, the blunt obturator is just forwarded by the spring-force and protrudes beyond the tip of the hollow needle, thus preventing from iatrogenic visceral and vascular injuries.

The reusable type should be preferred to reduce the costs of laparoscopic surgery. Verress needles are available in three lengths: 80 mm, 100 mm and 120 mm. In the thin patients, with scaphoid abdomen, an 80 mm Verress needle should be used. In obese patients, a 120 mm Verress needle is preferred. Disposable needles do not require cleaning or sterilization procedures. The Veress needle must be kept in perfect condition to ensure that the mandarin slides easily into the protective sleeve. The surgeon must have full knowledge of all safety features of the mandarin. The Verress needle should be held between the thumb and the index finger during insertion. When the needle is inserted through the abdominal wall, passage through the fascia into the peritoneal cavity can be recognized as a tactile "popping" sensation.

Trocars

The trocars establish a small interface between the surgeon and the surgical field. The trocars are the accesses through which the surgeon goes inside the abdominal cavity,

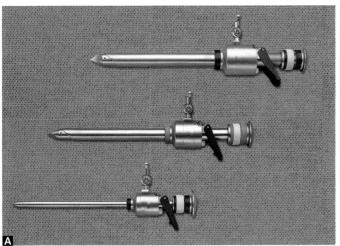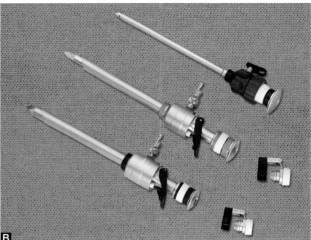

Figs 6A and B: Reusable trocars 3.5, 5.5, 11, 12 (Karl Storz)

establishing a shaft and support for different instruments. In the time of cost reduction, the use of disposable trocars is clearly diminishing. There are very high quality reusable trocars in the market that avoid the use of disposable ones (Figs 6A and B).

In general, trocars with various diameters are used in surgical endoscopy. The standard sizes are 3.5, 5.5, 11, 12, 15 and 22 mm but there has been a recent trend towards the use of smaller trocars, even for advanced procedures.

All trocars have a flapper or trumpet valve. Spherical and flap valves allow a quickly change of operating instruments, as this change can be carried out without activating the valve mechanism. Trumpet valves are mostly found in telescope trocars. The telescope is protected from contamination by tissue and blood particles during insertion by pressing the trumpet valve.

Trocars tips may be sharp or blunt, radially expanding, shielded and/or transparent. Sharp, pyramidal trocar tips can be positioned relatively easily; however, the sharp edges can sometimes damage smaller blood vessels and other organs. By using spherical, blunt, trocar tips, the blood vessels are pushed aside and protected to a large degree. Sometimes, however, greater pressure has to be exerted during insertion. Since the skin incision for the auxiliary puncture is carried out under transillumination and the puncture itself is in full view, the choice of trocar tip here can be regarded as being of secondary importance. Better protection to prevent the trocar slipping out of the intraperitoneal space is provided by sheaths with screw threading. However, these cause increased trauma to both the abdominal wall and the peritoneum. Trocar reducers may facilitate the surgery in case you use smaller instruments.

▌INSTRUMENTS

Dissection and grasping instruments: Dissect means "methodically cut up (a body or plant) in order to study its internal parts". Dissection is probably the finest part of a surgery. Almost all standard instruments available for laparotomy are available in a specialized form to fit through an endoscopic 3–20 mm port.

Grasping forceps have been designed for tissue manipulation, and may be locking (ratcheted) and no locking (nonratcheted). Some forceps are broad and flat, while others are finer and made for delicate tissue handling (Figs 7A and B).

Atraumatic stabilization of structures is achieved by fine grasping forceps multiserrated and with a round tip. With an atraumatic forceps the surgeon is able to expose and perform the countertraction needed to dissect and to suture. For example, prehension of the Fallopian tube or the ureter. A Babcock-type atraumatic grasper with a ratcheted scissors handle can be particularly useful in handling the mesentery or adnexal structures.

Toothed forceps (claw forceps) are used to grasp and liberate solid organs. In a laparoscopic cyst extirpation, to fix the ovary properly and remove the cystic capsule, it is crucial strong grasping forceps. Forceps with pointed ends are used for tissue dissection and surgical plane development.

Dissecting and grasping instruments are available in either reusable or disposable forms. The disposable instruments are typically less cost-effective, although they have the advantage of being available (when properly stocked), and the cutting edges are always sharp, whereas no disposable instruments may be in the process of cleaning

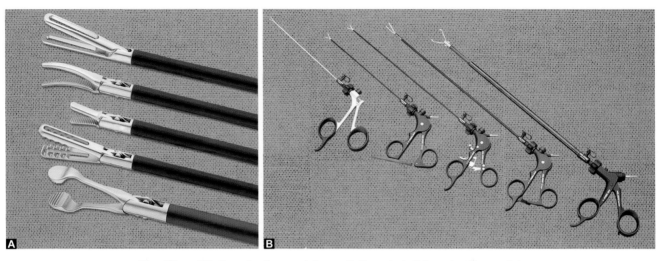

Figs 7A and B: Grasping forceps (atraumatic/fenestrated/dissectors/traumatic)

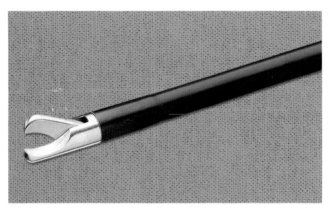

Fig. 8: Hook scissors

and resterilization, particularly where many laparoscopic surgeries are performed. Most of the dissectors and graspers have the availability of electrosurgery connection.
Biopsy forceps: They are used during diagnostic laparoscopy to sample suspected endometriosis implants, or in ovarian suspicious malignancy (before chemotherapy or during second-look laparoscopy).
Scissors: These instruments may be straight, curved or hooked. Delicate dissection can be carried out with straight scissors. Curved scissors, in general, have the same features as for straight scissors. In some cases, they are easier to dissect with, because the curvature changes the viewing angle. Hook scissors are particularly suitable for transecting ligature fibers and for tissue transection (Fig. 8). Scissors can be used to adhesiolysis, section of coagulated tissue and sutures cutting. Some have an electrical adapter so they can be combined with unipolar or bipolar electrocoagulation.
Coagulation instruments: Most devices used for coagulation during operative laparoscopy are adapted from open

surgery. More details about electrosurgery were described in the chapter *"Principals and use of electrosurgery in laparoscopy"*.

Concerning monopolar instruments there are different tips available (Fig. 9A). There is a monopolar high-frequency needle that can be retracted into the sheath (Fig. 9B). Also a vast armamentarium of bipolar forceps with various tips is seen with a coagulating probe (Fig. 10).
Needle holders: The figure below shows 5 mm needle holders. These instruments are essential to perform suture and knots. There are different types of needle holders. They may have a straight or curved handle, as well as straight and curved tips. The co-axial types with a locking system are preferred to the pistol type needle holders (Figs 11A and B). There are also automatic needle holders that after being charged, put the needle in a 90° angle. In extracorporeal sutures, the aim is to apply tension under a controlled way (myomectomy, promontofixation, vaginal cuff closure), a knot pusher is needful.
Suture passer devices: There are various types of sutures passers available for closure of ports and transfacial ligature (Fig. 12). The thread passer has a side slit to carry the thread into the peritoneal cavity on one side to the trocar. Once the thread is in the peritoneal cavity, the instrument is introduced on the other fascia side and the thread is pulled out closing the fascia defect caused, for example, by the trocar insertion. This procedure should be performed under laparoscopic view and guidance.
Intestinal probe: The intestinal probe is used to push back the bowel in order to achieve a good view. It may be important for endometriosis surgery to expose the rectum or in sacrocolpopexy to deviate laterally the rectum and sigmoid during the procedure.

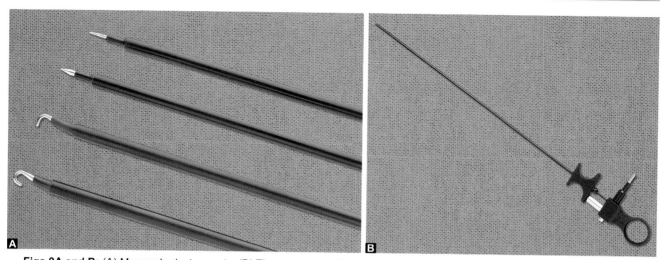

Figs 9A and B: (A) Monopolar instruments; (B) The monopolar high-frequency needle (Karl Storz): The tip of the needle can be retracted into the sheath

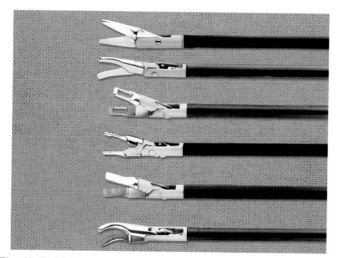

Fig. 10: RoBi: New generation of rotating bipolar forceps and scissors

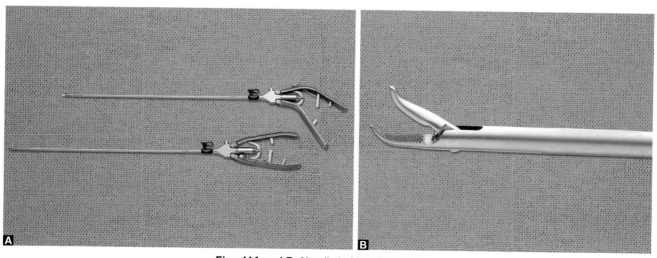

Figs 11A and B: Needle holders by Karl Storz

Vaginal probe: It is very useful for exposing the vagina mainly during deep endometriosis and prolapse surgeries (Fig. 13).

Myomas holder: During a laparoscopic myomectomy, it is difficult to stabilize a smooth, hard fibroid. Myoma screws (5 mm and 10 mm) allow the surgeon to maneuver the

myoma and apply traction with improved exposition and access (Figs 14A and B). Another alternative for myoma fixation is the use of a strong *tenaculum* offering you more mobility in the myoma traction points.

Tissue removal: In the past, laparoscopic surgeons were faced with the difficult problem of tissue extraction, and were often obliged to perform a suprapubic mini-laparotomy or a transvaginal extraction.

There are several good alternatives available for the surgeon to remove large volumes of tissue without increasing the size of the laparoscopic access incisions. Morcellators grasp, core and cut the tissue to be removed into small pieces. These fragments are forced into the hollow part of the instrument. Manual and automatic morcellators are available. Steiner developed the electromechanical morcellator, consisting of a motor-driven cutting tube. The speed can be selected in three stages. It is possible, with the aid of this morcellator, to extract even large amounts of tissue from the abdomen, using the size 11 trocar, in a short period of time. With 12 mm and 15 mm trocars, large quantities of tissue can be extracted in this way within a few minutes.

Automatic morcellators are more expensive but are very effective and save time when large amounts of tissue need to be removed (Figs 15A and B). It is obligatory to observe the tissue that will be removed from the moment it is divided from other tissues to its delivery through the abdominal wall regardless of whether or not it is removed in a tissue bag to prevent injury to adjacent tissues. Because of the good cutting quality of the rotating morcellator, the tissue structure is minimally damaged. It also enables a reliable histological examination to be carried out.

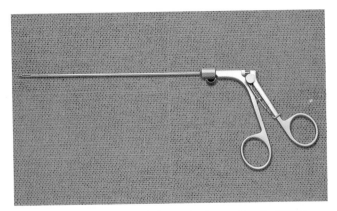

Fig. 12: BERCI® fascial closure instrument by Karl Storz

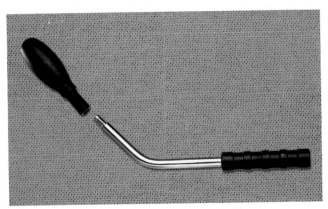

Fig. 13: Vaginal probe

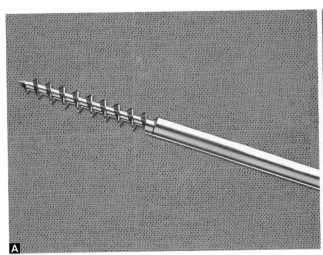
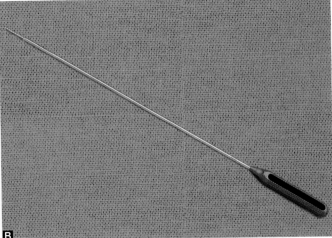

Figs 14A and B: Myoma screw

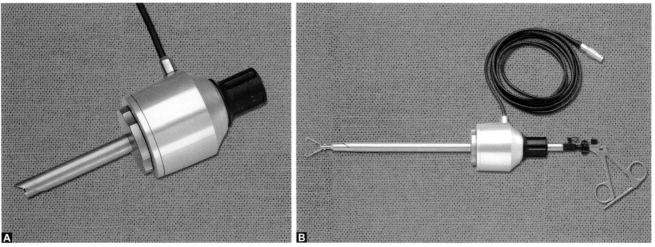

Figs 15A and B: Rotocut® myoma morcelator

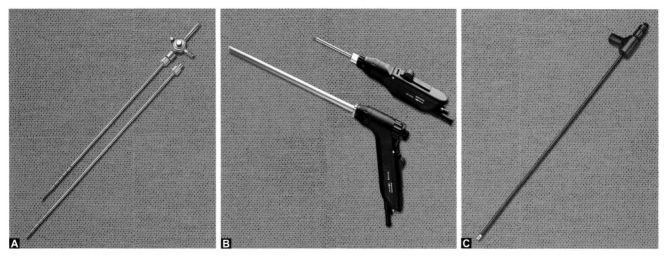

Figs 16A to C: (A and B) Suction-irrigation devices; (C) The GORDTS/CAMPO—coagulating suction and irrigation cannula by Karl Storz

Tissue bags can be used to isolate tissue (e.g. tumor, infected appendix) prior to removal with or without morcellation. The tissue bag can be removed through a secondary port site or through the infraumbilical port once the camera has been removed. For some (e.g. appendectomy), but not all types of laparoscopic surgeries, the use of a tissue bag may decrease the risk of surgical site infection or oncological dissemination. The tissue bag can also be removed through the *cul-de-sac* after a culdotomy (in alternative to a trocar port size enlargement).

Irrigation-suction: During diagnostic and surgical laparoscopy, it is commonly necessary to drain fluids and irrigate wound surfaces until they are clean and can be viewed adequately. Irrigation is used to clear debris or blood when bleeding is encountered, if a strong irrigation pressure is applied it can be helpful to clearly identify the origin of a bleeding. Some surgical teams defend that irrigation can also be used for hydrodissection and creation of tissue planes. On other hand, many surgeons say that irrigation should be avoided because it may interfere with the CO_2 pneumodissection of the retroperitoneal spaces. It is important that these solutions are used at body temperature.

Suction is performed either by means of a central vacuum supply system or with an additional suction pump that works usually better. Different laparoscopic suction instruments have been designed to remove irrigation fluid or intraperitoneal air and smoke. Combination suction/irrigation devices are also available (Figs 16A and B). A larger 10 mm suction-irrigation instrument is ideal for removing blood clots when brisk bleeding is encountered (e.g. severe hemoperitoneum after an ectopic pregnancy rupture).

In the market, there is available a suction-irrigation device with a bipolar current tip that may be useful in case of ovarian endometriomas and deep endometriosis.

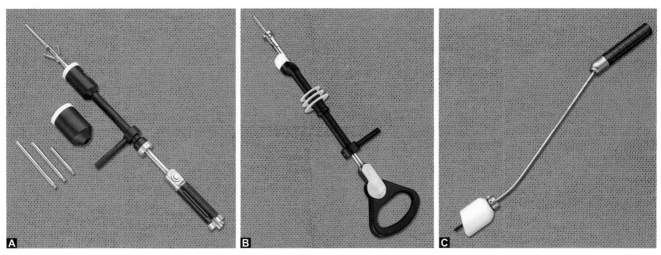

Figs 17A to C: Uterine manipulators (Mangheskiar®, Clermont-Ferrand® and Donnez®)

It is a more versatile device allowing blunt dissection, coagulation, irrigation and fluids suction, simultaneously (Fig. 16C).

Uterine manipulators: Safe, effective endoscopy, requires adequate mobilization and stabilization of the uterus and associated organs. Various combinations of uterine sounds, cannulas, and dilators are available (Figs 17A to C). They are very useful for the uterus exposition during procedures like hysterectomy, myomectomy, adnexal surgery and endometriosis. Some surgeons even say that *"...if an uterine manipulator is properly used, it makes half of the hysterectomy..."*

Key Points

- Almost all instruments available for laparotomy are now available in a specialized form for laparoscopy.
- The good knowledge of surgical instruments and equipment is an important condition for the biggest success of a surgery and avoidance of complications.

■ REFERENCES

1. Shah J, Buckley D, Frisby J, et al. Depth cue reliance in surgeons and medical students. Surg Endosc. 2003;17(9):1472-4.
2. Breedveld P, Wentink M. Eye-hand coordination in laparoscopy—an overview of experiments and supporting aids. Minim Invasive Ther Allied Technol. 2001;10(3):155-62.
3. Schurr MO, Breitwieser H, Melzer A, et al. Experimental telemanipulation in endoscopic surgery. Surg Laparosc Endosc. 1996;6(3):167-75.
4. Bholat OS, Haluck RS, Murray WB, et al. Tactile feedback is present during minimally invasive surgery. J Am Coll Surg. 1999;189(4):349-55.
5. Brydges R, Carnahan H, Dubrowski A. Surface exploration using laparoscopic surgical instruments: The perception of surface roughness. Ergonomics. 2005;48(7):874-94.
6. Reynolds W Jr. The first laparoscopic cholecystectomy. JSLS. 2001;5(1):89-94.
7. Cicione A, Autorino R, Breda A, et al. Three-dimensional vs standard laparoscopy: Comparative assessment using a validated program for laparoscopic urologic skills. Urology. 2013;82(6):1444-50.

CHAPTER 2

Peritoneal Access in Laparoscopy

Artin Ternamian

■ INTRODUCTION

Ever since antiquity, humans have devised different methods and instruments to access body cavities for several reasons; such as understand body functions, remedy ailments, ready corpses in preparation for the afterlife, among others.

Ancient Egyptian funerary embalmers developed deft "minimally invasive" methods and instruments to eviscerate internal organs of the deceased, through small and concealed ports, in preparation for mummification.

This unfortunate female died around 2,400 years ago, at the young age of 40 years and now rests in the Archaeological Museum of Zagreb, Croatia. An ancient Egyptian embalmer used a bamboo or palm *cannula* to evacuate her cerebral tissue, through the nostril or base of the skull, not to distort her facial appearance. However, their minimally invasive attempt must have failed, as a broken bamboo *cannula* remains lodged in her emptied skull (Fig. 1).

Contemporary surgery thrives to offer patients less disabling methods and endoscopists more enabling technologies, to diagnose and cure ailments. In doing so, surgeons along with industry, have been successful in minimizing size and number of surgical access incisions (decrease access trauma) and miniaturizing surgical tools (decrease operative trauma); with the net result of an overall lessening of tissue injury and patient disability.

This chapter describes different peritoneal access methods, access instruments, and abdominal access sites to help endoscopists achieve the first of the previously mentioned objectives; safe access into and exit from the peritoneal operative environment with the least collateral tissue injury or hurt.

Generally, visually directed endoscopic procedures are performed through natural body orifices (Hysteroscopy, Falloposcopy), through surgically created temporary access ports (Laparoscopy, Transvaginal hydrolaparoscopy) or through hybrid conduits (NOTES, natural orifice transluminal endoscopic surgery).

The first and most critical step of laparoscopic surgery is creation and maintenance of a robust and safe peritoneal operative compartment. Successful establishment of secure abdominal ports recruits three fundamental aspects of port creation (access method, access instrument and access location); these three determine success or failure of the intended endoscopic surgery (Fig. 2).

These tasks, (peritoneal cavity access, insufflation and exit) represent one of the fundamental core competencies, required for safe performance of all abdominal laparoscopic operations.

All surgeries, including endoscopic operations, are associated with some patient risk and although procedure-based analysis of serious laparoscopic access injury is low, 3–5 per 10,000, large *aggregate-based* studies, indicate them to be more common than reported in *procedure-based* studies.[1-3]

As more laparoscopies are performed globally in different disciplines, the cumulative public health impact of these "*uncommon*", yet potentially catastrophic misadventures remain substantial.

Peritoneal port creation is associated with risk to intraperitoneal and retroperitoneal tissues (gastrointestinal organs and major blood vessels), and at least 50% of these serious complications happen before commencement of the intended surgery.[4]

Peritoneal access-related complication rates have not changed over the last several decades and most serious port

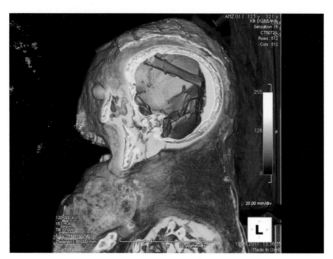

Fig. 1: Egyptian embalmers used minimally invasive methods to prepare deceased; broken bamboo cannula emptied in skull
Source: Archaeological Museum of Zagreb, Croatia

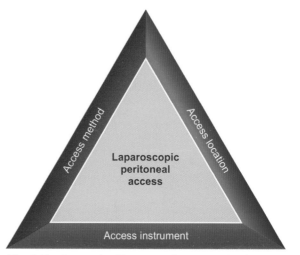

Fig. 2: Fundamentals of laparoscopic port creation (access method, access instrument and access location)

accidents occur during insertion of a primary umbilical port.

Push-through trocar and cannula designs remain the most common type of laparoscopic access devices used, causing injuries; regrettably more than two-thirds of these mishaps are not recognized until sometime after conclusion of the operation.(*http://www.piaa.us/Laparoscopic Injury Study/pdf/PIAA_2000*)

Accordingly, the US Food and Drug Administration (FDA), in a laparoscopic trocar injuries report, recommends surgeons performing endoscopic operations to be well versed in alternate laparoscopic access methods and instruments to address evolving patient expectations and societal safety requirements.[5]

Health regulators and gynecologists recognize the importance of less hazardous laparoscopic primary access options, especially in high-risk instances, and methods that can anticipate, avoid, or at the very least recognize task error are advocated; where injury recovery is possible before permanent patient harm develops.[6]

Endoscopy requires surgeons to remain skillful when using both hands, adept with hand-eye coordination and versed by constantly acquiring new motor skill dexterity that entails a steep learning curve.[7]

Gynecologists must thrive to adopt evolving access technologies, in addition to methods and instruments that they are schooled in, as an increasing variety of gynecological conditions are now treated endoscopically. Besides, repeated peritoneal access through the same abdominal location, may in itself create added risk (port site adhesions, hernia) that needs to be addressed and considered when planning future laparoscopic operations on these same patients.

As risk of grave unintended peritoneal access injury is low, no single gynecologist's personal experience, offers meaningful statistics to establish relative risk of alternate access methods. So far, no study has been remotely large enough to show any small but potentially important difference between access techniques or instruments.[8]

In reality, to demonstrate a 33% reduction in access bowel injury rate, from 0.3 to 0.2 per 1,000, requires a study population of more than 828,204 laparoscopic operations. Given these numbers, it is extremely unlikely to foresee a randomized trial to establish beyond doubt, advantage of one entry method over another.[9] Consequently, endoscopists can carry on using their preferred access technique, as there is no evidence favoring any one port creation technique.[10]

LAPAROSCOPIC PERITONEAL PORT FUNDAMENTALS

Whenever discussing peritoneal port creation, it is important to remember the three variable aspects mentioned earlier (Fig. 2), access method, access instrument design and access location, as each will present its unique challenges, advantages and applications.

Peritoneal access *method*s can be with or without preinsufflation, blind or visual, radially expanding, open, gasless, single port access or others.

Access instrument design can comprise a twin trocar with cannula or a single cannula; they may be single use or reusable, sharp or blunt tipped, threaded or smooth, visual or blind, single port or robotic.

Laparoscopic Peritoneal Access

Access method	With pre-insufflation access
	High pressure trocar access
	Visual/Blind access
	Radially expanding trocar access
	Gasless/Direct trocar access
	Open Hasson's trocar access
	Single-port access
Access instrument	Single/Multiple use
	Trocar with Cannula/Trocarless Cannula
	Threaded or smooth cannula
	Sharp/Blunt Trocar/Cannula
	Visual/Blind Trocar/Cannula
	Single-Port Trocar less Cannula
	Robotic
Access location	Supra-intra-sub umbilical
	Upper quadrant Left/right
	Lower quadrant Left/right
	Suprapubic

Fig. 3: Laparoscopic access method, location and instrument

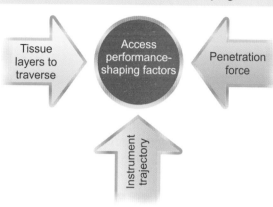

Fig. 4: Performance-shaping factors, irrespective of method, instrument and access location, determines outcome

Access location can be supra-, infra- or intraumbilical, suprapubic, left/right upper or lower quadrant, primary or ancillary port, among others (Fig. 3).

Safe placement of peritoneal access ports achieves a number of important functions, including introduction of carbon dioxide (CO_2) distending gas, preservation of a sealed leak-proof operative compartment, introduction of laparoscope, repeated insertion of operative instruments, conduit for tissue morcellation and retrieval and maintenance of port-competence by the end of surgery.

To avert repeated access injury and to better understand mishap causation; *port-dynamics* at tissue-instrument-force interface must be observed, archived, recalled and analyzed. When accident causation is examined in real time, more error tolerant and comparatively less dangerous laparoscopic access systems and access instruments are designed to offer method, instrument and access location redundancy.[11]

It is generally accepted that endoscopists, like all surgeons, need to be knowledgeable in anatomy, pathology and surgical skills, to safely navigate instruments during operations. In addition they must be aware of the different peritoneal access *performance shaping factors* (PSF), that irrespective of method, instrument and access location, left alone surgeon's experience, determines outcomes (Fig. 4).

In effect, there are three important variables to ponder during laparoscopic primary port creation; First is to consider the different anterior abdominal tissue layers to traverse, en route to the target peritoneal cavity (intra-, supra-, intraumbilical, left upper quadrant access, lower abdominal, other), second is the instrument trajectory design used to access (visual, blunt, sharp, threaded, single port, robotic), and third is the penetration force (amount, direction, control, recruitment) required to safely deploy the port.

The interposed anterior abdominal wall tissue layer is a dynamic body organ that offers essential trunk containment. It forms a stable platform on which primary, ancillary, and hybrid temporary ports remain anchored to perform extra-, intra-, or retroperitoneal endoscopic operations.

Knowledge of this important anatomical environment and understanding of the functional anatomy of every component from skin, subcutaneous fat, fascia, muscle, peritoneal membrane, vessel, nerve, and osseous scaffolding will guarantee effective and safe port application irrespective of method, instrument, and port site.

Some of the more important difference between open and laparoscopic surgery include size of surgical wound, visual fidelity (magnification, illumination, depth perception), and haptic (force + tactile feedback).

Additionally, a fixed access port creates a significant ergonomic challenge for surgeon and assistant alike while negotiating the dynamic surgical field.[12-14]

The fulcrum effect of laparoscopic fixed ports, when using straight instruments, requires paradoxical field and instrument movement, limits excursion, alters haptic, creates suboptimal work ergonomics, and alters the operator's body posture relative to the surgical target.

This dynamics becomes further altered when using curved operative instruments during single-port surgery and robotically assisted endoscopy.

Whereas open surgery allows the surgeon's hand two degrees of freedom (DOF) of movement, for each of the nine interphalangeal joints, conventional laparoscopic operative instruments, with the exception of contemporary robotic arms, offer only four DOFs.

Additionally, surgeon's body allows six trunk DOF activities, three rotations at the shoulders, one at the elbow and one in the forearm, with two at the wrist. Long straight or curved operative instruments hinge at access sites to generate force transmission variances according to the extra- or intracorporeal instrument length ratio.

Furthermore, short extracorporeal length decreases mechanical advantage, while long extracorporeal length induces surgeons to assume uncomfortable nonergonomic forearm and shoulder positions.[15]

Laparoscopic instrument tip movement differs from that of instrument handle, unless the instrument pivots exactly at its midpoint.[16]

As laparoscopic operative instruments have smaller grasping surfaces and reduced mechanical advantage, force necessary to securely grip tissue is estimated to be six times greater than force required to operate with conventional surgical instruments. In this current suboptimal operating room ergonomic physical environment and endoscopic instruments, endoscopists regularly struggle with needless technical difficulty, avoidable overuse fatigue, and unneeded operative morbidity, more so than during conventional open surgery.[17]

As a result, endoscopic surgeries are usually appreciably more stressful and necessitate added operator attentiveness compared with conventional laparotomy.[18]

Unlike other professionals operating under equally demanding, stressful and safety critical environments, surgeons are less inclined to acknowledge the effects of stress on their operative performance.[19]

Although it is recognized, a suboptimal surgical environment and other stressors (such as sleep deprivation) can impede surgical dexterity and increase the likelihood of inadvertent error.[20,21]

Primary peritoneal access methods can either be visual or nonvisual (Fig. 5). Visual access requires a zero-degree laparoscope mounted into the access instrument during port creation, whereas nonvisual blind access requires no laparoscope during placement. Peritoneal primary entry is also described as Closed (applied after CO_2 insufflation) or Open-Direct none preinsufflated access.[22]

When using visual access, identification of the anterior abdominal wall tissue layers is very important, as a real-time navigational compass to safe port placement and offers

Laparoscopic Access Methods

Nonvisual access

Insufflated	Closed trocar access
	High-pressure trocar access
	Radially expanding trocar access
Non-insufflated	Direct trocar access
	Open Hasson's trocar access

Visual access	Visual trocar access Endopath Optiview VISIPORT
	Visual veress trocar mini-laparoscope
	Visual cannula ENDOTIP Endoscopic Threaded Imaging Port
	Single-port visual cannula

Fig. 5: Primary peritoneal access methods: Visual or nonvisual

a singular opportunity for recognizing unintended access harm if and when they occur. The peritoneal cavity is a vacuum sealed envelope, described as a "virtual cavity" in which viscera dwell with a few milliliters of peritoneal fluid.

Surgeon's palm the conventional push-through trocar and cannula with their dominant hand and apply considerable, steady, linear penetration force, generated by their shoulder and trunk muscles, toward the abdominal wall.

The linear thrust requirement dictates instrument design, to have a pointed or sharp trocar tip, to lessen penetration force needed to transect several anterior abdominal wall layers during port placement.[23]

It is apparent that in more than 30 commercially available different access systems, all have a specific reproducible quality and predictable linear *penetration force* profile that is necessary to penetrate the loosely bound thin peritoneal membrane; compared with that of the taught thicker anterior rectus fascia, causing considerable tissue deformation. In addition, once the peritoneal layer is transfixed, a sudden loss of resistance is registered, causing overshoot.[24]

When the trocar loss of entry resistance is sudden (200–300 milliseconds) and uncontrolled, the trocar tip overshoot excursion is farther, and the likelihood of loss of control causing entry injury is more. Conventional trocars are blind with a smooth outer cannula surface, with no ability to avoid trocar overshoot, no mechanism to anticipate, avoid, or recognize injury; and no means to control penetration.[11]

In effect, successful primary port insertion represents a fundamental core competencies required for safe endoscopic surgery. This single task remains the most important and potentially dangerous first step in laparoscopy, irrespective of discipline or specialty.[25,26]

Failure of satisfactory peritoneal access or strategic port placement can undermine the laparoscopic approach or render the procedure unsafe for patient and surgeon alike.[27]

Conventional push-through trocar and cannula application at primary and ancillary access, offers limited safety redundancy, as applying uncontrolled linear penetration force to a sharp nonvisual trajectory toward the viscera, with no mechanism to control penetration force, gage insertion depth, and avoid sudden uncontrolled overshoot.

In high reliability industries, when human error is analyzed and accident causation is examined, industry-specific performance shaping factors are identified that render task performance less forgiving and set the stage for inadvertent injury, irrespective of human skill and experience.

When this PSF concept is applied to penetration force during primary push-through peritoneal port insertion, specific characteristics become evident, that once identified, deconstructed and re-engineered, a less error prone system can be introduced where uncontrolled, excessive, sharp, linear, blind penetration force is controlled, minimized, blunted, redirected to radial torque, and rendered visible, where tissue layers traversed is archived in real time (Fig. 6).

Assemblage of these potentially hazardous PSFs during primary access renders nonvisual port creation less forgiving and sets the stage for inadvertent injury.

When conventional push-through laparoscopic port creation is deconstructed and re-engineered after deleting the identified access PSFs, intuitively increments of access redundancy is introduced that individually and collectively render peritoneal access less hazardous.[28,29]

CLASSIFICATION OF LAPAROSCOPIC ACCESS METHODS

Primary peritoneal access methods can be classified as either nonvisual or visual (Fig. 5); in addition, they are further subdivided into those that are applied after Veress insertion and CO_2 insufflation (closed entry) and those that are deployed without Veress insertion (direct or open entry). Visual access systems require a zero degree laparoscope sheath into the primary access instrument during port creation, irrespective of entry instrument used, whereas nonvisual access systems entail no laparoscope during port insertion.[22]

❑ Closed laparoscopic access method
❑ High pressure laparoscopic access method
❑ Radially expanding laparoscopic access method
❑ Direct laparoscopic access method
❑ Open laparoscopic access method
❑ Visual laparoscopic access method.

CLOSED CONVENTIONAL LAPAROSCOPIC ACCESS METHOD

Conventional primary push-through closed access methods use a central spike (trocar) and outer sheath (cannula) to transect different anterior abdominal wall layers toward a vacuum-sealed peritoneum; 0–3 mm Hg.

This method has served gynecologists well over the years, however, given recent patient safety awareness initiatives, recurring incidence of serious access errors and mounting medicolegal concern, it is necessary to re-examine the fundamentals of peritoneal access in general and primary access in particular.

Most gynecologists first preinsufflate with the Veress needle to distend the virtual peritoneal cavity with a noncombustible CO_2 gas and then insert a push-through trocar and cannula to establish a primary laparoscopic access port (*also called the Closed method*).

A survey of 155,987 gynecologic surgeries and 17,216 general surgical operations, the Veress needle was used in 78% of them. More than 80% of gynecologists preinsufflated with the Veress needle, and used the closed push through access method as opposed to 48% of general surgeons, who preferred the open access methods, using the Hasson trocar and cannula.[30]

In 1932, a Hungarian respirologist, Dr Janos Veress (Fig. 7), invented a spring-loaded needle designed to induce pneumothorax when treating pulmonary tuberculosis, without puncturing the lung (Fig. 8).[31,32]

Dr Veress's needle was popularized again in 1947, when a Swedish-born French gynecologist, Dr Raoul Palmer (Fig. 9), used it to induce pneumoperitoneum for laparoscopy and recognized the importance of gauging the intraperitoneal insufflation pressure. Additionally, he recognized the benefits of the Trendelenburg position and uterine manipulator.

Access Principles

Insufflation is intended to counter the linear penetration force generated by the trajectory of conventional push-through trocars during port insertion. This is also intended to distance the retroperitoneal tissues from the advancing sharp primary trocar tip to mitigate unintended access injury, by overshoot; though, complications related to their use are well-documented.[33-35]

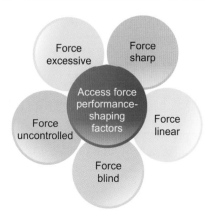

Fig. 6: Laparoscopic access penetration force performance-shaping factors

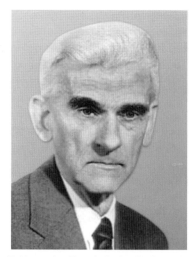

Fig. 7: Hungarian Respirologist, Dr Janos Veress

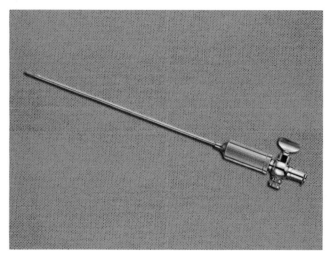

Fig. 8: The Veress needle

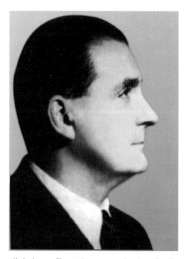

Fig. 9: Swedish-born French gynecologist, Dr Raoul Palmer

Most surgeons will lift the skin or anterior rectus fascia to offer counter pressure to the advancing needle trajectory or push-through trocars during port insertion. Usually, the Veress needle is inserted in the midline, sub- or intraumbilical region of the abdomen.

Alternate CO_2 insufflation sites include cul-de-sac, transuterine or ninth intercostal space insufflation. The needle is usually held by the dominant index and thumb at the hub and advanced toward the pelvic hollow. The angle of the Veress needle insertion should vary according to the body mass index of the patient; 45° in nonobese women and 90° in morbidly obese women.[36]

Correct placement of the Veress needle is very important and different tests are described to ascertain its placement. The peritoneal cavity is layered by a continuous layer of moist mesothelial cells, with an approximate surface area of 1.5 m².[37] Generally, the intraperitoneal pressure is 0–3 mm Hg, while supine, at 37°C.[38]

By far the most reliable and evidence-based measure of correct Veress placement is the initial intraperitoneal pressure reading.[39]

Some gynecologists prefer inserting the Veress needle while connected to the CO_2 and the gas flowing at a low rate; once the entry pressure is measured, the insufflation rate is increased.[40,41]

HIGH PRESSURE LAPAROSCOPIC ACCESS METHOD

Abdominal palpation to gage sufficient insufflation is sometimes preferred to determine adequacy of distension, as instilled gas volume measurement can be unreliable. Generally, obesity does not adversely affect insufflation volume for a given intra-abdominal pressure as the actual intra-abdominal volume is a finite value, and 94% of this capacity is attained at an abdominal pressure of 55 mm Hg.[42]

The high CO_2 insufflation pressure ($\geq$25–30 mm Hg) technique is an alternate closed entry method, where the elevated intraperitoneal pressure braces the anterior abdominal wall to counter axial penetration force and inevitable overshoot that accompanies all push through trocar and cannula entry methods, by interposing a larger gas envelope between the advancing trajectory and great vessels, viscera or retroperitoneum.[43,44]

A Canadian gynecologist's survey demonstrated that 45% of practitioners claimed to use 25 mm Hg of CO_2 insufflation pressure at primary port insertion, 28.8% of respondents use 20–25 mm Hg and 16.2% use 16–19 mm Hg.[45]

During laparoscopic surgery, CO_2 gas is used to create and maintain a working surgical space as it is readily available, safe to use in the operating room environment and cheap. However, it is important to remember that it is generally insufflated at 14°C lower than normal resting body temperature (21°C), at almost zero percent humidity, with considerable consequences that remain underestimated.[46,47]

Once the primary port is inserted, the central trocar is removed and a laparoscope with camera and light cable attached are advanced into the insufflated peritoneal cavity. The very first objective is inspection of the primary access site for inadvertent insufflation or trocar-related injury, then the upper and lower abdomen is carefully observed and a decision is made to place additional ancillary operative ports, prior to assumption of the Trendelenburg position.

If high peritoneal insufflation pressure access method is used, then the intraperitoneal and insufflation pressure must be readjusted to a safe 15 mm Hg maintenance level to avoid inadvertent untoward complications; temporary high insufflation pressures have been shown not to have adverse cardiovascular effects.[48]

When the operation is completed, the access ports removed under vision and peritoneal cavity is disinsufflated. Port competence remains an important aspect of safe laparoscopy as the true incidence of port hernia remains unknown.

Moreover, it is understood that when large cannulas are used (more than 10 mm in diameter), or if morcellated tissue is extracted through a given port site, or if the patient is immune compromised, among other high risk situations, the port site needs to be reinforced by a fascial suture, to avoid port site hernias.

RADIALLY EXPANDING LAPAROSCOPIC ACCESS METHOD

In 1994, a new peritoneal access instrument and method was introduced called Step, by a California company (InnerDyne, Sunnyvale, CA). The original instrument design consisted of a 1.9 mm, radially expanding polymeric cannula sleeve, sheathed around a conventional Veress needle (Fig. 10).

The method involves conventional peritoneal insufflation using this modified radially expandable sheath with Veress needle. Once peritoneal insufflation is achieved, the central Veress needle is withdrawn leaving the outer sleeve in situ, to act as a conduit through the anterior abdominal wall layers, toward the peritoneal cavity. Then a second larger diameter obturator trocar is shoved with considerable penetration force, through the radially expanding outer sheath; when this second blunt obturator trocar is intraperitoneal, it is withdrawn and the operating laparoscope with attached camera is introduced.[49]

The penetration force required to thrust this second, larger diameter trocar through the anterior abdomen wall layers is significantly higher than the penetration force required placing a laparoscopic peritoneal access device using a conventional single-use, sharp trocar and cannula.[50]

Several small case series and randomized studies have reported no serious injury to major vessels and no deaths. Patients appeared to demonstrate less postoperative pain and more patient satisfaction with this access system compared with the conventional trocar and cannula entry

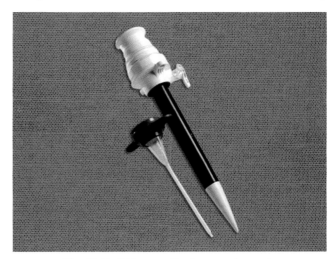

Fig. 10: Radially expanding trocar and cannula

methods. However, most studies were small and abdominal wall bleeding and Veress injury to mesentery has been encountered.[51-53]

DIRECT LAPAROSCOPIC ACCESS METHOD

In 1978, Dingfelder first published on direct primary peritoneal trocar insertion in a non-preinsufflated peritoneum for laparoscopic surgery.[54]

He suggested that advantages of this peritoneal access method include elimination of Veress needle related complications: unsuccessful insufflation, preperitoneal insufflation, visceral insufflation, or the more serious and extremely rare incidence of CO_2 embolization.[55]

Although the direct trocar and cannula primary peritoneal access method is the most rapid method, compared to other available techniques, it remains the least performed laparoscopic entry method in clinical practice to date.[30,56]

An infra- or intraumbilical skin incision is made using a 15 surgical blade, wide enough to accommodate the entry of cannula's outer diameter. The anterior abdominal wall is then elevated by hand or, by two towel clips placed on either side of the umbilical incision, then the trocar and cannula unite is palmed by the dominant hand of the surgeon and considerable linear penetration force is generated to propel the sharp, pointed and blind access port directly into the peritoneal cavity, toward the pelvic hollow; then the sharp trocar is retracted and laparoscope inserted to ascertain correct and safe placement.[57]

Although entry is achieved with only one step, avoiding preinsufflation with the Veress, it is required that a sharp and blind trocar is used with direct access, where considerable uncontrolled linear penetration force is applied, while significant strength is recruited to adequately elevate the abdominal wall, to offer counter traction to the uncontrolled advancing sharp and blind trocar toward a noninsufflated peritoneal cavity; each one of these aspects of direct blind access more hazardous as they all present important performance shaping factor in laparoscopic access that individually, left alone in combination make primary port insertion more injury prone.

It is recognized that a high percentage of women surgeons experience difficulty in inserting primary and ancillary access trocars compared to male endoscopists. Injuries appear to happen twice as often among those who experienced difficulty with port insertion ($P = 0.04$); when primary port insertion was considered alone, correlation is more significant ($P = 0.02$).[58]

Several retrospective studies are published regarding safety of this method, with comparatively small number of patients, with only three (n = 664 patients) randomized papers.[59-64]

Few of the papers were prospective, and some publications used this method only in low-risk patients; high-risk patients with suspected adhesions were excluded from the studies. These papers purported fewer minor access complication rates with direct trocar entry than with the Veress needle methods, with no major complications occurring in either group. Fewer injuries were found with direct trocar and cannula access, but there were no differences with respect to frequency of several access attempts or ease of port insertion (n = 200 patients).[65]

In 1989, Byron et al. used this direct access method in unselected patients (n = 937 women), where a total complication rate of 4.2% (39/937) was recorded, with a significant increased risk of minor complications ($P < 0.001$). They reported more than three entry attempts in 2.7% of cases and failed access technique in 1.4% of cases; they surmised that history of previous abdominal surgery was not associated with an increased risk of access complications.[66]

Later, they randomized 252 women with Veress needle pre insufflation entry (n = 141) and direct trocar and cannula access (n = 111) for laparoscopy; they discovered a fourfold increase in minor access complication rates with the former method over the latter entry method (11.3% vs 2.7%, $P < 0.05$) and a longer port insertion time (5.9 vs 2.2 minutes, $P < 0.01$).[56]

When Molloy et al. reviewed 51 laparoscopic access publications (134,917 Veress/trocar-cannula, 21,547 open, and 16,739 direct entry), visceral-bowel injury rates were 0.04% (Veress/trocar-cannula), 0.11% (open), and 0.05% (direct access); whereas corresponding vessel injury rates were 0.04%, 0.01%, and 0%, respectively.

Their overall mortality rate with laparoscopic port insertion is 1 per 100,000 procedures; visceral-bowel injury is more frequent in general surgical cases than in gynecological patients 0.15% versus 0.04% ($P = 0.0001$) and vascular injury when using open and direct access methods have the same 0.0% incidence.

These authors are convinced that the present literature, "there is no clear evidence as to the optimal form of laparoscopic entry in the low-risk patient. However, direct entry may be an under-utilized and safe alternative to the Veress needle and open entry technique".[30]

A number of publications describe major vessel injuries when using the direct access method,[30] with five deaths occurring among those where conventional closed Veress/trocar/cannula method was used to create the primary laparoscopic port. Two deaths were ascribed to delayed realization of visceral-bowel injury-perforation and three purported to be attributed to CO_2 gas embolization during insufflation.[67]

Likewise, Borgatta et al. included patients with previous abdominal surgery and revealed a two-fold increase in unintended omental injury with the Veress needle over the direct trocar insertion with an obvious longer insertion time of 2 minutes 10 seconds when the Veress needle closed method is used.[58]

When Copeland et al. examined 2,000 unselected patients where direct primary peritoneal access was used, eight (0.4%) required conversion to conventional closed Veress insufflation access where one patient sustained and inadvertent visceral-bowel injury; whereas the two additional visceral-bowel injuries occurred when the direct laparoscopic port access method was used (0.1%).[62]

Other publications encountered a considerably higher omental injury rate, 26 of 542 patients (4.8%), with direct trocar access application.[68]

OPEN LAPAROSCOPIC ACCESS METHOD

This method was first described in 1971 and the purported benefits include prevention of extra-peritoneal insufflation, gas embolism and possibly decrease in visceral and major vascular injury.[69]

This method entails use of a smooth cannula with a side CO_2 gas insufflation spout, a mobile cone-shaped sleeve with two stay sutures holding wings and a blunt obturator (Fig. 11).

This access method is essentially a minilaparotomy, performed at the umbilical area where a 2 cm supra-, intra- or subumbilical incision is made transversely, and the subcutaneous fatty tissue is dissected off the anterior abdominal rectus fascia; the fascia is then incised and the peritoneal cavity is entered blindly using a pointed hemostat.

Once intraperitoneal, the surgeon inserts the index finger to ascertain absence of port site adhesions and viscera, then two anterior rectus fascial stay sutures are applied and held ready to tie around the cannula's stay suture holding wings.

The cannula and sheathed trocar are then inserted into the peritoneal cavity, without preinsufflation, the mobile cone-shaped sleeve is lowered into the access wound to offer an air-tight seal, while the two fascial sutures are snuggly secured to the con's suture holding wings. Insufflation is commenced, central trocar retrieved and laparoscope sheathed.

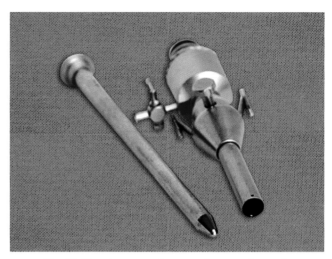

Fig. 11: Open laparoscopic access trocar and cannula

Occasionally, a purse-stringed anterior rectus fascial suture is required in addition to discourage CO_2 gas leakage around the cone-shaped cannula's seal.

By the end of the surgery, the laparoscope is removed, peritoneal cavity disinsufflated, stay sutures unraveled off the cone and cannula retrieved; the fascial defect is then secured by the fascial stay sutures and the skin incision is closed.

This access method is popular with general surgeons and is indicated by some to be a preferred access method in high-risk patients where abdominal wall adhesions are suspected or known to exist, especially those having previous abdominal surgery, through a vertical abdominal wall incision.

Several studies on the benefits and complications of the various laparoscopic access techniques have been published.

Hasson examined 17 publications on open laparoscopic access by general surgeons (9 publications, 7,205 laparoscopic procedures) and gynecologists (8 publications, 13,486 laparoscopic procedures) and compared them with closed conventional laparoscopic access, performed by general surgeons (7 publications, 90,152 patients) and gynecologists (12 publications, 579,510 patients).

He observed that during open laparoscopic access, the rate of umbilical infection was 0.4%, bowel injury 0.1%, and vascular injury 0%. The rates during closed laparoscopic access were 1% umbilical infections, 0.2% bowel injury, and 0.2% vascular injury. Hasson consequently advocated his open access method to be a preferred method for laparoscopic surgery.[70]

However, closer analysis of his publication suggests that the prospective studies and surveys indicate that general surgeons experience higher complication rates than gynecologists when using the closed access method, but experience similar complication rates with the open access method.

When using the closed laparoscopic access method, visceral and vascular complication rates were found to be 0.22% and 0.04% for general surgeons and 0.10% and 0.03% for gynecologists. In a published paper of his own 29-year endoscopic experience, with laparoscopy (5,284 patients), Hasson reported only one bowel injury during his first 50 cases.[71]

A surgical paper described their experience in general surgery and reviewed publications up to 1996 on closed (6 series, n = 489,335 patients) and open (6 series, n = 12,444 patients) laparoscopic access methods, to discover the rates of visceral and vascular injury were respectively 0.08% and 0.07% after closed laparoscopic access, and 0.05% and 0% after open laparoscopic access (P = 0.002). Mortality rates following closed and open laparoscopic access were 0.003% and 0% respectively.[72]

In a different European study, the Swiss Association for Laparoscopic and Thoracoscopic Surgery (SALTS) collected prospective data on 90.3% low-risk patients having different laparoscopic operations 1995 to 1997 (14,243 patients, M/F ratio 0.7).[73]

Umbilical trocar insertion resulted in eight visceral injuries: six following closed access and two following open Hasson access. They observed that in contrast to general surgery publications by Sigman et al.[74] Bonjer et al.[72] and Zaraca et al.[75] in their series, the open access method used clearly did not demonstrate any superiority over the closed laparoscopic access method.

Upon reviewing six publications (n = 357, 257) on conventional closed laparoscopic access and six papers with one survey (n = 20,410) on open laparoscopic access, performed by gynecologists, Garry observed that the closed laparoscopic access method, revealed major vessel and bowel inadvertent injury rates of 0.02% and 0.04%, respectively; the open laparoscopic access method, revealed 0% and 0.5%, respectively. When one excludes the survey report (n = 8000), bowel injury rates with open laparoscopic access method was 0.06%.

He suggests that open laparoscopic access is an adequate option that appears to avoid risk of inadvertent injury, almost completely in normal risk surgical patients where intra-abdominal structures are not altered by previous surgery, infection, etc.[9]

The European Association for Endoscopic Surgery in its clinical practice guideline observes that insertion of the primary port with the open technique appears to be faster, as compared to the conventional closed access method (grade A).

Admittedly, all randomized controlled trials, comparing conventional closed versus open laparoscopic access methods have insufficient sample-size to demonstrate a difference in serious access-related complications.

Larger outcomes studies demonstrated a lower complication rate with closed access (grade B); in effect, RCTs determined the open access approach to be faster and causing less minor complications (grade A), their panel also revealed that they cannot support use of a specific laparoscopic access technique. Moreover, use of either one of these methods will have advantages in specific patient groups (grade B).[76]

The recent French College of Gynaecologists and Obstetricians Clinical Practice Guideline on laparoscopic entry also supports this assumption.[77]

The Canadian Clinical Practice Guideline on laparoscopic entry also supports this assertion where use of the open, visual and direct access systems were also carefully evaluated; however, one has to be clear that all these reports lumped the published complications of the visual single-use trocar and cannulas, with the entirely different safety record of the threaded visual cannula.[78]

Studies reporting injury rates with open laparoscopic access demonstrates 23 bowel injuries in 21,547 laparoscopies (0.1%) and one vascular injury in 21,292 laparoscopies (0.005%). Regrettably, most studies present level III evidence only, as these publications were mainly chart reviews or surveys. Findings of this English language meta-analysis, from both gynecological and general surgical literature, showed that vascular injuries are almost entirely preventable by using the open laparoscopic access method (4.7/100,000).[30]

Irrespective, several vascular injury case reports are available in the European literature with the open laparoscopic access method use.[75,79,80]

The Australian paper also reports a statistically significant difference in visceral-bowel complication rates: 0.4/1,000 (gynecologists) as opposed to 1.5/1,000 (general surgeons) (P = 0.001). When open laparoscopic access cases are extracted from the examination, incidence of visceral-bowel injuries is 0.3/1,000 in gynecological surgeries and 1.3/1,000 in general surgical surgeries (P = 0.001). They wonder if the difference could be due to several difficult variables, including underreporting, patient selection bias, retrospective data, clinical practice differences and they note that gynecologists at the time were more skilled than general surgeons with laparoscopic port insertion.[30]

Visceral injuries are more prevalent in open laparoscopic accessing than with other accessing methods (0.11%: 0.04% with conventional closed-Veress needle access,

0.05% with direct entry). It is important to consider that patient selection bias influences this data as generally open laparoscopic access is more used in patients who have had previous umbilical or abdominal operations. Besides, these figures may also be potentially biased as the number of open laparoscopic access reports is much smaller than the number of conventional closed Veress needle laparoscopic access reports (open: 21,547 patients, closed-Veress: 134,917 patients). This paper also concludes that an optimal method of laparoscopic port insertion, in a normal risk patient, remains elusive.[30]

A French nonrandomized study compared open versus closed laparoscopic access, used by university-affiliated endoscopists. Visceral-bowel and major vascular injury rates were 0.04% and 0.01% with closed access (n = 8,324) and 0.19% and 0% with open access.

(n = 1,562), respectively. They reckoned that open laparoscopy access does not lessen the risk of major complications during laparoscopic port creation.[81]

In a systematic review of the different methods of establishing peritoneal ports during laparoscopic surgery by general surgeons and gynecologists. Merlin et al. determined that retrospective studies tend to compare high-risk with low-risk patient population, whereas prospective studies examine unselected patient population. They indicated an evident tendency toward reduced danger of major complications in unselected patients having open laparoscopic port insertion.[82]

However, they stressed that the most common major complications related to laparoscopic access were bowel injury and risk of visceral injury in nonrandomized patients is higher when the open laparoscopic access method is used as opposed to the conventional closed method. They reason that relative safety and effectiveness of the two laparoscopic access methods is not definitively settled and requires carful further analysis.[82]

A different multicenter general surgical survey (57% responding) discovered an unexpectedly high rate of major injuries; highest in single-use optical trocar and cannula use *(not the multiple use threaded visual cannula)* (0.27%), second highest in conventional closed (0.18%, used 82% of the time), and lowest in open trocar and cannula use (0.09%).[55]

However, when Jansen et al. compared different port creation methods in clinical trials, port-related complication rates were 0.07% and 0.17% for closed and open laparoscopic access methods, respectively; a significantly different result.[8]

Hasson et al. conclude that "there is no evidence to support abandoning the closed entry technique in laparoscopy; however, the selection of patients for an open or alternative procedure is still recommended".[4]

When Chandler et al. examined 566 patients inadvertently injured during laparoscopic access; they observed that visceral-bowel injuries were no less common when the primary port was created using the open method. Eighteen open access attempts were associated with small bowel injury in four patients, two were recognized late and patients succumbed, and four other patients sustained retroperitoneal large vessel injury with one patient's death. Of the other 10 patients, there were four large bowel injuries, three abdominal wall vessel injuries, and one urinary bladder, liver, and mesenteric vessel injury.[83]

The literature attests that 30–50% of visceral-bowel injuries and 13–50% of vascular injuries are undiagnosed intraoperatively.[7,29] As visceral-bowel injury is more common than vascular injury, it is more likely to create sinister consequences, especially because of delayed injury recognition; consequently mortality rate from laparoscopic access visceral-bowel injury is extremely high (2.5–5%).[84]

A French study demonstrated delayed recognition can occur even when optical trocar and cannulas are used to create the primary laparoscopic port; however, their study did not include mishaps with the use of the EndoTIP visual cannula method. Of 25/52 (48%) visceral-bowel injuries, close to half injuries went undiagnosed.[85]

A general surgical publication described how of the six visceral-bowel injuries in 12,444 laparoscopic open access, two (33%) were not diagnosed intraoperatively; in addition, they detected a 0.001% (489,335) CO_2 embolism rate during conventional closed access.[72]

Other publications have also described such incidences when catastrophic if not fatal coronary, cerebral, or other CO_2 gas embolism occurred, when inadvertently the Veress needle tip is lodged intraviscerally; clearly this serious complication is never reported with the open method for obvious reasons.[43,70]

As it stands now, despite assertion by our general surgical colleagues, there is not definitive scientific evidence to prove that open laparoscopic primary port insertion is superior or inferior to the conventional closed trocar and cannula access method.

Though the open access method has a lower vascular injury rate, however, this is countered by a marginally higher visceral-bowel injury occurrence; consequently an alternate primary access site or method is advised, such as the left upper quadrant, the ninth/tenth intercostal spaces, or visual access in high-risk patients.[5]

VISUAL LAPAROSCOPIC ACCESS METHOD

Visual primary laparoscopic access adds redundancy to task performance and offers endoscopists additional real-time interactive feedback during peritoneal port insertion; by definition, visual laparoscopic access methods display *port dynamics* (intersection of penetration force, access instrument, and anterior abdominal wall), on to the operating room monitor.

This added dimension during primary peritoneal access *(situational awareness)*, becomes an important tool that can anticipate access error and offer an opportunity for all to learn from inadvertent access mishaps.

Visual primary access methods are incapable of avoiding all primary port access incidents; they can however offer an invaluable opportunity to archive, replay and analysis of laparoscopic port dynamics, without recall or hindsight bias.

They can avert, predict, or at least, recognize primary access injury when and if inadvertent mishaps occur. It affords an important chance to repair access injury before error evolves to irreparable patient harm.

This particular attribute renders visual access methods more desirable, especially in high-risk patients, when peritoneal adhesions are anticipated and when access under visual control is highly desirable.[86,87]

Moreover, behavioral psychologists and others who have studied human behavior and inadvertent error established that routine videotaping improves outcomes. A system that captures and displays error details in real time is essential to scientifically enhance our ability to analyze error, understand accident causation and improve our risk recognition capabilities. Human reliability assessment techniques can identify, analyze, and categorize surgical error during endoscopic surgery and introduce risk aversion mechanisms.[88]

Mackenzie et al. demonstrated that interactive real-time video capture and recall allows thorough causation analysis and medical error aversion studies. Anesthetists have demonstrated that video analysis of performed tasks identifies performance deficiencies and discloses contributing factors.[89]

Furthermore, safety critical industries, such as the transportation, nuclear or mining industries have established that data collected concurrently at error point, increases safety.[90]

In addition, visual peritoneal access methods improve laparoscopic entry, safety awareness and raises error recording and reporting compliance.[91]

All visual access methods require operators to have knowledge in anatomy, have a solid understanding of navigational cues *(perceptual blindness)* and be able to correctly recognize displayed monitor images *(situational awareness)*; essential competencies for safe deployment of the port instrument.[11]

Patients with known or suspected abdominal adhesions present a higher risk for peritoneal entry complications. When consenting patients with previous abdominal surgery, they must be informed of the likelihood of using a different peritoneal access method (visual or open entry), the possibility of a different access site (LUQ), or the odds of conversion to a laparotomy.[92]

In high risk acute instances, a visual Veress access method may be used, where a 1.2 mm diameter semirigid fiberoptic microlaparoscope, sheathed into a 2.1 mm diameter modified visual Veress needle method may be required to use.[93]

These can be inserted in the left upper quadrant, which is generally adhesion free, even in those who have had previous lower abdominal open operations. An umbilical "primary" ancillary ports can subsequently be safely placed under direct visual control, in an adhesion-free peritoneal area. Special care must be exercised in those patients with hepatosplenomegaly, portal hypertension, previous left upper quadrant or gastric surgery.[94-97]

These small caliber microlaparoscopes are generally available for conscious pain mapping, trauma units or diagnostic outpatient facilities where peritoneal visualization procedures may be required under conscious sedation.[98]

First to extol advantages of visual peritoneal access was Professor K. Semm of the University of Kiel, where his group advocated use of a beveled reusable cannula to navigate the primary port under visual control. His teaching proscribed blind penetration of the peritoneal cavity at all costs to improve patient safety.[99]

Several single use visual access methods were introduced (Optiview XCEL; Ethicon Endo-Surgery, Cincinnati, OH, USA, VisiPort; Tyco, Norwalk, CT, USA, other trocars) to improve primary laparoscopic peritoneal port placement safety. These visual access methods traded the blind sharp trocar/cannula for a hollow trocar with a transparent crystal tip at its distal end; when a zero degree laparoscope is sheathed into the hollowed central trocar, the distal crystal tip transmits entry images, as it transects abdominal tissue layers during insertion (Figs 12 and 13).

These visual access methods maintain a *push-through* trocar and cannula design where the central *spike principle* is employed to thrust a clear tipped trajectory across abdominal wall layers. Insertion requires significantly more penetration force, applied axial to anterior abdominal wall tissue layers, that tent towards the viscera; tissue compression at the distal crystal tip renders recognition of the different tissue layers during insertion difficult.[87,100]

Second generation reusable visual access cannula systems were then introduced to safeguard against human access error, through system redesign and elimination of

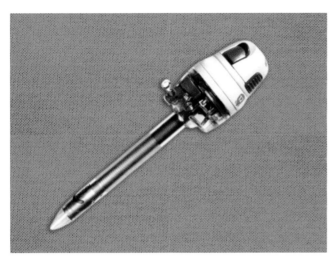

Fig. 12: Single-use visual trocar and cannula (Optiview XCEL™; Ethicon Endo-Surgery, Cincinnati, OH)

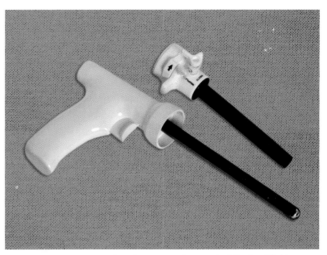

Fig. 13: Single-use visual trocar and cannula (VisiPort™; Tyco, Norwalk, CT, USA)

identified PSFs. As these specific access PSFs *(blind, sharp, forceful, uncontrolled, linear entry)* of conventional push-through trocar/cannula peritoneal entry are eliminated, port insertion becomes less hazardous. Error recognition is likely when mishaps occur and recovery is possible; interactive and real-time visual access avoids application of excessive axial penetration force at port site, requires no sharp or pointed trocar and allows visual and controlled port placement without overshoot.[101]

The Endoscopic Threaded Imaging Port (*EndoTIP™ Karl STORZ GmbH, Tuttlingen, Germany*) is a reusable visual access cannula that may be used during closed or open laparoscopy. It can be applied as a primary or ancillary port, and may be used to perform intra- or retroperitoneal operations.

It has a proximal valve and a stainless steel hollow distal cannula section. A single thread winds diagonally on its outer surface, which ends distally in a blunt notched tip. These are available in several lengths and diameters for different endoscopic applications. A retaining ring, telescope stopper is sheathed on to the 0° laparoscope to keep the distal end of the laparoscope 1 cm inside, short of the cannula's end during insertion (Fig. 14).

CLOSED Laparoscopic Access with the Threaded Visual Cannula: EndoTIP™

As recommended, all port insertions should be with the patient lying supine, with the operating table horizontal, since the Trendelenburg tilt position rotates the sacral promontory sliding the aortic bifurcation closer to the umbilicus, consequently increasing the likelihood of inadvertent vascular primary access injury.[102]

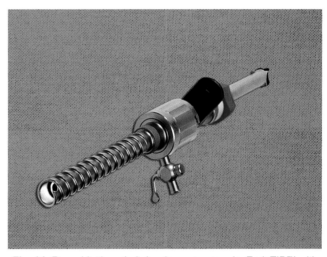

Fig. 14: Reusable threaded visual access cannula: EndoTIP™ with Telescope Stopper (Karl STORZ GmbH, Tuttlingen, Germany)

A generous sub-, intra- or supraumbilical skin incision is made, using a 15 surgical blade to accommodate the access cannulas outside diameter to avoid skin dystocia and obviate use of excessive penetration force at port site. Clearly CO_2 leak around a cannula has very little to do with skin incision size and everything to do with the anterior rectus fascial incision size, relative to the cannula's diameter and tissue recoil. Ribbon retractors and "peanut sponges" are used to expose the white anterior rectus fascia, as insertion starts at fascial level; then a Veress needle is inserted as described previously.

During insufflation, a 0° laparoscope is white balanced and defogged (*UltraStop sterile anti-fog solution. Sigmapharm, Wien*); then the telescope stopper ring, followed by the threaded visual cannula are mounted. The

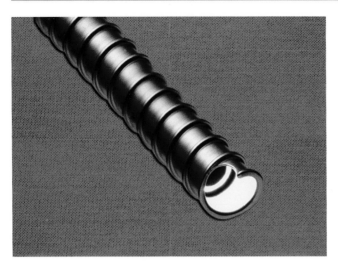

Fig. 15: Reusable threaded visual access cannula: EndoTIP™ with zero degree laparoscope, 1 cm short of the cannula's distal end

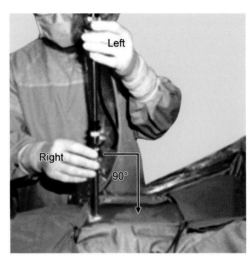

Fig. 16: How to hold the threaded visual access cannula: EndoTIP™ during application at primary umbilical site in an insufflated peritoneum

telescope stopper ring holds the laparoscope 1 cm short of the cannula's distal end and the camera is focused to the visual cannula's tip (Fig. 15).

When insufflation is complete, the Veress needle is retrieved; the cannula with mounted laparoscope is held vertical to the patient's supine abdomen, using the surgeon's nondominant hand and is lowered into the umbilical well with the CO_2 stopcock in the closed position.

Using the surgeon's dominant hand wrist muscles, the cannula is rotated clockwise, while keeping the forearm horizontal and shoulders in a comfortable resting position facing the monitor (Fig. 16). The bladeless blunt cannula's tip engages the anterior rectus fascia and lifts to transpose successive tissue layer sequentially onto the cannula's outer thread. The white anterior rectus fascia, red rectus muscle, pearly white posterior fascia, and yellowish pre-peritoneal fat are observed in sequence (Figs 17A to D).

The laparoscope's intense light traverses the thin taut peritoneal membrane and the CO_2-filled peritoneal cavity appears gray-blue in color. Vessels, bowel or adhesions are recognized and inadvertent injury avoided.

Further clockwise rotation, parts the thin peritoneal membrane radially to advance the cannula intraperitoneal, under direct visual control, without requiring a sharp trocar or applying axial excessive axial penetration force; the visual cannula and laparoscope has to remain perpendicular to the horizontal anterior abdominal tissues at all times to avoid tunneling.

OPEN Laparoscopic Access with the Threaded Visual Cannula: EndoTIP™

Surgeons, who are not familiar with the visual threaded access cannula, must first familiarize themselves with its use with pre-insufflation (Closed method), before attempting to use it without pre-insufflation (Open method). In addition, it is essential for the operator to clearly recognize tissue image transition off the monitor and not apply perpendicular penetration force toward the supine abdominal wall during insertion.

A generous skin incision is made using a 15 surgical blade; ribbon retractors are used to expose the anterior rectus fascia, the laparoscope is defogged and camera white-balanced. Then the telescope stopper ring and cannula are mounted, keeping the laparoscope's end 1 cm short of the visual cannula's distal tip (Fig. 15). The camera is focused to the cannula's blunt end and laparoscope held vertical to the patient's supine abdomen using the surgeon's nondominant hand.

The visual threaded access cannula EndoTIP™, with the CO_2 stopcock in the OPEN position, is lowered into the umbilical well and rotated clockwise, using the wrist muscles of the dominant hand while keeping the forearm horizontal and shoulders square in resting position, facing the monitor (Fig. 16).

The cannula's bladeless tip engages the anterior abdominal fascia, stretches it radially and then lifts to transpose successive tissue layers on to the visual cannula's outer thread. The white anterior rectus fascia, red rectus muscle, then pearly white posterior fascia and yellowish preperitoneum are pulled up in sequence along outer pitch. It is very important for the surgeon to identify and recognize each layer to avoid unintended overshoot and visceral injury (Figs 18A and B).

Given the intense light and magnification of the laparoscope, viscera, bowel or omentum can be observed moving across a transparent thin peritoneal membrane

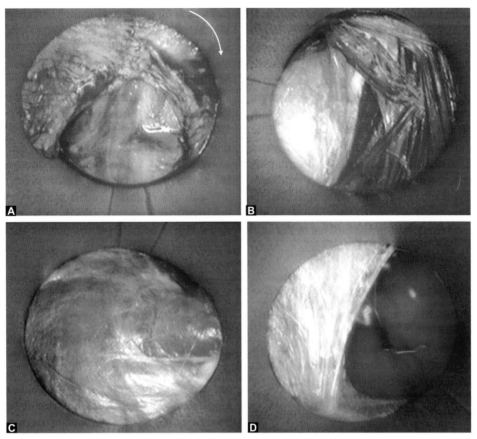

Figs 17A to D: Anterior abdominal wall layer sequencing during closed application of the threaded visual-access cannula: EndoTIP™

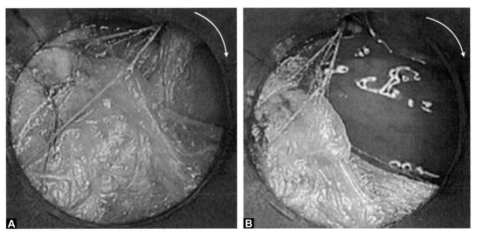

Figs 18A and B: Anterior abdominal wall layer sequencing during open application of the threaded visual-access cannula: EndoTIP™

with respiratory movements of the patient; bowel peristalsis is also clearly seen across the peritoneal membrane.

Upon peritoneal entry, room-air streams through the visual cannulas' open CO_2 stopcock, into the virtual peritoneal cavity, interposed between presenting organ and cannula. At this point, clockwise rotation is stopped and CO_2 insufflation initiated through a partially parted peritoneal membrane under visual control.

During closed preinsufflated laparoscopy, a CO_2-filled buffer zone is interposed between access device tip and intra-abdominal organs. Whereas, during open laparoscopy, the visual access cannula encounters abdominal contents directly upon peritoneal entry. It is, therefore, *very important* to identify location of the cannula at all times *(situational awareness)*, and distinguish access images at all times during port insertion. Surgeons must be familiar with normal anterior abdominal wall anatomy at entry site, learn when to stop rotation and know when to initiate insufflation.

Care must be exercised to minimize application of perpendicular penetration force as excessive axial force may cause unintended visceral injury. Tissue sequencing at port site during open insertion of laparoscopic access instruments in general is different from closed laparoscopic access. Therefore when applying the EndoTIP™ visual cannula in open laparoscopy, the surgeon must exercise extreme caution until well-versed in closed application of EndoTIP™ and fully familiar with anatomic image sequencing at access site.

Ancillary Laparoscopic Access with the Visual Threaded Cannula: EndoTIP™

Successful ancillary port insertion remains a very important step during laparoscopic surgery, as through these strategically placed ports, various specialized operative instruments are introduced to perform complex endoscopic operations.

Several important factors determine their insertion site, number and method of access; patient's weight, abdominal girth, anatomy, type of procedure performed and surgeon's preference will be taken into account.

As the abdomen is already distended with CO_2 gas and laparoscope-camera inserted, it is vital that all ancillary ports be observed visually through the primary port during their insertion, so as to minimize inadvertent injury.

Careful attention to vascular anatomy is also important, as injury to the deep epigastric vessels is the single most common vascular accident during operative laparoscopy.

Course of the epigastric vessel can be identified through laparoscopic inspection (inferior epigastric—last branch of the external iliac vessels) and abdominal transillumination (superficial epigastric—first branch of the femoral vessels); invariably, applying axial abdominal pressure with the

advancing instrument tip indents access-site. Access direction and penetration force axis can then be modified when vessels are suspected to lurch along a cannula's path to avoid injury.

Occasionally the inferior epigastric vessels are difficult to identify by abdominal transillumination, especially in overweight patients, those with abdominal adhesions and who have had previous surgical scars. Generally, they are easily identified laparoscopically on either side of the bladder, just medial to the internal inguinal ring, as they course lateral to the umbilical ligaments.

So as to avoid vascular injury, ancillary ports must be inserted lateral to the internal inguinal ring or medial to the umbilical ligaments. The triangular area between these two demarcating lines should be avoided when possible. Vessels encountered along the threaded visual cannula's path, move radially out of harm's way and are not transected (Figs 19A to C).

Application of the visual access cannula at ancillary sites requires a skin incision along Langer's lines and subcutaneous tissue dissection; an ancillary telescope is not necessary. As with all ancillary port insertions, ancillary threaded visual access cannulas must also be introduced under direct laparoscopic visual control. So as to avoid peritoneal tenting or tunneling, the threaded visual access cannula insertion must remain at right angle to skin surface until the abdominal cavity is entered and as usual, the urinary bladder should always be emptied before suprapubic port insertion.[101]

SINGLE-PORT LAPAROSCOPIC ACCESS WITH THE THREADED VISUAL CANNULA ENDOCONE™

Recently, the threaded visual access cannula method has been adapted to offer ergonomic single port access opportunities where a shorter and wider version

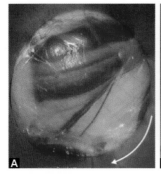 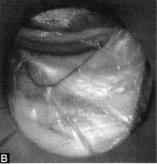 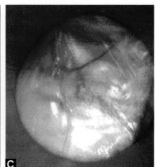

Figs 19A to C: Vessels encountered along the threaded visual-access cannula: EndoTIP's entry paths are not transected; they move laterally out of harm's way

(EndoCone, Karl STORZ GmbH, Tuttlingen, Germany), is applied at the umbilicus with several ancillary instrument conduits at its proximal end (Fig. 20).

At The Cleveland Clinic consensus meeting on single-port laparoscopic access surgery, there was general agreement to use the acronym LESS (Laparoendoscopic single-site surgery) to describe this contemporary form of laparoscopic operations.[103]

The evolutionary progress of minimally invasive surgery now offers four different and distinct approaches to achieve safe and less disabling endoscopic operations: conventional laparoscopic surgery, robotically assisted surgery, LESS and NOTES (natural orifice transluminal endoscopic surgery).

Single-site surgery in turn has three applications where through a single skin incision, different laparoscopic port methods are used to access the peritoneal cavity. The first method is application of a single conventional port and use of a laparoscope with an inline operative channel, the second method is applications of several smaller ports through a single skin incision with several fascial incisions, and the third method is application of a single port through a single anterior fascial incision, designed to accommodate several ancillary portals that accommodate several laparoscopic operative instruments.[104]

To this date, the threaded visual cannula method has been successfully used with all above three applications, however, insertion of several smaller cannulas through the anterior fascia in such close proximity through a single skin incision must be regarded with caution, as the collective effect of several fascial wounds in the same vicinity may undermine tissue recoil and the ability to restore port competence; once port shutter mechanism is compromised, the likelihood of incisional hernia becomes real.

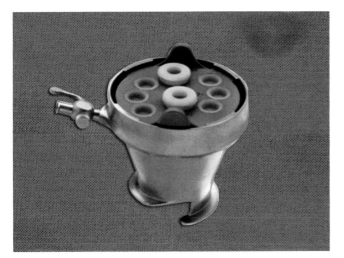

Fig. 20: Single-port access with the threaded cannula EndoCone™

One must remember that present scientific evidence regarding emerging port technologies, including some of these more contemporary LESS applications in general, is lacking and too limited to draw any firm conclusions regarding their long-term outcomes and benefits.[105]

Importance of Port Removal

Gradually more endoscopists are appreciating the importance of safe cannula removal to maintain port competence and avoid implantation of malignant cells along port tract, following oncological procedures. Introduction of the visual laparoscopic access systems allows surgeons to understand tissue dynamics at port-site during cannula removal as well; it helps to determine and maintain integrity of different tissue planes that preserve port competence.

Without the ability to visually observe port tract during insertion and removal of cannulas, surgeons are unable to identify compromised access sites; consequently, appropriate pre-emptive measures are not taken. Considering that the incidence of ventral hernia after laparotomy ranges between 11% and 20% versus the purported postendoscopic port site herniation of 0.02%;[106,107] although, some authors have published a port herniation rate of about 0.3–1.3%.[108]

Sharp pyramidal, bladed or cutting, trocars transect tissue layers along their path, disrupting the shutter mechanism at port site; their fascial defect is significantly larger, compared to the noncutting, bladeless visual cannula tip's fascial window.[50]

The threaded visual access cannula; EndoTIP™ is designed to address port competence concerns, such that the radially displaced tissue layers regain their normal gridiron orientation and restore the shutter mechanism at access site upon cannula removal.

Besides, entry point at the anterior rectus fascia, muscle, posterior fascia and peritoneal membrane are not stacked along a straight vertical axis, instead they are dispersed along the cannula's perimeter, thereby maintaining port competence (Figs 21A to C).

Glass et al. demonstrated in a randomized trial, that a smaller fascial wound area and less muscle damage, requiring less force when applying the threaded visual access cannula EndoTIP™, compared with the Ethicon Endopath TriStar Pyramidal Cutting Trocar of the same diameter.[109]

As the operation is completed, the stopcock is closed, CO_2 gas tubing disconnected, and laparoscope's end retracted 1 cm into the cannula, telescope stopper locked and camera focused to the visual cannula's tip.

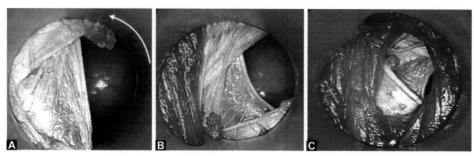

Figs 21A to C: Anterior abdominal wall layer sequencing during removal of the threaded visual-access cannula: EndoTIP™

Ancillary ports are removed under visual control, then peritoneal cavity dis-insufflated and finally the primary umbilical port is removed under visual control as well. The laparoscope is held perpendicular to the patient's abdomen with the nondominant hand, and cannula rotated counter clockwise with the dominant hand.

Since threaded cannula removal is visual, incremental and controlled, tissue injury or entrapment along the cannula's tract is avoided. When fascia is extended to retrieve surgical specimens; fascial reinforcing stay sutures are applied to that cannula entry site to further secure port competence.[110]

Anterior rectus fascial defect closure is particularly important in high risk patients where predisposing factors may exist. Several direct port-site fascial closure instruments are available; however, it has been shown that fascial suturing of laparoscopic entry sites decreases but does not eliminate incidence of all hernias.[34]

LAPAROSCOPIC ACCESS SITES

When umbilical placement of the Veress needle or primary port is deemed unsafe, such as in patients known to have umbilical adhesions, alternate access sites must be entertained. Palmer's point, located 3 cm below the left costal margin at midclavicular line is a popular and safe alternative, irrespective of access instrument or method used.[111]

First a nasogastric tube is inserted to prevent inadvertent gastric injury, as sometimes, the stomach may get distended with anesthetic gases during bagging and intubation. Surgeons must be particularly careful in patients with portal hypertension, gastric or pancreatic masses, splenomegaly or when left upper abdominal pathology is suspected.[112]

Patients who are considered high-risk, a preliminary umbilical inspection is possible with the optical Veress microlaparoscope, the threaded visual cannula, or other visually guided trocar-cannula systems; when peritoneal adhesions are mapped and additional ports inserted accordingly.

Safe and successful peritoneal access on first passage of a Veress needle through conventional sites does not exclude the possibility of umbilical adhesions or inadvertent subsequent bowel injury upon insertion of conventional trocars. The clinical burden of postoperative adhesions is well-documented in the SCAR study and it is clear that 60–90% of women who have undergone major gynecologic surgery will have some adhesions.[113]

Umbilical adhesion incidence is quoted to be less than 0.03%; however, it may be as high as 68 percent in certain patients with previous laparotomy, especially in those where a midline surgical scar extends to the umbilical region.[114]

Those patients with known peritoneal adhesions, those with a history of more than one previous laparoscopy, the morbidly obese patients, those with history of previous failed laparoscopy or insufflation and others with special circumstances may be candidates for alternate access techniques, with specialized laparoscopic visual access instruments.[5]

LAPAROSCOPIC ACCESS INSTRUMENTS

Regardless of model or make, conventional access instruments comprise two parts, a removable central trocar *[Origin: 1700–10. French trocart: trois, three (Old French, from Latin tres; Indo-European roots) + carre, side of an object (Old French, from carrer, square, from Latin quadrare; Indo-European roots), quadrum, square]* and an encasing outer sheath or cannula.[115]

Over the years a multitude of models and shapes of access instruments have appeared, however, the great majority conform to accommodate the traditional push through, spike and cannula entry concept, where linear force is recruited to propel the instrument into the peritoneal cavity; the only different system is the threaded visual cannula EndoTIP method where radial torque is used instead and the instrument is designed to access without requiring a central trocar.

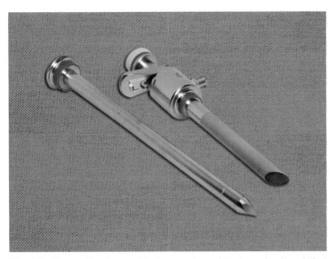

Fig. 22: Conventional reusable trocars have blunt proximal end that accommodates a surgeon's dominant palm and a distal sharp pointed tip

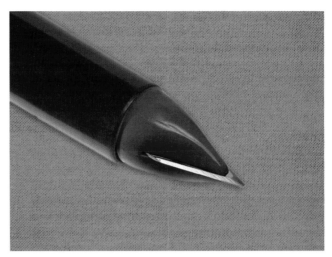

Fig. 23: Shielded single-use trocars have higher complication rates than multiple-use trocars

Generally conventional trocars have a blunt proximal end that accommodates a surgeon's dominant palm to create the required penetration force that is transmitted to the distal sharp, pointed tip at the instrument-tissue interface (Fig. 22).

The significant PF generated by the endoscopist's dominant arm and trunk muscles, is aligned axial at port site to drive the trajectory across different tissue layers toward the peritoneal cavity; then the trocar is withdrawn to sheath a laparoscope or operating instruments.

The distal trocar tip is frequently designed to comprise a piercing, sharp, conical, beveled, cutting, pyramidal or bladed end. Cutting pyramidal or bladed trocars are commonly used as their extremely sharp pointed tips make trajectory propulsion recruit less PF, which is theoretically intended to offer better trocar and cannula control.[23]

Moreover, excessive sharpness of single use trocars is purported by some to be advantageous to transect anterior abdominal myofascial tissue layers, risk of unintentional bowel or vessel injury cannot be overlooked; generally because of uncontrolled overshoot and blind insertion.

Some publications suggest risk of bowel injury with single use shielded trocars to be three times that previously reported for reusable trocars and 87% of deaths from vascular injuries involve use of shielded single use trocars (Fig. 23).[116]

Trocar tip shape is an essential ingredient when investigating access accident causation, as it determines entry method, application and propensity to unintended harm. Conical trocars have pointed sharp tips with no transecting edges; consequently considerably more PF is applied as tissue layers are not transected but parted to accommodate cannula's outer diameter.

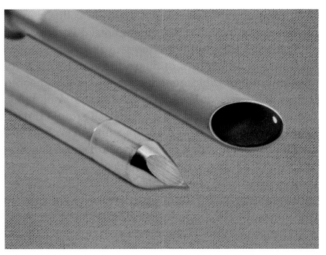

Fig. 24: Cannulas ends either horizontally or in an oblique slant with a small venting window at their distal end

The radially expanding Versa Step access device (Covidien, Mansfield, MA, USA) requires the most Penetration Force, as additional force is recruited to radially expand the outer encasing polymeric sheath in addition to abdominal wall layers, during trocar placement (Fig. 10).[50]

Surgeons with smaller hands and musculature should exercise additional caution when using these comparatively large gripped access instruments, as these are not generally designed to be gender compatible.[117]

Whereas blunt-tipped trocars are generally more risk averse and conical tips have to inflict a "direct hit" on a vessel to cause vascular injury as only the pointed tip is sharp, same sized bladed or cutting pyramidal trocars will cause significant injury, when it encounters any vessel along its entry path. [118]

While theoretical and intuitive advantages of these trocars appear to be clear, practical clinical application must be weighed against the considerable added PF required during insertion.[50]

It has been shown that the risk of port site incisional hernia is 10 times greater when single use cutting pyramidal trocars are used instead of a multiple use conical trocar (1.83 versus 0.17%).[119]

Open laparoscopic access trocars have a blunt tip, as peritoneal entry is not achieved by the trocar itself; instead access is established by "thrusting *blindly* a small pointed hemostat against the transversalis fascia and peritoneum".[70]

The cannula portion of access devices has a proximal valve section to allow insertion and removal of telescope or laparoscopic instruments without losing insufflated gas. They also offer a CO_2 insufflation stopcock, particularly those used at primary port. The shaft's outer surface is generally smooth and ends either horizontally or in an oblique slant with a small venting window at their distal end (Fig. 24).

There are several types of valves; some have pliable silastic seals to accommodate instruments of different diameters (5–15 mm) and are more user-friendly, while others have a fixed seal diameter to house instruments of one diameter at a time. The seal creates friction and dampens haptic feedback that distorts surgical performance.

Recently threaded cannulas have gained popularity as they fasten securely at port site and discourage inadvertent intraoperative slippage, requiring reinsertion and loss of insufflated gas.

The *Open* laparoscopy cannula has a cone-shaped anchoring sleeve that secures the cannula to anterior rectus fascia and discourages inadvertent displacement or CO_2 leakage (Fig. 11).

Laparoscopic entry instruments are either intended for single or multiple uses. Moreover, environmental concerns and escalating health care costs generally encourage reusable instrument use. Certainly, multiple uses of *single-use* designated instrument, especially trocars, is frowned upon and strongly discouraged as reliable re-sterilization is not possible and safe application not guaranteed.[120,121]

Single-use access trocars with automatic extending shields were initially designed to reduce risk of unintentional access harm, but recurring serious trocar related injuries continue to occur. According to the US FDA Office of Device Evaluation data, over the last 10 years, there have been more than 40,000 trocar-related injuries. These include several trocar-related deaths every year; consequently, the FDA ordered single use shielded trocar manufacturers and distributors to delete all such claims as no added "safety" is inferred and they have failed to decrease access injuries.[122]

Several publications suggest that serious access related injury to major vessels and bowel are not reported and the real accident incidence could be higher. [72,80,123-126]

Laparoscopic access injury is best understood when tissue dynamics at port site is studied in real-time. Careful error analysis is required to appreciate interaction between surgeon, instrument, and tissue. It has been published that a minimum of 25% of practicing Canadian gynecologists have experienced Veress needle or trocar injuries.[58]

A similar study surveyed about 2,000 US gynecologists, where 46% acknowledged trocar vessel injuries and 8% recognized major vessel or bowel trocar injuries.[127]

■ CONCLUSION

This chapter attempts to describe different peritoneal access methods, access instruments, and abdominal access sites available to laparoscopists, to help them achieve safe access into and exit from the peritoneal operative environment, with the least collateral tissue injury or hurt.

Undoubtedly all humans err, and endoscopists are no exception; those who claim to perform error-free are destined to repeatedly fail without learning from their mistakes. In doing so, they disregard the most important and fundamental tenet of safety; harness the ability of predicting accidents and learning from mistakes. As President JF Kennedy once said "An Error does not become a mistake until we refuse to correct it".[128]

Unlike the health care sector, high reliability organizations in business and industry appreciate and accept the reality that conditions inherent in task performance will and can occasionally lead to unintended human failure, with untoward serious consequences.

When faced with serious but very infrequent devastating industrial accidents such as chemical spills, mining incidents, or nuclear disasters, the luxury of conducting randomized controlled trials is unavailable. Instead, industry manages rare and devastating adverse events by applying tested and proved accident causation strategies and error analysis knowhow, to deconstruct events and re-engineer tasks to render them less hazardous.

Contemporary endoscopists need to learn from industry and invest in peritoneal access modeling and simulation studies to better understand recurring primary and ancillary peritoneal access injury; this is only possible when visual ports are used to capture, recall and review events at port, tissue and force interface.

Primary peritoneal access using the threaded visual cannula method creates a Zero Fault Tolerance Environment as it introducing three important patient safety redundancies that render laparoscopic port creation less perilous; allows real-time recognition of port injury (heightened situational awareness), offers mishap archiving opportunities for objective accident causation analysis (eliminates hind-sight bias) and develops error aversion techniques (warning annunciation) that other trocar and cannula access methods fail to offer.

As the US FDA recommends, endoscopists will also have to be versed in alternate peritoneal entry methods, learn how to apply other access instruments and be familiar with different port placement sites, for those patients where conventional port placement is not advisable.[5]

▌REFERENCES

1. Chapron C, Fauconnier A, Goffinet F, et al. Laparoscopic surgery is not inherently dangerous for patients presenting with benign gynaecologic pathology. Results of a meta-analysis. Hum Reprod. 2002;17:1334-42.

2. Harkki-Siren P, Kurki T. A nationwide analysis of laparoscopic complications. Obstet Gynecol. 1997;89:108-12.

3. Jansen FW, Kapiteynnn K, Trimbos-Kemper T, et al. Complications of laparoscopy: a prospective multicentre observational study. Br J Obstet Gynaecol. 1997;104:595-600.

4. Jansen FW, Kolkman W, Bakkum EA, et al. Complications of laparoscopy: an inquiry about closed versus open-entry technique. Am J Obstet Gynecol. 2004;190(3):634-8.

5. Laparoscopic Trocar Injuries: A report from a U.S. Food and Drug Administration (FDA) Center for Devices and Radiological Health (CDRH) Systematic Technology Assessment of Medical Products (STAMP) Committee. Cited 2003 Nov 7. [online] Available from: URL:http://www.fda.gov/cdrh/medicaldevicesafety/stamp/trocar.html. [Accessed January, 2015].

6. Bogner MS. "Medical Devices and Human Error" in Human Performance in Automated Systems: Current Research and Trends. In: Mouloua M, Parasuraman R (Eds). Hillsdale, NJ: Lawrence Erlbaum; 1994. pp. 64-7.

7. Lekawa M, Shapiro SJ, Gordon LA, et al. The laparoscopic learning curve. Surg Laparosc Endosc. 1995;5:455-8.

8. Garry R. Complications of laparoscopic entry. Gynecol Endosc. 1997;6:319-29.

9. Garry R. Editorial. Towards evidence-based laparoscopic entry techniques: clinical problems and dilemmas. Gynaecol Endosc. 1998. pp. 315-26.

10. Garry R. Letter to the Editor. Surgeons may continue to use their chosen entry technique; Laparoscopic entry techniques. Cochrane Database Syst Rev. 2008 Apr 16;(2): CD006583. Gynecol Surg. 2009;6:87-92.

11. Ternamian A. Laparoscopic Access. In: N Jain (editor). State-of-the-Art Atlas of Endoscopic Surgery in Infertility and Gynecology. Laparoscopic Access. 2nd edition. Chapter 3. New Delhi: Jaypee Bros; 2010. pp. 20-33.

12. Patkin M, Isabel L. Ergonomics, engineering and surgery of endosurgical dissection. J R Coll Surg Edinb. 1995;40:120-32.

13. Cuschieri A. Whither minimal access surgery: tribulations and expectations. Am J Surg. 1995;1:9-19.

14. Hanna GB, Shimi SM, Cuschieri A. Optimal port locations for endoscopic intracorporeal knotting. Surg Endosc. 1997;11:397-401.

15. Quick NE, Gilette JC, Shapiro, et al. The effect of using laparoscopic instruments on muscle activation patterns during minimally invasive training procedures. Surg Endosc. 2003;17:462-5.

16. Emam TA, Hanna GB, Kimber C, et al. Effect of intracorporeal-extracorporeal instrument length ratio on endoscopic task performance and surgeon movements. Arch Surg. 2000;135:62-5.

17. Beurger R, Forkey D, Smith WD. Ergonomic problems associated with laparoscopic surgery. Surg Endosc. 1999;13:466-8.

18. Beurger R, Smith WD, Chung YH. Performing laparoscopic surgery is significantly more stressful for the surgeon than open surgery. Surg Endosc. 2001;15:1204-7.

19. Sexton JB, Thomas EJ, Helmreich RL. Error, stress, and teamwork in medicine and aviation: cross-sectional survey. BMJ. 2000;320:745-9.

20. Moorthy K, Munz Y, Dosis A, et al. The effect of stress-induced conditions on the performance of a laparoscopic task. Surg Endosc. 2003;17:1481-4.

21. Taffinder N, McManus IC, Gul Y, et al. Objective assessment of the effect of sleep deprivation on surgical psychomotor skill. Lancet. 1999;353:1191.

22. Ternamian A. In Endoskopische Abdominalchirurgie in der Gynäkologie. In: L. Mettler. Stuttgart, Schattauer, 2002, Chapter 9, 175-80.

23. Corson SL, Batzer FR, Gocial B, et al. Measurement of the force necessary for laparoscopic trocar entry. J Reprod Med. 1989;34(4):282-4.

24. Passerotti CC, Begg N, PennaFJ, et al. Safety profile of trocar and insufflation needle access systems in laparoscopic surgery. J Am Coll Surg. 2009;209(2):222-32.

25. Singh SS, Marcoux V, Ternamian A. Core competencies for gynecologic endoscopy in residency training: a national consensus project. J Minim Invasive Gynecol. 2009;16(1):1-7.

26. Raymond E, Ternamian A, Tolomiczenko G. Endoscopy teaching in Canada: a survey of obstetrics and gynecology program directors and graduating residents. J Minim Invasive Gynecol. 2006;13:10-6.

27. Munro MG. Laparoscopic access: complications, technologies, and techniques. Curr Opin Obstet Gynecol. 2002;14(4):365-74..

28. Ternamian A. Port creation during laparoscopic hysterectomy. In: Mettler L, (Ed). New Delhi, India: Jaypee Brothers Medical Publishers (P) Ltd; 2007. pp. 175-80.

29. Ternamian AM. Laparoscopy without trocars. Surg Endosc. 1997;11:815-8.

30. Molloy D, Kaloo PD, Cooper M, et al. Laparoscopic entry: a literature review and analysis of techniques and complications of primary port entry. Aust NZJ Obstet Gynaecol. 2002;42:246-53.

31. János Veress. Neues Instrument zur Ausführung von Brust- oder Bauchpunktionen und Pneumothoraxbehandlung. Deutsche Medizinische Wochenschrift - DEUT MED WOCHENSCHR. 01/1938; 64(41):1480-1.

32. Wolfart W. Surgical treatment of tuberculosis, its modifications, collapse therapy, resection treatment and present-day sequelae. Offent Gesundheitswes. 1990;52(8-9):506-11.

33. Richardson RE, Sutton CJ. Complications of first entry: a prospective laparoscopic audit. Gynaecol Endosc. 1999;8:327-34.

34. Leonard F, Lecuru F, Rizk E, et al. Perioperative morbidity of gynecological laparoscopy, a prospective monocenter observational study. Acta Obstet Gynecol Scand. 2000;79:129-34.

35. Härkki-Sirén P. The incidence of entry-related laparoscopic injuries. Finland Gynecol Endosc. 1999;8:335-8.

36. Pickett SD, Rodewald KJ, Billow MR, et al. Avoiding major vessel injury during laparoscopic instrument insertion. Obst Gynecol Clin of North America. 2010;37(3):387-97.

37. Albanese A, Albanese E, Mino J, et al. Peritoneal surface area: measurements of 40 structures covered by peritoneum: correlation between total peritoneal surface area and the surface calculated by formulas. Surg Radiol Anat. 2009;31:369-77.

38. Ott DE. Desertification of the peritoneum by thin-film evaporation during laparoscopy. JSLS. 2003;7:189-95.

39. Teoh B, Sen R, Abbott J. An evaluation of four tests used to ascertain Veress needle placement at closed laparoscopy. J Minim Invasive Gynecol. 2005;12:153-8.

40. Vilos GA, Vilos AG. Safe laparoscopic entry guided by Veress needle CO_2 insufflation pressure. J Am Assoc Gynecol Laparosc. 2003;10:415-20.

41. Vilos GA, Vilos AG, Abu-Rafea B, et al. Three simple steps during closed laparoscopic entry may minimize major injuries. Surg Endosc. 2009;23:758-64.

42. McDougall E, Figenshau RS, Clayman RV. J Laparoscopic Surgery 1994;4:6. Mary Ann Liebert, Inc.Publishers.

43. Phillips G, Garry R, Kumar C, et al. How much gas is required for initial insufflation at laparoscopy? Gynaecol Endosc. 1999;8:369-74.

44. Reich H, Robeiro SC, Rasmussen C, et al. High-pressure trocar insertion technique. J Soc Laparoendosc Surg. 1999;3:45-8.

45. Kroft J, Aneja A, Ternamian A, et al. Laparoscopic peritoneal entry preferences among Canadian gynaecologists. J Obstet Gynecol Can. 2009;31:641-8.

46. Sammour T, Kahokehr A, Hill A. Meta-analysis of the effect of warm humidified insufflation on pain after laparoscopy. Br J Surg. 2008;95:950-6.

47. Binda M, Molinas C, Hansen P, et al. Effect of desiccation and temperature during laparoscopy on adhesion formation in mice. Fertil Stertil. 2006;86:166-75.

48. Abu-Rafea A, Vilos GA, Vilos AG, et al. High-pressure laparoscopic entry does not adversely affect cardiopulmonary function in healthy women. J Minim Invasive Gynecol. 2005;12:475-9.

49. Turner DJ. Making the case for the radially expanding access system. Gynaecol Endosc. 1999;8:391-5.

50. Tarnay CM, Glass KB, Munro MG. Entry force and intra-abdominal pressure associated with six laparoscopic trocar cannula systems: a randomized comparison. Obstet Gynecol. 1999;94:83-8.

51. Yim SF, Yuen PM. Randomized double-masked comparison of radially expanding access device and conventional cutting tip trocar in laparoscopy. Obstet Gynecol. 2001;97:435-8.

52. Lam TY, Lee SW, So HS, et al. Radially expanding trocars: a less painful alternative for laparoscopic surgery. J Laparoendosc Adv Surg Tech A. 2000;19(5):269-73.

53. Bhoyrul S, Payne J, Steffes B, et al. A randomized prospective study of radially expanding trocars in laparoscopic surgery. J Gastroint Surg. 2000;4:392-7.

54. Dingfelder JR. Direct laparoscopic trocar insertion without prior pneumoperitoneum. J Reprod Med. 1978;21:45-7.

55. Catarci M, Carlini M, Gentileschi P, et al. Major and minor injuries during the creation of pneumoperitoneum: a multicenter study on 12,919 cases. Surg Endos. 2001;15:566-9.

56. Byron JW, Markenson G, Miyazawa K. A randomized comparison of Veress needle and direct trocar insertion for laparoscopy. Surg Gynecol Obstet. 1993;177:259-62.

57. Borgatta L, Gruss L, Barad D, et al. Direct trocar insertion vs Veress needle use for laparoscopic sterilization. J Reprod Med. 1990;35:891-4.

58. Yuzpe AA. Pneumoperitoneum needle and trocar injuries in laparoscopy: a survey on possible contributing factors and prevention. J Reprod Med. 1990;35:485-90.

59. Kaali SG, Barad DH. Incidence of bowel injury due to dense adhesions of direct trocar insertions. J Reprod Med. 1992;27:617-8.

60. Jacobson MT, Osias J, Bizhang R, et al. The direct trocar technique: an alternative approach to abdominal entry for laparoscopy. J SLS. 2002;6:169-74.

61. Copeland C, Wing R, Hulka JF. Direct trocar insertion at laparoscopy: an evaluation. Obstet Gynecol. 1983;62:655-9.

62. Saidi SH. Direct laparoscopy without prior pneumo-peritoneum. J Reprod Med. 1986;31:684-6.

63. Jarett JC. Laparoscopy: direct trocar insertion without pneumoperitoneum. Obstet Gynecol. 1990;75:725-7.

64. Woolcot R. The safety of laparoscopy performed by direct trocar insertion and carbon dioxide insufflation under vision. Aus NZ J Obstet Gynaecol. 1997;37:216-9.

65. Silfen SL, Evans D, Nezhat C. Comparison of direct insertion of disposable and standard reusable laparoscopic trocars and previous pneumoperitoneum with Veress needle. Obstet Gynecol. 1991;78:148-50.

66. Byron JW, Fujiyoshi CA, Miyazawa K. Evaluation of the direct trocar insertion technique at laparoscopy. Obstet Gynecol. 1989;74:423-5.

67. Mintz M. Risks and prophylaxis in laparoscopy: A survey of 100,000 cases. J Reprod Med. 1977;18:269-72.

68. Hill DJ, Maher PJ. Direct cannula entry for laparoscopy. J Am Assoc Gynecol Laparosc. 1996;4(1):77-9.

69. Hasson HM. A modified instrument and method for laparoscopy. Am J Obstet Gynecol. 1971;110:886-7.

70. Hasson HM. Open laparoscopy as a method of access in laparoscopic surgery. Gynaecol Endosc. 1999;8:353-62.

71. Hasson HM, Rotman C, Rana N, et al. Open laparoscopy: 29-year experience. Obstet Gynecol. 2000;96:63-6.

72. Bonjer HJ, Hazebroek EJ, Kazemier G, et al. Open versus closed establishment of pneumoperitoneum in laparoscopic surgery. Br J Surg. 1997;84;599-602.

73. Schafer M, Lauper M, Krahenbuhl L. Trocar and Veress needle injuries during laparoscopy. Surg Endosc. 2001;15:275-80.

74. Sigman HH, Fried GM, Garzon J, et al. Risks of blind versus open approach to celiotomy for laparoscopic surgery. Surg Laparosc Endosc. 1993;3:296-9.

75. Zaraca F, Catarci M, Gosselti F, et al. Routine use of open laparoscopy: 1,006 consecutive cases. J Laparoendosc Adv Surg Tech A. 1999;9:75-80.

76. Neudecker J, Sauerland S, Nengebauer F, et al. The European Association for Surgery Clinical Practice Guideline on the pneumoperitoneum for laparoscopic surgery. Surg Endosc. 2002;16:1121-43.

77. Deffieux X, Ballester M, Collinet P, et al. Risk associated with laparoscopic entry: guidelines for clinical practice from the French College of Gynaecologists and Obstetricians. Euro J Obstet Gynaecol Repro Bio. 2011:158;159-66.

78. Vilos GA, Ternamian A, Dempster J, et al. Laparoscopic entry: a review of techniques, technologies and complications. J Obstet Gynecol Can. 2007;29:433-47.

79. Hanney RM, Carmalt HL, Merrett N, et al. Use of the Hasson cannula producing major vascular injury at laparoscopy. Surg Endosc. 1999:13;1238-40.

80. Vilos GA. Litigation of laparoscopic major vessel injuries in Canada. J Am Assoc Gynecol Laparosc. 2000;7:503-9.

81. Chapron C, Cravello L, Chopin N, et al. Complications during set-up procedures for laparoscopy in gynecology: open laparoscopy does not reduce the risk of major complications. Acta Obstet Gynecol Scand. 2003:82:1125-9.

82. Merlin T, Hiller J, Maddern G, et al. Systematic review of the safety and effectiveness of methods used to establish pneumoperitoneum in laparoscopic surgery. Br J Surg. 2003;90:668-70.

83. Chandler JG, Corson SL, Way LW. Three spectra of laparoscopic entry access injury. J Am Coll Surg. 2001;192:478-91.

84. Magrina J. Complications of laparoscopic surgery. Clin Obstet Gynecol. 2002;45:469-80.

85. Marret H, Harchaoui Y, Chapron C, et al. Trocar injuries during laparoscopic gynaecological surgery. Report from the French Society of Gynecological Laparoscopy. Gynaecol Endosc. 1998;7:235-41.

86. Cuschieri A, Berci G. Laparoscopic Biliary Surgery. 1992;34-6.

87. Mettler L, Schmidt EH, Frank V, et al. Optical trocar systems: laparoscopic entry and its complications (a study of case in Germany). Gynaecol Endosc. 1999;8:383-9.

88. Joice P, Hanna GB, Cuschieri A. Errors enacted during endoscopic surgery—a human reliability analysis. Appl Ergo. 1998;29:409-14.

89. Mackenzie C, Jefferies N, Hunter W, et al. Comparison of self-reporting of deficiencies in airway management with video analyses of actual performance. Human Factors. 1996;38:623-35.

90. Krizek T. Surgical error: reflections on adverse events. Bull Am Coll Surg. 2000;85:18-22.

91. Wanzel K, Jamieson C, Bohnen J. Complications on a general surgery service: incidence and reporting. Can J Surg. 1999;43:113-7.

92. Fuller J, Ashar BS, Carey-Corrado J. Trocar-associated injuries and fatalities: an analysis of 1399 reports to the FDA. J Minim Invasive Gynecol. 2005;12:302-7.

93. Audebert AJ. The role of micro-laparoscopy in the diagnosis of peritoneal and visceral adhesions and in the prevention of bowel injury associated with blind trocar insertion. Fertil Steril. 2000;73:631-5.

94. Janicki TI. The new sensor-equipped Veress needle. J Am Assoc Gynecol Laparosc. 1994;1(2):154-6.

95. Noorani M, Noorani K. Pneumoperitoneum under vision—a new dimension in laparoscopy. Endo World. 1997;39-E:1-8.

96. Schaller G, Kuenkel M, Manegold BC. The optical Veress needle initial puncture with a mini-optic. Endosc Surg Allied Technol. 1995;3:55-7.

97. Parker J, Reid G, Wong F. Micro-laparoscopic left upper quadrant entry in patients at high risk of periumbilical adhesions. Aust NZJ Obstet Gynecol. 1999;39(11):88-92.

98. Okeahialam MG, O'Donovan PJ, Gupta JK. Micro-laparoscopy using an optical Veress needle inserted at Palmer's point. Gynaecol Endosc. 1999;8:115-6.

99. Semm K, Semm I. Safe insertion of trocars and the Veress needle using standard equipment and the 11 security steps. Gynae Endosc. 1997;6:319-29.

100. Meltzer A, Weiss U, Roth K, et al. Visually controlled trocar insertion by means of the optical scalpel. Endosc Surg Allied Technol. 1993;1:239-42.

101. Ternamian AM. A trocarless, reusable, visual-access cannula for safer laparoscopy; an update. J Am Assoc Gynecol Laparosc. 1998;5(2):197-201.

102. Garry R. A consensus document concerning laparoscopic entry: Middlesbrough, March 19 –20 1999. Gynaecol Endosc. 1999;8:403-6.

103. Gill IS, Advincula AP, Aron M, et al. Consensus statement of the consortium for laparoscopic single-site surgery. Surg Endosc. 2010;24:762-8.

104. Uppal S, Frumovitz M, Escobar P, et al. Laparoscopic single-site surgery in gynecology: review of literature and available technology. J Minim Invasive Gynecol. 2011;18(1):12-23.

105. Romanelli JR, Earle DB. Single-port laparoscopic surgery: an overview. Surg Endosc. 2009;23:1419-27.

106. Luijendijk RW, Hop WC, van den Tol MP. A comparison of suture repair with mesh repair for incisional hernia. N Engl J Med. 2000;343:392-8.

107. Montz FJ, Holschneider CH, Munro MG. Incisional hernias following laparoscopy: a survey of the American Association of Gynecologic Laparoscopists. Obstet Gynecol. 1994;84:881-4.

108. Mayol J, Garcia-Aguilar J, Ortiz-Oshiro E, et al. Risks of the minimal access approach for laparoscopic surgery: multivariate analysis of morbidity related to umbilical trocar insertion. W J Surg. 1997;21:529-33.

109. Glass KB, Tarnay CM, Munro MG. Intra-abdominal pressure and incision parameters associated with a pyramidal laparoscopic trocar-cannula system and the EndoTIP cannula. J Am Assoc Gynecol Laparosc. 2002;9:508-13.

110. Ternamian AM. How to improve laparoscopic access safety: EndoTIP. Min Invas Ther & Allied Technol. 2001;10:31-9.

111. Palmer R. Safety in laparoscopy. J Reprod Med. 1974; 13(1):1-5.

112. Chapron C, Pierre F, Harchaoui Y, et al. Gastrointestinal injuries during gynaecological laparoscopy. Hum Repro. 1999;14:333-7.

113. Lower AM, Hawthorn RJ, Ellis H, et al. The impact of adhesions on hospital readmissions over ten years after 8849 open gynaecological procedures: an assessment from the Surgical and Clinical Adhesions Research Study 2000. Brit J Obstet Gynecol. 2000;107:855-62.

114. Childers JM, Brzechffa PR, Surwit EA. Laparoscopy using the left upper quadrant as the primary trocar site. Gynaecol Oncol. 1993;50:221-5.

115. The American Heritage® Dictionary of the English Language, 4th edition. Houghton Mifflin Harcourt Publishing Company. 2010.

116. Nezhat F, Nezhat C, Levy JS. A report of laparoscopic injuries and complications over a 10-year period. Presented at the 41st annual clinical meeting of the American College of Obstetricians and Gynecologists, Washington DC, 1993.

117. Brill AI, Cohen BM. Fundamentals of Peritoneal Access. J Am Assos Gynecol Laparosc. 2003;10(2):287-97.

118. Hurd WW, Wang L, Schemmel MT. A comparison of the relative risk of vessel injury with conical versus pyramidal laparoscopic trocars in a rabbit model. Am J Obstet Gynecol. 1995;173:1731-3.

119. Leibl BJ, Schmedt CG, Schwarz J, et al. Laparoscopic surgery complications associated with trocar tip design: review of literature and own results. J Laparosc Adv Surg Tech. 1999;9:135-40.

120. Hurd WW, Diamond MP. There's a hole in my bucket, the cost of disposable instruments. Fertil Steril. 1997;67:13-5.

121. Chan AC, Ip M, Koehler A, et al. Is it safe to reuse disposable laparoscopic trocars. Surg Endosc. 2000;14:1042-4.

122. Department of Health and Human Services FDA Division of Enforcement II, Center for Devices and Radiological Health. (www.fda.gov/cdrh/mdrfile).

123. Deziel DJ. Avoiding laparoscopic complications. Int Surg. 1994;79:361-4.

124. Deziel DJ, Millikan KW, Economou SG, et al. Complications of laparoscopic cholecystectomy: a national survey of 4,292 hospitals and an analysis of 77,604 cases. Am J Surg. 1993;165:9-14.

125. Wherry DC, Marohn MR, Malanoski MP, et al. An external audit of laparoscopic cholecystectomy in the steady state performed in a medical treatment facility of the Department of Defense. Ann Surg. 1996;224:145-54.

126. Champault G, Cazacu F, Taffinder N. Serious trocar accidents in laparoscopic surgery: a French survey of 103,852 operations. Surg Laparosc Endosc. 1996;6:367-70.

127. Feste JR, Winkel CA. Is the standard of care what we think it is? JSLS. 1999;3:331-4.

128. The President and the Press: Address before the American Newspaper Publishers Association. [online] Available at www.jfklibrary.org/Historical 1Resources/Archives/Reference1Desk/Speeches/JFK/003POF03News paper-Publishers04271961.htm. [Accessed January 7, 2015].

CHAPTER 3

Port Placement in Laparoscopy

Ibrahim Alkatout, Liselotte Mettler

■ INTRODUCTION AND OUTLINE

Although the anatomy of the human being has not changed, technical developments in operating materials and methods demand a simultaneous development in operative management. Developments in electronic and optical technologies permit many gynecological operations to be performed laparoscopically. One fundamental distinction between any other operating method and laparoscopy is the hurdle that the initial entry, whether with a needle, cannula, or trocar, is mostly performed blind. Blind entry may result in vascular or organ damage. One of the difficulties associated with entry complications is that any damage may not be immediately recognized, leading to major abdominal reparative surgery and at worst a temporary colostomy. Therefore, the technical and operative quality of laparoscopic surgery begins with port placement and trocars. Visual access systems are available but are not yet widely used.

The aim of this chapter is to introduce the different port placement and trocar systems as well as their correct and professional usage.

■ COUNSELING AND INFORMED CONSENT

Patients undergoing a laparoscopic procedure have to be informed of the risks and potential complications as well as the alternative operating methods. Counseling before laparoscopy should include discussion of the entry technique used and the different risks associated with laparoscopic entry: Injury of the bowel, urinary tract, blood vessels, omentum and other surrounding organs and, at a later date, wound infection, adhesion associated pain, and hernia formation.

Counseling needs to integrate the individual risk dependent on the body mass index (BMI) and obesity or significant underweight of the patient. Depending on the medical history, it is important to consider anatomical malformations, midline abdominal incisions, a history of peritonitis or inflammatory bowel disease.[1]

■ EXTRA-ABDOMINAL RELEVANT ANATOMY

Relevant Anatomy

Anatomical basis: The anterior abdominal wall has four muscles which are penetrated at all entries: rectus abdominis, external obliquus abdominis, internal obliquus abdominis, and transversus abdominis. At laparotomy the incision possibilities are transversal with the conventional, Pfannenstiel "incision in the lower abdomen, a little higher than the fascial opening called, Misgav-Ladach cesarean section incision" as described by Joel Cohen and Michael Stark, and the longitudinal incision up to the umbilicus or around it.

Although at laparoscopy, the penetrating areas are variable, the usual trocar placement uses similar inserting areas. Therefore, it is obligatory for any surgeon to be experienced in the anatomy of the abdominal wall and its consecutive relevant anatomical structures.

There are no significant vascular structures that need to be respected on insertion of the subumbilical trocar. Solely, strict attention has to be given to holding to the median line to avoid any accidental damage to paramedian structures.

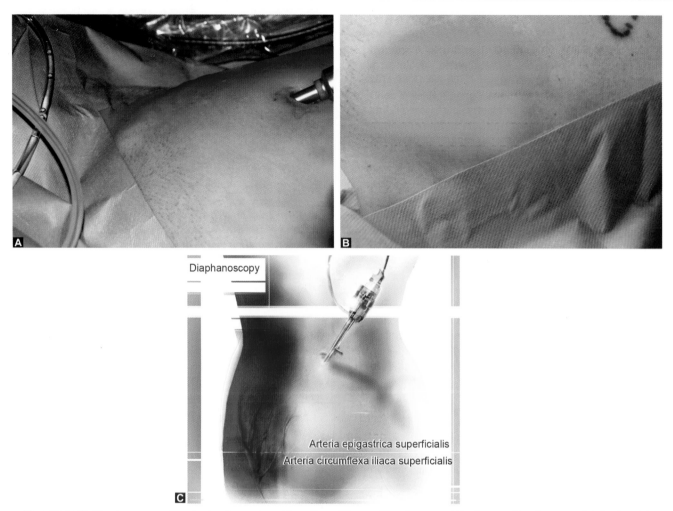

Figs 1A to C: Diaphanoscopy illuminates the region of insertion of the ancillary trocars while demarcating the superficial epigastric artery and the circumflex iliac superficial artery

There are two arteries in the superficial abdominal wall that should be visualized. Damage to these arteries should be avoided as even superficial incisions can lead to severe bleedings that require the conversion from laparoscopy to laparotomy. Both vessels can be visualized by diaphanoscopy (Figs 1A to C). Trocar placement is performed, dependent on the corresponding internal site, at a 90° angle to the abdominal wall once the aiming point has been located. The *superficial epigastric artery* arises from the femoral artery about 1 cm below the inguinal ligament through the fascia cribrosa, turns upward in front of the inguinal ligament, and ascends while spreading out between the two layers of the superficial fascia of the abdominal wall, nearly as far as the umbilicus. The *circumflex iliac superficial artery* originates from the femoral artery close to the superficial epigastric artery. After perforating the fascia lata, it runs parallel to the inguinal ligament and laterally to the iliac crest while spreading into smaller branches.

Places for Trocar Insertion

The laparoscope and optic trocar should be inserted, whenever possible, in the subumbilical region using a semilunar or straight incision (Figs 2A and B). Only if trocar placement is not possible, due to severe adhesions or large intra-abdominal tumors, are alternative entry sites negotiated, e.g. above the umbilicus or Palmer's point (Figs 3A to C) as a precursor entry site.

The placement for the working trocars depends on the operation. If the operative focus is located in the pelvis and no large tumor is expected to be touching the umbilical region, the two working trocars can be inserted in the lower abdominal wall in a vessel-free area confirmed by diaphanoscopy. Any auxiliary trocar can be placed in the midline suprasymphysically. Apart from the obliterated urachus and the bladder in the lower region, no remarkable anatomical structures are to be found (Figs 4A and B).

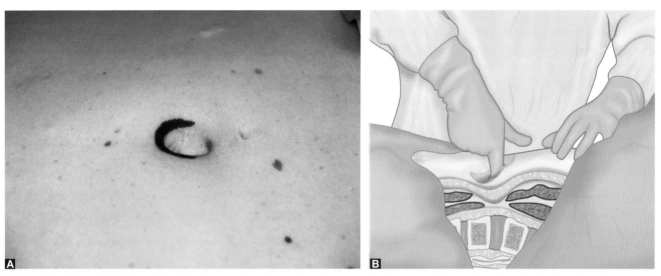

Figs 2A and B: Subumbilical incision and local palpation demonstrate the short distance from the skin to the spine. The retroperitoneal vessels are visible

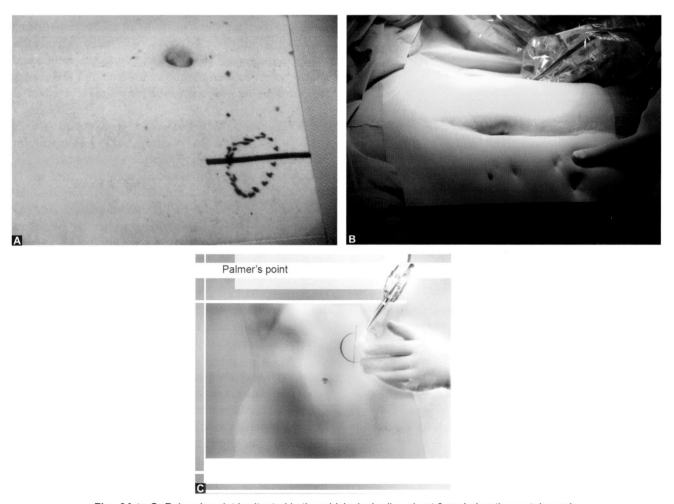

Figs 3A to C: Palmer's point is situated in the midclavicular line about 3 cm below the costal margin

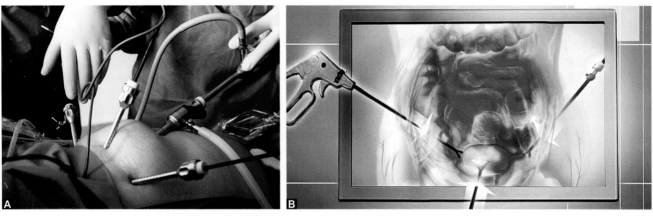

Figs 4A and B: Overview after insertion of the laparoscope and 3 ancillary trocars

INTRA-ABDOMINAL RELEVANT ANATOMY THROUGH THE EYE OF THE TROCAR

Anatomical Landmarks

Before any additional trocar to the optic trocar is inserted, the area of insertion has to be examined carefully with the laparoscope. Assuming a standard operation, the placement of two additional working trocars in the lower abdomen alongside an auxiliary trocar in the midline can be performed. It is important to identify the different landmarks of the abdominal wall. Beginning in the midline, the *plica umbilicalis mediana* contains the obliterated urachus and requires no further attention besides a hoisted bladder, e.g. after cesarean section. Moving laterally, the paired *plica umbilicalis medialis* contains the obliterated umbilicalis artery in the ligamentum umbilicale mediale that carries fetal blood through the umbilical cord to the placenta before it obliterates after birth and is therefore hazard-free, too. The next step leads to the plica umbilicalis lateralis with the integrated vasa epigastrica inferiors. The *inferior epigastric artery* originates at the inguinal ligament of the external iliac artery. It cuts along the subperitoneal tissue ventrally and then moves upward oblique—alongside the medial edge of the anulus inguinalis profundus. Afterward, it perforates the fascia of the musculus transversus abdominis and climbs upward between the musculus rectus abdominis and the rectus wall, thereby moving ventrally of the linea arcuata. Above the umbilicus, it divides into many small branches that anastomose with the superior epigastric artery. In contrast to the superficially spreading vascular branches, the inferior epigastric artery cannot be visualized by diaphanoscopy.

Places for Trocar Insertion

Once the cutaneous region has been determined from the outside with the aid of diaphanoscopy, the safe distance to the plica umbilicalis lateralis can be verified by palpation (Figs 5A to D). The correct point of insertion is usually about two thumbs medial of the spina iliaca anterior superior (Figs 6A and B). Being distant to the plica, the trocar is placed at a 90° angle and pushed forward until the tip of the trocar can be seen with the laparoscope (Figs 7A to C).

PORTS AND TROCARS

Development of Ports and Trocars

The word "trocar" is of French origin and is derived from *trois* (three) + *carré* (edge). A trocar is a medical instrument with a mostly sharply pointed end, often three-sided, that is used inside a hollow cylinder (cannula) to introduce ports into the abdomen.

Types of Ports and Trocars

Trocars are available in different sizes, from 3 mm up to 12 mm and larger. In standard procedures, the optic trocar is placed in the lower part of the umbilicus and its size varies depending on the operative procedure. For easy procedures, such as diagnostic laparoscopies or adnectomies, a 5 mm optic trocar is usually sufficient and provides enough light and precision. More pretentious procedures demand a brighter light source and a better picture which is provided by a 10 mm optic trocar. Standard procedures use two working trocars on each side of the

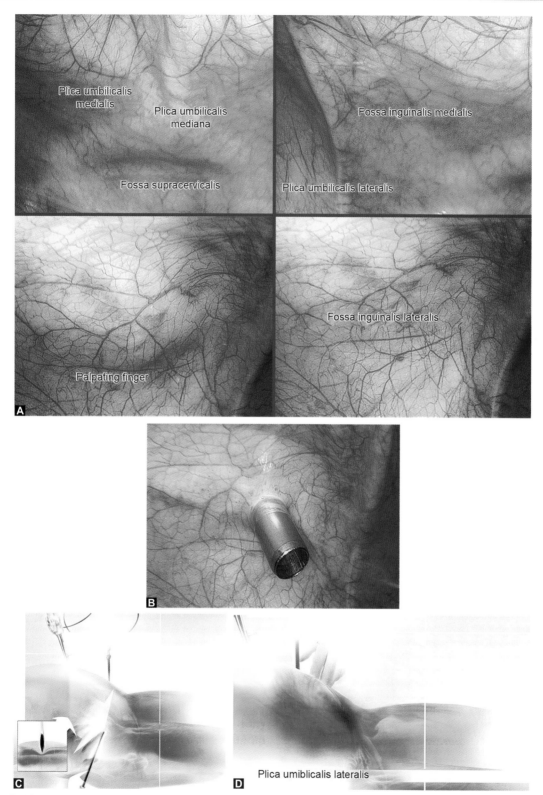

Figs 5A to D: Abdominal wall inside view demonstrating the plica umbilicalis lateralis containing the epigastric vessels. The point of insertion needs to be lateral to this structure

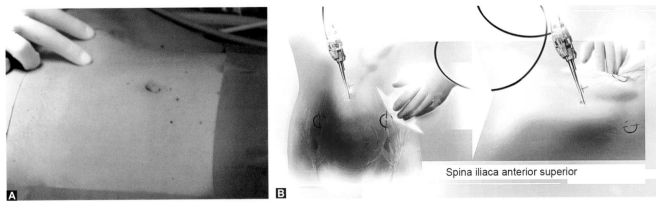

Spina iliaca anterior superior

Figs 6A and B: Point of insertion from the outside (two thumbs medial of the anterior superior spine), at a 90° angle to the surface with penetration of all abdominal wall layers

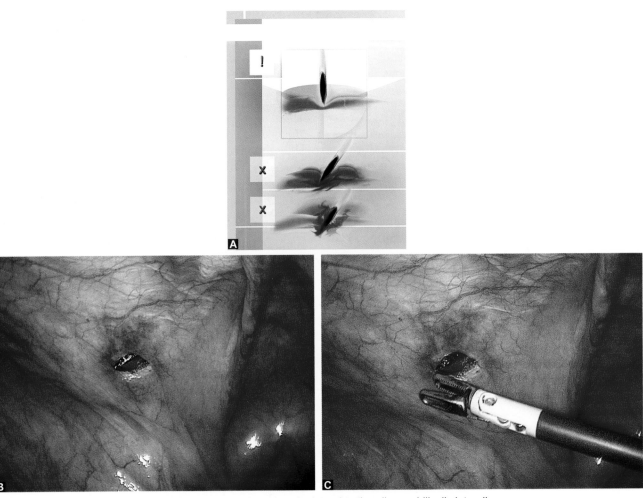

Figs 7A to C: Trocar insertion site lateral to the plica umbilicalis lateralis

lower abdomen for secondary instruments and 5 mm ports are usually sufficient. Smaller trocars, up to 3 mm, can be used for unproblematic procedures. Trocar entries for the laparoscope and instruments can be dilated to 12 mm or larger, e.g. if a morcellator has to be utilized or larger tumors need to be extracted through an endoscopic bag.[2]

Disposable versus Reusable Trocars

Disposable Trocars

With the decrease in production costs, disposable trocars have become popular in many countries. The advantage of disposable material is that the tips are always sharp and therefore, less manual energy is necessary for the trocar insertion. The disadvantages are higher expenses and the environmental stress (Fig. 8).

Reusable Trocars

Reusable trocars are available with two different types of inserting tips—pyramidal and conical (Fig. 9). Today, the most popular tip is the pyramidal as this tip is sharper than the conical one. Sharpness, therefore, is the most important factor in the closed entry technique.

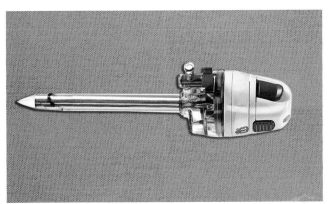

Fig. 8: Endopath™, a disposable entry port under view

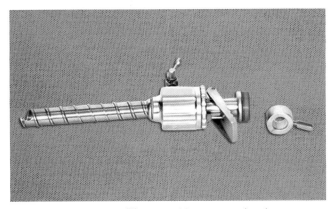

Fig. 9: Endotip™, a reusable trocar under view

In economic terms, reusable trocars seem to be more cost-effective than disposable instruments. However, the disadvantages of reusables are the time required for cleaning and sterilizing and the necessity of frequent sharpening and technical service.[2]

▌ ENTRY TECHNIQUES

Brief Manual of Port Placement

The technique of entering the abdominal cavity can be separated into three different approaches:
1. The open technique.
2. The classical closed technique via Veress needle.
3. The modified closed technique via direct trocar insertion.

Most gynecologists use the classical closed entry technique whereas most general surgeons still use the open (Hasson) method. Only a minority of surgeons use the modified closed technique.

Prearrangement Before Creation of the Pneumoperitoneum

Before laparoscopic procedures begin, the place and type of trocar positioning have to be evaluated carefully. The correct positioning of the patient is essential no matter what type of operation is performed. For procedures that include or require manual aid through the vagina by means of a uterine manipulator, the patient must be positioned in the dorsolithotomy position with the buttocks extended over the end of the table. The thighs are flexed at about 120° to allow a good instrument manipulation. For longer procedures maximum care has to be given to the proper positioning as the risk of postural damage, e.g. compartment syndrome or nerve compression with neural damage, rises with the operation time and the patient's weight. For operations that do not require intraoperative vaginal manipulation, the patient can be positioned in the beach chair position.

In the neck zone, shoulder braces should be used to allow a steep Trendelenburg positioning during surgery. Nerve injury in this region can be avoided, if braces are placed over the acromion and the neck is free of compression. Furthermore, both arms should be placed in a stretched position along the patient's trunk to provide more space for the surgeons and avoid brachial plexus injury. For electrosurgery, a return plate for unipolar instruments is placed with full surface contact over the patient's thigh. Short operations only require a straight bladder catheterization whereas longer operations or operations with a higher risk for ureter or bladder injury require a Foley catheter, at least for the time of operation. The risk of bladder injury is minimized after draining.[3]

Povidone-iodine or any other legalized disinfectant medium is applied 3 times to the abdominal area extending from the nipple line to the inner thighs. The patient is then draped with chausses and a laparoscopy sheet.

In all cases of establishment of a pneumoperitoneum, the use of a nasogastric or orogastric tube is essential to avoid gastric injury during primary insufflation.

There is a controversy as to the prophylactic use of antibiotics. For small operations with a low risk of infection, the prophylactic dose of an antibiotic seems to be avoidable. This has to be seen in context with the increasing number of antibiotic side-effects, development of resistant bacteria and increasing incompatibilities. The use of a single shot of prophylactic antibiotics is recommended for operations with an increased risk of infection, e.g. longer operations or operations during which the uterine cavity is opened or neighboring organs are injured. The most tolerable and broad-spectrum antibiotics are cephalosporins of the second generation.[3]

Creation of the Pneumoperitoneum

The most critical moments in laparoscopy, independent of operating competence, are the creation of the pneumoperitoneum and the insertion of the primary trocar whether by Veress needle and trocar insertion under sight or blindly or by minilaparotomy (Hasson technique).

Patients with a higher than average risk for complications in between the first steps:

Obese Patients

The thicker abdominal wall decreases tactile sensation and the insertion of the Veress needle is more difficult. At minilaparotomy vision is likewise restricted so that the section is often more than mini and the risk for organ damage and postoperative complications, such as wound infection or hernia formation, is higher due to the limited overview and the larger wound. Once the trocar is inserted, the required insufflation pressure is set.

Very Thin Patients

The distance between the umbilicus and the main vessels is no more than 2 cm since the abdominal wall lies very close to the retroperitoneal situated structures. To prevent the wrong insertion angle, the inserting instrument has to be at a 45° angle to the back of the patient and, after elevating the abdominal wall, at a 90° angle to the wall surface. Before needle or trocar insertion, the anatomic route of the major vessels can be identified by palpating the pulse of the vessel track.

Patients with Previous Laparoscopies or Laparotomies

A history of previous abdominal operations significantly increases the risk for omental or bowel adhesions to the abdominal wall. In the case of scars or a history of previous operations, an alternative entry site or entry method has to be considered.

Patients with Previous Failed Insufflations

Previous preperitoneal insufflation is associated with an artificial space that extends all the way to the peritoneal cavity and makes the entry for the Veress needle or for any other entry method difficult. An alternative insufflation site should be considered.[3]

Open Entry Technique

The open entry technique was invented by Harrith Hasson in 1974 and is still used extensively worldwide as the direct alternative to the closed entry technique. The open entry technique is favored by general surgeons; although, its advantages over other entry techniques cannot clearly be proven. This entry technique begins with opening the peritoneal cavity prior to CO_2 insufflation. After performing a minilaparotomy in the subumbilical region, the optic trocar is placed intraperitoneal under sight (Figs 10A to D).[1,3-12]

Advantages and Disadvantages of Open Laparoscopy (Hasson Technique)

This technique supersedes the blind puncture of the abdominal cavity by either the Veress needle or a sharp trocar. The open technique is less likely to cause major vessel injury and if any injury does occur, it is easier to recognize and to repair at the same time. The technique has an equivalent risk of bowel and vessel injury as the closed technique; however, the operative process to dissect the different layers of the abdominal wall can be quite time consuming. Furthermore, open access leads to irritating air leaks because of the large incision, especially in obese patients. Additionally, due to the larger skin incision and the faster surgical preparation, the open technique is associated

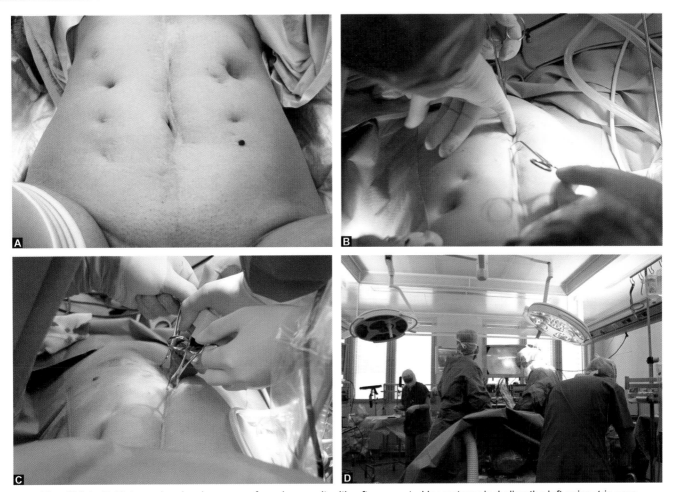

Figs 10A to D: Entry under view in a case of previous peritonitis after repeated laparotomy including the left epigastric area

with a higher rate of wound infection. Several randomized trials and a Cochrane analysis do not indicate a significant safety advantage to either technique.[1,4-7,13-15]

Technique of Open Entry

Direct access or entry by the open technique, without creating pneumoperitoneum and without use of an insufflator, was described by Hasson in 1974. It is also called the Scandinavian or Fielding technique.

This technique is still popular among general surgeons and to a minor degree among gynecologists. Especially patients with suspected adhesions can profit from the open technique.

After penetrating the peritoneum, the intra-abdominal space can be verified by confirmation of bowel or omentum before inserting the blunt-tipped cannula.

Insertion technique: A small, half-moon-shaped skin incision is made under the umbilicus and the different layers of the abdominal wall are prepared by minilaparotomy with the help of Kocher clamps. After dissecting the skin,

subcutaneous tissue, muscle, fascia, and peritoneum under direct vision, a blunt trocar is inserted through which the laparoscope is introduced.[1,5-7]

Closed Entry Technique

This is a blind entry and the most commonly practiced worldwide by surgeons and gynecologists since the invention of the spring-loaded needle by the Hungarian gynecologist "Veress". It is easy to insert the Veress needle and create the pneumoperitoneum mainly through the umbilicus or at alternative entry sites; however, lacerations of vessels and more seldom bowel loops do occur as the instruments used for the closed entry technique are usually sharp (Figs 11A to C).

Veress Needle Technique and CO_2 Gas

To insert the Veress needle, the operating table needs to be in a horizontal position. The Trendelenburg tilt is carried out after having created the pneumoperitoneum. The most

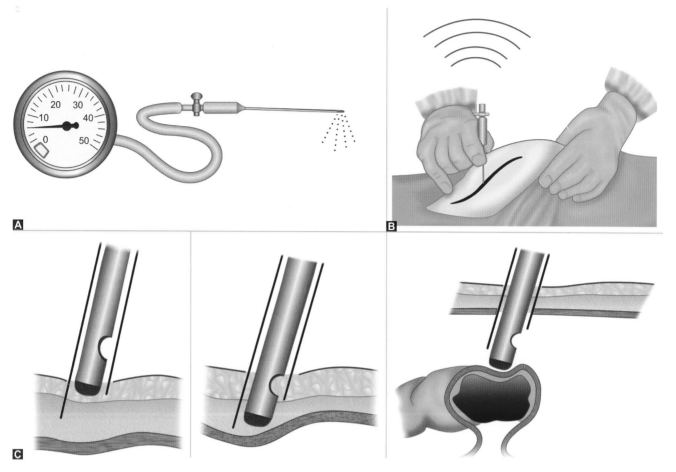

Figs 11A to C: Veress needle and its insertion

common site for the Veress needle entry is the umbilical area. The skin incision in the lower part of the umbilicus is between 0.5 cm for the use of a 5-mm optic trocar and 1.5 cm for the use of a 10-mm optic trocar. The incision is made horizontally with an 11-scalpel blade after carefully lifting the skin underneath so that the risk of damaging organs lying under the peritoneum in extremely thin patients is minimized. As the wall layers are at their thinnest at this level, a deep incision might enter the peritoneal cavity. Before incising the skin, it is recommended to palpate the aorta in its course and identify the iliac bifurcation. This allows the abdomen to be inspected and palpated for any extraordinary masses.[16]

All instruments need to be checked before use. The Veress needle needs to be tested to check that the valve springs and the gas flow is between 6 and 8 mm Hg. A sharp needle with a good spring action is necessary. Disposable needles fulfill these criteria. For the insertion of the primary trocar, the patient is still in the flat position. In this position, the insertion of the primary instrument at a 45° angle towards

the uterus is associated with the lowest risk of damaging the major vessels running retroperitoneally downward. Before inserting the instrument, the abdominal wall is lifted. The abdominal wall can either be lifted medially with one hand or with two hands on both sides depending on the obesity of the patient. In obese patients, the inserting angle is close to 90° whereas in thin patients the angle is close to 45°. If the first entry attempt fails, a second attempt is made before choosing an alternative entry site. Before placing the Veress needle, different safety checks should be performed to guarantee the lowest risk of complication.

❑ *Needle flow*: To ensure flawless insertion of the Veress needle, the manometer should be set to a maximum resistance of 4–6 mm Hg with a gas flow rate of 1 L/minute. If the resistance is high, there is some obstruction inside the Veress needle.

❑ *Palpation of aorta*: If the abdominal aorta can be palpated directly below the umbilicus, the bifurcation must be situated further toward the lower pelvis. It cannot be injured by oblique insertion of the Veress needle. If the bifurcation is felt above the umbilicus, perpendicular insertion after lifting of the anterior abdominal wall is recommended.

❏ *Most times "two clicks" can be heard*: The first click is heard after perforation of the muscle fascia and the second click after perforation of the peritoneum. The proper needle placement is ensured by keeping the Veress needle between thumb and index finger.

❏ *Aspiration test*: Injection of 5–10 mL of normal saline solution results in negative aspiration if the Veress needle is correctly placed and blood-tinged aspirate or aspirate with intestinal contents if the needle is placed in a blood vessel or intestine.

❏ *Hanging drop test and "fluid-in-flow"*: With the Veress needle placed in the abdominal cavity, lifting the abdominal wall creates a negative intra-abdominal pressure. A drop of water is then positioned on the open end of the Veress needle. If the needle is correctly positioned, the water should disappear down the shaft. The drop is only sucked in if the intra-abdominal pressure is negative. For *"fluid-in-flow"*, a 5-mm syringe is filled with a saline solution. The piston is removed; the syringe is connected to the Veress cannula and by lifting the abdominal wall, the saline solution level drops rapidly as it enters into the free abdominal cavity.

❏ Before insufflation with CO_2 gas begins, the initial pressure must be below 9 mm Hg to confirm the correctly placed needle. The initial gas pressure (<9 mm Hg) reflects the correct intraperitoneal Veress needle placement; although, this pressure is not a precise reflection of the intraperitoneal pressure. The Veress needle is connected to the insufflator and the pressure is measured continuously as the needle traverses the various layers of the abdominal wall. A pressure below 9 mm Hg confirms the correct needle placement.

Any movement of the needle after placement must be avoided as this may convert a small needlepoint injury into a complex and threatening tear. After ensuring that the Veress needle has been positioned correctly, the insufflation of CO_2 gas is started. CO_2 gas is used because room air is not soluble in blood and may cause an air embolism if it is pumped into a blood vessel accidentally. Before starting the intra-abdominal insufflation, the gas hose is flushed with about 1 L of CO_2 gas to purify any room air. The initial intra-abdominal insufflation pressure should not exceed 10 mm Hg and is started with only 1 L of CO_2 gas flow per minute. Once a good gas flow and an appropriate pressure have been achieved, the influx can be raised so that 2–3 L CO_2 gas can be insufflated per minute until 3–6 L is insufflated depending on the patient's size and obesity.

❏ After an insufflation volume of about 300 mL, the percussion of the liver region confirms the *loss of liver dullness*. This sign indicates the intra-abdominal insufflation and the distribution of the gas in the whole abdominal cavity.

After having created the pneumoperitoneum in the usual manner, the abdominal pressure should be built up to 20–25 mm Hg before inserting the primary trocar as this maximizes the distension of the abdominal wall from all underlying structures. Once the layers of the abdominal wall are compressed, trocar incision becomes easy and the risk of injury minimal as the inflated distance between abdominal wall and intra-abdominal structures further reduces the risk of damage. Distension pressure should be reduced to 12–15 mm Hg for ventilation reasons once trocar placement has been verified. During gas insufflation, symmetric distension of the lower abdomen and the disappearance of liver dullness can be observed. Once the insufflation pressure reaches 20–25 mm Hg, the distension of the abdominal wall should be sufficient for safe insertion of the trocar. This can be tested by the:

❏ *Aspiration and sounding test (after CO_2 insufflation)*: CO_2 is aspirated in a syringe containing 20 mL of normal saline solution and the result examined. When the tip lies free in the abdominal gas, CO_2 bubbles are visible in the normal saline solution during respiration indicating the position in the free abdominal cavity. When planning a Z insertion, the aspiration must be carried out horizontally toward the right or left and caudally depending on the preparation.

The 5-mm trocar is then placed in a Z technique superficially and brought through the abdominal wall orthogonally.

❏ *Hiss phenomenon*: After successful perforation of the anterior abdominal wall with the primary trocar, a soft hissing sound is produced as a result of negative pressure in the abdominal cavity.

The correct position of the trocar can be checked with a 5-mm optic in cases of small operations or the entry site can be dilated to 10 mm after validation that there are no remarkable adhesions. Panoramic viewing reveals any pathological changes in the vicinity of the abdomen, e. g. in the intestines, liver, gallbladder and spleen.[1,7,17-19]

It is recommended to use heated and humidified CO_2 gas for insufflation. Various types of small machines can be attached to the electronic pneuautomatic to fulfill this purpose. The advantage of heated, moist CO_2 gas can best be illustrated with an egg. If you spray the egg white and yellow yolk with a continuous flow of heated CO_2 gas (37°C), they dry out. If you spray them with cold CO_2 gas, they dry out. If you spray them with cold, moist CO_2 gas, they dry out; however, if you spray them with heated, moist CO_2 gas, they retain their original composition.[20-22]

Direct Blind Entry

Some surgeons perform blind trocar insertion without pneumoperitoneum. The rate of vascular and bowel lesions appears to be similar to other entry techniques. Nevertheless, this entry technique is mostly used by general surgeons and the indication is strictly for thin patients with a flaccid anterior abdominal wall.

After the incision in the subumbilical region, the abdominal wall is lifted with one hand and the trocar is pushed through the abdominal wall with the dominant hand in the same direction as the Veress needle. After visualizing the bowel loops, the pneumoperitoneum is created and the laparoscope inserted.

This technique is fast and cheap although reliability is given only in carefully chosen patients. Direct insertion of the trocar is associated with less insufflation-related complications, such as gas embolism, and it is a faster technique than the Veress needle entry. The disadvantage is the entry with a sharp trocar, which is much larger than a Veress needle, into an abdomen without a preliminary built pneumoperitoneum. This is associated with a higher risk of bowel and vascular damage if unexpected adhesions are situated beneath the abdominal wall. The increased risk of injury also results from the shorter distance to any intra-abdominal structure. Once any damage has occurred, it has been done with an unnecessary large instrument. Direct blind entry should not be performed in preoperated patients.

Innovations in trocars and entry techniques are leading to a safer method than blind entry trocars but without the necessity of performing a laparotomy. These vision-directed trocars try to combine the advantages of both methods while eliminating the disadvantages. The availability and continuous innovation of direct vision trocars may enhance the safety of this technique.[1,8,12]

Entry Under Vision

Entering the abdominal cavity under vision is more popular among general surgeons than among gynecologists but its use is increasing. Trocar insertion is performed with direct vision trocars that are available as single use or reusable instruments. Entry under vision can either be reached directly or after creation of pneumoperitoneum with the Veress needle.

The 5- or 10-mm laparoscope is placed directly into the trocar sheath so that the trocar end can be seen and followed. The trocar is then pushed with a twisting motion stepwise into the peritoneal cavity. Each layer of the abdominal wall is visualized and registered as the trocar is moved in.

Beside disposable trocars (Fig. 12), there is one nondisposable port system for this technique. It features a reusable, stainless steel-threaded cannula with no sharp components and requires no trocar. This port system can be screwed in without any physical effort (Fig. 13). Using the *Endotip*™ a 0° telescope is put into the trocar behind the aperture so that the whole circumference can be seen. The cannula is then rotated clockwise with low force with finger/wrist action. The trocar is inserted into the skin and fascia incision and held perpendicularly to the supine patient with the nondominant hand. The cannula is then rotated clock-wise with the dominant hand applying minimal downward force.[23] Only little force is needed to engage and transpose upward the various layers as it burrows through the either hyperdistended or soft and flat abdominal wall. Under continuous gentle rotation of the optic trocar, it passes through the sequential layers subcutaneous fat, anterior rectus sheath, preperitoneal fat and peritoneum. The different layers are easy to differentiate and the

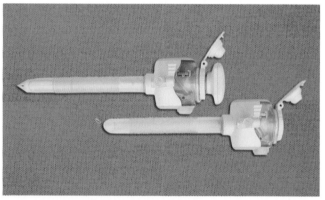
Fig. 12: Disposable optic trocar

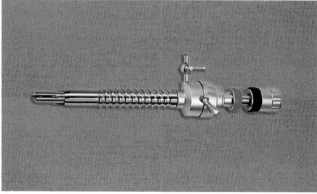
Fig. 13: Nondisposable optic trocar

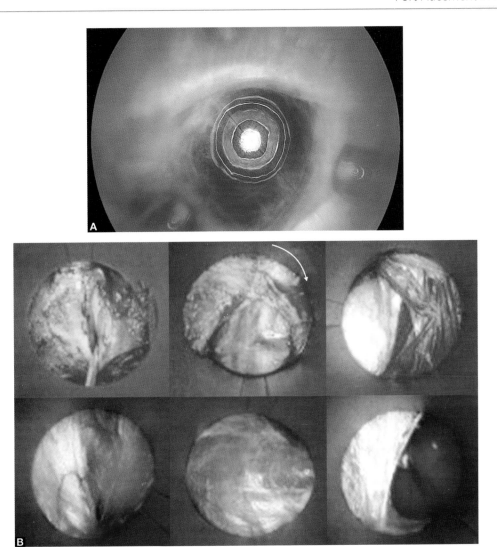

Figs 14A and B: Entry under sight—division in different layers

peritoneum is pierced only after it has been ascertained that the abdominal wall is free of adherent bowel (Figs 14A and B). The peritoneum is seen as a white ring. Accumulated subcutaneous fat and debris may be aspirated with the 5-mm suction/irrigation cannula. The cannula's blunt notched tip engages the tissue layers of the abdominal wall and transposes successive tissue layers onto the cannula's outer sheath in accordance with Archimedes' principle. The yellow fat, white anterior rectus fascia, red rectus muscle, white posterior rectus fascia, yellowish preperitoneal space and transparent dark-bluish peritoneal membrane are all observed sequentially on the monitor. The blunt tip of the cannula pushes aside abdominal wall blood vessels, adhesions and even bowel when adjacent to the anterior abdominal wall not, however, when really firmly adhered (Figs 15A and B).[14,19,24,25]

Endopath[TM] of Ethicon surgery (Fig. 16) has a cannula-integrated thread design that provides greater abdominal wall retention and minimal trocar slip-outs. It is compatible with a wide range of instruments (4.7 mm to 12.9 mm). The bladeless tip separates, rather than cuts along tissue fibers, pushing tissue and vessels away. Visualization through a plexiglas cannula eliminates blind entry by enabling visualization of tissue layers during insertion. The design requires a lower peak instrument insertion and extraction force.

Both methods have in common a laparoscope that is inserted into the trocar and once the trocar has penetrated the subcutis, it advances through the abdominal wall layers stepwise under permanent monitoring. By this method, bowel damage or blood vessel injury may be avoided.

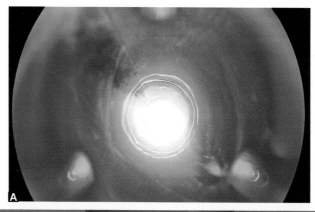

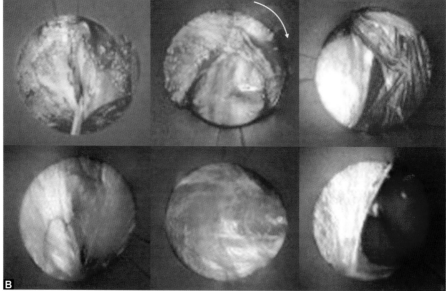

Figs 15A and B: Entry under sight preperitoneal

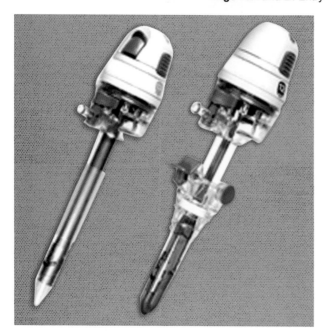

Fig. 16: Endopath™ insufflation access

Another bladeless trocar is the *VersaStep*™ (Covidien Surgical) (Fig. 17). This Veress needle-type instrument is inserted into the abdominal wall. Its sheath can be expanded to allow the passage of larger sheaths without any severe tissue damage as insertion is performed mainly by dilation rather than by cutting. The *Visiport* of Covidien allows a stepwise entry, again through a Plexiglas cannula.

▌ VAGINAL INSTRUMENTS

Uterus Manipulator

There are a number of different uterine manipulators (Figs 18 to 26). The use of a uterine manipulator is controversial. The auxiliary function of manipulating the uterus during the procedure is not required for small operations with good operative access, e.g. adnexal surgery. The indication for the use of a uterine manipulator has to be taken carefully as its use is associated with a certain intraoperative risk for

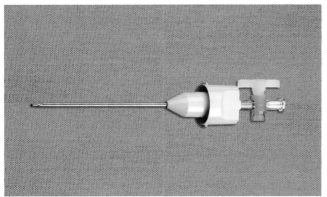

Fig. 17: Versastep™ insufflation access needle

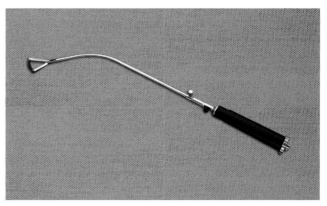

Fig. 21: Dionisi uterine manipulator (Storz)

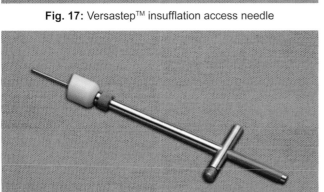

Fig. 18: Hohl manipulator (Storz)

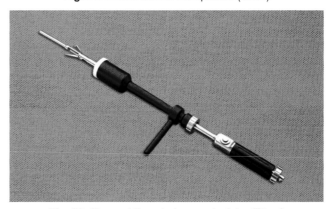

Fig. 22: Mangeshikar uterine manipulator (Storz)

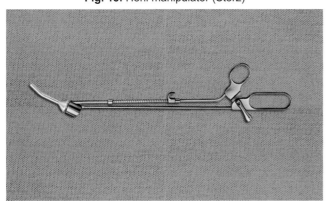

Fig. 19: Braun uterine manipulator

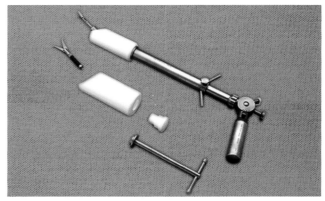

Fig. 23: Koninckx uterine manipulator (Storz)

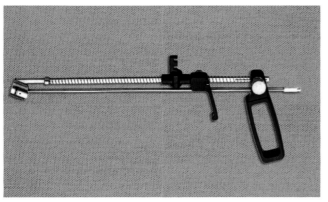

Fig. 20: Uterine manipulator

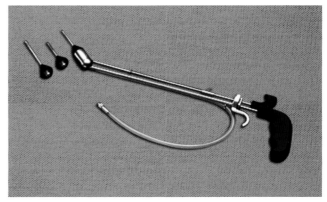

Fig. 24: Tintara uterine manipulator (Storz)

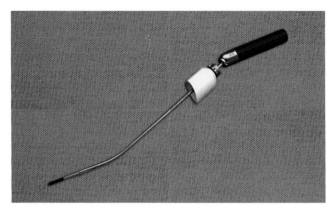

Fig. 25: Donnez uterine manipulator (Storz)

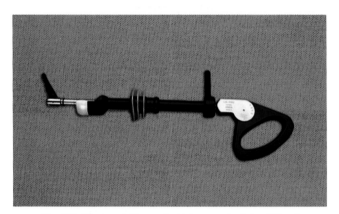

Fig. 26: Clermont-Ferrand uterine manipulator (Storz)

injury of the cervix, uterine cavity and other neighboring structures. On the other hand, the proper application of a uterine manipulator helps to improve vision, and therefore, provides better surgical preconditions.[3]

ADVANCEMENTS IN LAPAROSCOPIC ENTRIES

Single-port Entry

Natural orifice transluminal endoscopic surgery (NOTES) includes the transgastric and transvaginal approach and natural orifice surgery (NOS). Originating mainly in the field of general surgery, various systems with the entry point in the stomach and umbilicus are available and facilitate surgical interventions with only one incision [Single port entries: SILS, single port laparoscopic system (Covidien); LESS, laparoendoscopic single site surgical technique (Olympus), X-CONE (Storz)].

ALTERNATIVE ENTRY SITES

If the umbilical region is considered to be unsuitable for primary insertion, an alternative entry site has to be chosen depending on the planned operation and on the physiognomy of the patient.

Subcostal Insufflation Technique (Palmer's Point)

No entry technique can completely eliminate the risk for entry-related injury of the vascular, intestinal, and urinary tract and gas embolism. Palmer's point is the safest laparoscopic entry point as this place is known to be the least likely to be affected by adhesions (Figs 3A to C).

For all patients with a significantly increased risk for adhesions, with a history of abdominal surgery including cesarean section, a large fibroid uterus, an umbilical hernia, large ovarian cysts, preperitoneal gas insufflation or failed umbilical entry, Palmer described in 1974 an abdominal entry point in the midclavicular line about 3 cm below the costal margin. Palmer's point can be used for Veress needle entry as well as for small trocars.

The left upper quadrant is easily accessible and is mostly free of intra-abdominal adhesions. The rigid rib cage provides high tension and prevents the downward placement of the abdominal wall.

Indications for the use of Palmer's point are:
❏ After two failed attempts of subumbilical insufflation
❏ Primarily in selected very obese patients
❏ Primarily in selected patients with previous abdominal surgeries and suspicion of intra-abdominal adhesions
❏ In patients with previous longitudinal abdominal incisions.

When using this entry site, there is the risk of puncture of the left lobe of the liver, the spleen, the stomach, and the transverse colon; although, this can be prevented by inserting the needle at an angle slightly less than 90°. Creating a subcutaneous emphysema is awkward as the insertion is straight and unambiguous.

Insertion Technique

A Veress needle is placed in the midclavicular line two square fingers below the lowest rib. The angle is 90° and the skin is not lifted as described in the subumbilical region. There are three audible signals of the needle advancing toward the peritoneal cavity. The abdominal wall is usually less than 3–4 cm thick.

Having achieved pneumoperitoneum with this technique, the Veress needle can be replaced by a 5-mm trocar and a 5-mm scope can be introduced through this trocar. After inspection of the umbilical region, if there are no signs of adhesions, a 10-mm trocar can be inserted directly into the subumbilical region under sight. If adhesions are present, these can be removed before inserting the trocar into the usual area.[3,26-28]

Contraindications for the use of Palmer's point are splenomegaly and left upper quadrant surgery.

Transuterine Insufflation

This method of creating a pneumoperitoneum bypasses transabdominal entry and is restricted to selected cases, such as very obese patients with a large abdominal panniculus.

The transuterine insufflating technique involves entering the abdominal cavity with a longer Veress needle through the uterine fundus.

Extra precaution has to be taken for patients with large uterine fibroids and patients with a subsequent chromopertubation. The indication for this entry technique has to be considered carefully and includes severe obese patients and patients with failed transabdominal insufflation where an artificial preperitoneal space has been created.

In preparation for the operation a transvaginal ultrasound scan is performed to obtain information on size and direction of the cavity. The patient is placed in the Trendelenburg position and a speculum is placed in the vagina. After grasping the anterior cervical lip with an atraumatic grasper, the uterus is pulled forward to straighten its axis. A long Veress needle is passed through the cervix into the uterine cavity until a slight resistance is felt when the needle tip reaches the fundus. The needle is then pushed through the uterine wall into the peritoneal cavity, ascertained by a pop of the needle. The abdominal cavity is then insufflated in the same manner as described before.[3]

Transdouglas Insufflation

For transdouglas insufflation the patient is placed in the Trendelenburg position. The posterior cervix is grasped, the Veress needle is passed through the pouch of Douglas and the abdominal cavity is then insufflated.

■ TROCAR PLACEMENT

Precondition for safe trocar insertion is the elevation of the abdominal wall by means of a sufficient pneumoperitoneum (excluding blind entry without pneumoperitoneum). Therefore, an extensive insufflation pressure up to 25 mm Hg can be tolerated.

For correct handling, the trocar and sheath are held between the middle and index finger with the hub of the trocar against the palm of the hand.

Optic Trocar

Insertion of the optic trocar is performed in two steps. During the first step, a 5-mm optic trocar and laparoscope are inserted to confirm the correct pneumoperitoneum and the absence of local adhesions. In the second step, dilation to 10 mm occurs, either under sight or blindly, which guarantees an optimal overview during all operations. In low-risk operations and short operations that do not require a maximal light source, a 5-mm optic trocar and laparoscope may be sufficient.

First step: Entry is realized by a Z *technique* in the following manner—after stepping the trocar forward horizontally for about 1.5 cm, the tip of the trocar is moved to the right at a 90° angle for about 1.5 cm. After lifting the abdominal wall in the same manner as when inserting the Veress needle, the trocar is screwed with the dominant hand straight into the abdominal wall at a 90° angle, towards the hollow of the os sacrum. The index finger is extended under tension along the shaft of the trocar so that excessive penetration of the trocar through the abdominal wall can be prevented.

The sign for correct placement of the trocar is the hissing sound created when gas escapes through the open valve of the trocar [*see* page 45 under Veress needle head Veress needle technique and CO_2 gas]. The obturator is then removed and the trocar is held in place. Insertion must be stopped immediately once the intra-abdominal position has been attained. Before dilating to 10 mm, a 5-mm laparoscope is introduced and rotated through 360° to check visually for any bleeding, intra-abdominal abnormality and adherent bowel loops. If there is concern that the bowel might be adherent in the umbilical region, the primary trocar site needs to be visualized from a secondary port site, e.g. in the lower abdominal wall with a 5-mm laparoscope.

Second step (only if required): A blunt palpation probe is placed in the 5-mm trocar and the shaft is pulled over the palpation probe and taken out. A 10-mm trocar is then screwed into the abdominal cavity using the palpation probe as stylet. It is important to screw the trocar as the sheath is a nuance shorter, and therefore, needs high exertion of force. The risk of abrupt excessive penetration with injury of intra-abdominal organs is increased. It demands a lot of patience depending on the strength of the abdominal wall and its thickness to screw the 10-mm trocar inside.[1]

Ancillary Trocars

All ancillary trocars must be inserted with an intra-abdominal pressure of 20–25 mm Hg under direct vision. The inferior epigastric vessels are visualized laparoscopically whereas the superficial vessels can be visualized by diaphanoscopy. By this means, it can be ensured that the entry points are away from the vessel. It has to be kept in mind that in some cases an extension of the incision is needed during the operation (*see also* extra-abdominal relevant anatomy and intra-abdominal relevant anatomy through the eye of trocar).

Once the tip of the trocar has pierced through the peritoneum, it should be angled in the direction of the uterine fundus under visual control until the port is placed correctly and the sharp tip can be removed.

Before any ancillary trocars are inserted, the patient is moved into the Trendelenburg position. Premature Trendelenburg position can also increase the risk of retroperitoneal vascular injury as the iliac vessels lay right in the axis of a preconceived 45° insertion angle, especially in thin patients with minimal retroperitoneal fat. In the *Trendelenburg position,* the patient is on an elevated and inclined plane, usually at about 15°, with the head down and legs and feet over the edge of the table. The number of ancillary trocars is variable but they all must be inserted under direct view. If two working trocars are needed, they should be placed in the lower quadrant above the pubic hairline lateral to the deep epigastric vessels from the interior view. From the exterior view, the trocars are placed two fingers medial of the spina iliaca anterior superior. For safe insertion, the two major superficial vessels in this region have to be avoided. These are the arteria epigastrica superficialis and the arteria circumflexa iliaca superficialis. These two superficial vessels can be visualized by diaphanoscopy (Figs 1A to C). If a third ancillary trocar is needed, the suprapubic midline is the most common site (Figs 4A and B). Diaphanoscopy cannot be relied upon to locate the deep vessels, especially in obese patients.

Finger-tapping from the outside can identify the right area of trocar placement, and a small skin incision should be made before the trocar sleeve is inserted. The trocars must be inserted by the shortest route at a 90° angle to the skin surface so that the risk of injuring structures on the way to the abdominal wall is minimized. Once the trocar tip is seen under the peritoneum, the pressure on the trocar should be released and the trocar twisted until it enters the abdominal cavity. For the use of trocars in the midline the Foley catheter must be identified to avoid accidental bladder perforation. By this means, a false route in the subperitoneal tissues or damage to the large prevertebral vessels can be avoided.[1,3,28,29]

TERMINATION OF THE LAPAROSCOPIC PROCEDURE

After completion of the operation, the laparoscope should be used to check on the way out that there has not been a through-and-through injury of bowel adherent under the umbilicus by visual control during port and laparoscope removal. All ancillary ports are removed under direct vision to ensure that there is no unrecognized hemorrhage and if there is one, it can be treated immediately. Prior to the removal of the instruments, a last inspection of the abdominal cavity is essential to ensure absence of bleeding and retroperitoneal hematoma. Also, the area under the optic trocar has to be inspected for any unrecognized bleeding from this place of insertion. Once the working trocar on the left and possibly in the midline are taken out, the peritoneal gap is coagulated from the trocar in the right lower abdomen. The peritoneal gap of this trocar is coagulated bipolarly after the trocar has already been taken out and the gap is closed on the way out (Fig. 27). Fascial incisions of the ancillary trocars larger than 5 mm should be sutured to prevent hernia formation. A single stitch with an absorbable polyfilar suture 3-0 is applied under direct view using the pneumoperitoneum and the laparoscope to prevent peritoneal involvement or even injury of omentum or bowel. At the end of the operation, the patient is returned to the horizontal position to avoid brisk vascular changes. The pneumoperitoneum is then released slowly by opening the inserting valve. The laparoscope is taken out in the horizontal position to avoid a possible aspiration of air that is responsible for shoulder pain in the postoperative period. Before removing the optic trocar, reinsert the laparoscope and remove the trocar under sight so that the stepwise closure of the abdominal wall in a reverse Z technique is guaranteed. In this way, the fascial incision does not have to be sutured as it is functionally closed.

The skin incisions are closed with single inverted knots with an absorbable monofilar suture 4-0.

A certain amount of gas or irrigation fluid remaining in the abdominal cavity can be tolerated. This gas may irritate the peritoneum and the patients may feel discomfort and minor pain in the shoulder area up to 2 weeks after the operation.[1,3,28]

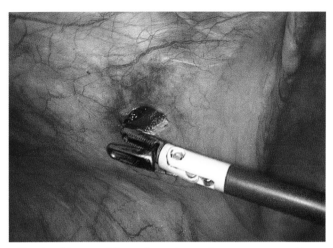

Fig. 27: Closure of the peritoneal gap after trocar removal but before releasing the pneumoperitoneum

COMPLICATIONS IN PORT PLACEMENT

Complications in laparoscopy in general can be divided into *early complications* that are recognized immediately and can be solved instantly, and *late complications* that occur after a time interval in the postoperative period. These late complications are more difficult to manage as patients have already been discharged from hospital or their symptoms are unspecific.

Laparoscopic entry lesions are classified as follows:

Type 1 Injuries

Damage to major blood vessels and normally located bowel by Veress needle or trocar (0.1–0.4%).

Type 2 Injuries

Damage to vessels in and bowel adherent to the abdominal wall by Veress needle or trocar. Type 2 lesions may occur whether the mode of access is by laparotomy or laparoscopy.

Complications associated with laparoscopy vary according to the experience of the surgeon and the medical staff as well as the wide range of operational demands. The rate of complications varies between 0.1% and 1.3%.

The establishment of laparoscopic surgery for routine procedures at university teaching hospitals as well as at small county hospitals has led to a higher quality of laparoscopic surgeons with a shorter learning curve. This advancement has been accompanied by a lower rate of complications. The development of laparoscopic instruments and optic

transmission has also contributed to this trend. It is well proven that more than 50% of all laparoscopic injuries occur during the initial entry steps: insertion of the Veress needle or blind entry, creation of pneumoperitoneum and insertion of the primary trocar. Accordingly, the incidence of injuries has decreased significantly in the last three decades. Injury to bowel occurs in 0.04% and to major vessels in 0.02–0.04% of all laparoscopic procedures. Most of these injuries occur at the insertion of the primary trocar. Nevertheless, 30–50% of bowel injuries and 13–50% of all vascular injuries are not diagnosed immediately during the operation, resulting in a respective morbidity and mortality rate. Furthermore, laparoscopic cases are scheduled in outpatient clinics lacking banked human blood, vascular operative instruments and expertize. Bowel injury is the third cause of death from a laparoscopic procedure after major vascular injury and anesthesia.[10,12,19]

Vascular and Visceral Lesions at Port Placement

Vascular lesions may occur in the abdominal wall (superficial and epigastric vessels) or intra-abdominal (vessels of the mesentery, omentum, vena iliaca and aorta). Vessel injury leads to parietal hematoma or intraperitoneal hemorrhage depending on the injury site. If the Veress needle even partly enters the lumen of any vessel, this can lead to a gas embolism. Also, CO_2 has a great solubility in plasma and higher volumes can be lethal and cause immediate death. Injury of the retroperitoneal space and the retroperitoneally situated structures can result after the use of excessive force to insert the Veress needle or the primary trocar, failing to follow the midline axis or using an incorrect angle relative to the abdominal wall to enter the peritoneal cavity. As the aorta and the inferior vena cava bifurcate and diverge before entering the pelvis, the risk of injury needs to be minimized. For this reason, the instruments are inserted in the midline and directed toward the hollow of the pelvis at a 45° angle to the horizontal line. Insertion in a too oblique a manner often results in a preperitoneal insufflation, especially in obese patients. The safety of this insertion technique depends on the relationship of the subumbilical entry site to the aortic bifurcation and other major vessels. In nonobese patients, the aortic bifurcation is at or caudal to the umbilicus, therefore the insertion angle should be 45°. The mean distance from the umbilicus to the aorta at 90° is only 6 cm. In overweight and obese women, the bifurcation of the aorta is above the umbilicus and the mean distance from the umbilicus to the aorta at 90° is up to 13 cm. The insertion at a 45° angle in obese patients rarely results in intraperitoneal placement and the angle can safely be increased toward vertical. The advantage of an almost vertical entry angle is the minimized risk for preperitoneal insufflation with an only negligible risk of severe organ damage. This method is primarily applied in obese patients but can be transferred to thin patients.[29-31]

Visceral Lesions

Visceral lesions include injury of the omentum majus, the stomach, the bowel, the liver or the spleen depending on the entry site and the fill of the hollow organs.

Penetration of the bowel may be recognized during the first security step by the aspiration of gas or unclear or malodorant fluid. Injury of the liver or the spleen would lead to the aspiration of blood during the first security step. Depending on the interdisciplinary team, injuries to visceral organs can either be solved laparoscopically or, if necessary, by immediate laparotomy.[28,30]

False Route of the Gas

If the insufflating instrument has been correctly placed, the correct filling of the pneumoperitoneum can be confirmed by a regular and symmetrical distension of the abdominal wall. The right hypochondrium becomes tympanic after an insufflation volume of about 300 mL [*see* pages 45 and 47 Veress needle technique and CO_2 gas]. The false route of the gas can be subcutaneous, subperitoneal, or between dense intra-abdominal adhesions, intraomental, in the bowel or in the stomach. *Subcutaneous* insufflation is predominant in obese patients. If the abdominal distension is asymmetrical, a crepitation can be felt superficially. This false route is harmless, as the resorption of the gas is very rapid and the needle can be reinserted at the same sight immediately without difficulty. *Subperitoneal* emphysema is recognized later because there are no superficial signs such as crepitation. The distension is asymmetrical and inserting the optic trocar is often not possible as the distance from the skin to the peritoneal cavity is extended. Subperitoneal insufflation often occurs in obese patients when the needle is inserted in too oblique a manner. *Localized* pneumoperitoneum may occur in cases of dense adhesions. The diffusion of the gas throughout the entire abdominal cavity is prevented and manometric anomalies soon become evident. An alternative entry sight has to be chosen for the creation of the pneumoperitoneum. *Omental* emphysema is caused by the insertion of the Veress needle into the partially fixed omentum majus. This harmless but impressive phenomenon disappears in a few minutes; however, it may contribute to some reflex cardiorespiratory disturbances. Insertion into the *bowel* or *stomach* is associated with aspiration of gas or feces. The

danger results from the risk of inserting the trocar through the organ wall.[28]

Open laparoscopy offers no advantage in avoiding these lesions. Immediate action upon recognition of complications guarantees the safety of the patient. As already mentioned by Kurt Semm, in every laparoscopic procedure special vascular clamps such as "right angled" Kelly clamps, Adson-Schmidt, hemostat DeBakey or Crawford clamps have to be nearby. No attempt should be made to grasp any injured vessel with nonvascular instruments.[11,32-34]

Early Complications

Early complications occur during surgical interventions as bowel, vessel, bladder and ureter lesions as well as anesthesia-related or general complications, such as pulmonary embolism, massive bleedings, consecutive to major vessel injuries or intravascular insufflation and heart arrest. Even with the most experienced laparoscopic and laparotomic surgeon early complications are not always avoidable. The quality of a surgeon is recognized by the speed and skill with which he diagnoses and deals with any complications.

Vascular Lesions

Major vessel injury can also occur during the operative part of the surgery, particularly at retroperitoneal dissection. Regardless of whether the various controversial Veress needle safety tests or checks are performed or not, if the insufflation rate is varying and the right needle placement doubtful, waggling of the tip of the needle must be avoided. A potential 1.6 mm puncture of a vessel or intra-abdominal organ can easily enlarge to an injury of up to 1 cm.[12] According to the normal anatomical situation, the distal abdominal aorta and the common, as well as the external and internal, iliac arteries lie in the retroperitoneal space. Lacerations of these vessels luckily occur rarely. Most venous injuries, other than to the vena cava, are accompanied by injury of the overlying arteries. The number of injuries to the aorta and vena cava is somehow surprising as these vessels are above the umbilicus in most women. In most aortic or vena cava laceration cases, periumbilical trocars were placed at angles greater than 45° from the plane of the spine.

The first step in effective management of major vessel injury is early recognition, minimization of bleeding and conversion to laparotomy, if the bleeding cannot be laparoscopically compressed or stilled. A vascular surgeon is needed to complete the operation.

Bowel Lesions

Abdominal access and the creation of a pneumoperitoneum carry a significant risk of bowel injuries. Such injuries are more frequent in laparoscopic surgery and are often avoided in open surgery. Although these injuries are uncommon, they represent a major reason for mortality from laparoscopic procedures, and a significant source of the morbidity associated with any laparoscopic procedure. Many intraoperative bowel lesions can be sutured; a partial excision and suturing as well as resections of lacerated areas can be necessary, including end-to-end anastomosis and temporary ileostoma. Unlike major vascular injuries where the risk and presentation are immediate, many bowel injuries go unrecognized at the time of the procedure. Consequently, patients present postoperatively, often after discharge, with specific or unspecific symptoms of peritonitis. Persistent pyrexia, tachycardia or ileus in the postoperative period should raise the index of suspicion for bowel injuries. This delay makes it a significant cause of morbidity and mortality. The experience of the surgeon is an important factor in the overall complication rate and in the incidence of intestinal injury. A sound knowledge of laparoscopic anatomy is essential to understand the distorted anatomy often present in the disease. Failure to keep to tissue planes, blunt dissection, diathermy in close proximity to the intestine, excessive traction and poor visualization account for most injuries. Previous surgery, endometriosis, chronic pelvic inflammatory disease, malignancy or radiotherapy may distort anatomy and obliterate tissue planes. Bowel preparation is no longer advisable before major pelvic surgery. Injuries with healthy edges can be repaired primarily using tension-free, single-layer, interrupted sero-submucosal 3-0 vicryl or 4-0 polydioxanone (PDS) sutures. For more extensive injuries, resection and primary anastomoses are required.

Bladder and Ureter Injuries

The intraoperative demonstration and dissection of the ureter is often necessary and required if the surgery is performed in the ureteric area. Routine intraoperative cystoscopies after many major gynecological operations allow an early recognition and repair at the primary surgery with less morbidity for the patient. An open bladder is, of course, also detected by direct emission of urine. Sometimes the Foley catheter bag fills with CO_2 and indicates a bladder lesion.

Urinary tract injuries associated with laparoscopic surgery differ substantially from laparoscopic major vessel or intestinal iatrogenic injury. The former rarely results in the death of the patient, whereas the latter two are associated with mortality. Urinary complications are seldom the result of needle or trocar trauma (i.e. entry-related). The most cogent factors related to ureteral damage are: (1) Suboptimal knowledge of pelvic anatomy; (2) Failure to open the peritoneum and dissect retroperitoneally; (3) Employment of energy devices with marginal knowledge relating to the physics as well as the tissue interaction of these devices; (4) Imprecise application of stapling devices; (5) Pelvic adhesions, particularly dense adhesions located in and around the ovarian fossa. Injury sustained to the ureter is egregiously compounded by late postoperative recognition. Failure to order suitable diagnostic tests (e.g. indigo carmine dye injection, cystoscopy, intravenous pyelogram, retrograde pyelograms) will accrue additional damage. Bladder injuries may be less serious than ureteral injuries, particularly if lacerations are recognized intraoperatively and are repaired appropriately in a timely manner. As with ureteral injury, the instillation of a dye (e.g. methylene blue) into the bladder will lead to early diagnosis as will intraoperative cystoscopy. Injury to the trigone may be avoided by performing a cystoscopy before or during bladder laceration closure. Resecting a significant portion of the bladder during a gynecologic surgical procedure reflects a deficit in pelvic anatomical knowledge. Failure to secure the ureters by exposing the retroperitoneal space and deficient anatomical knowledge of the bladder and ureters, including their relationships, are critical factors associated with complications. The presence of adhesions and particularly a history of abdominal surgery or cesarean section as well as the presence of significant endometriosis and accompanying inflammation place the patient in a high-risk category for bladder injury. Similarly, the creation of a vesicovaginal fistula or ureterovaginal fistula is clearly a recognition failure and is associated with a compromise of the blood supply to the bladder or ureter. Although urinary tract injuries are rarely lethal, they can and do lead to significant morbidity, sometimes chronic. The risk of injuries, especially to the ureter, is increased with the laparoscopic approach and particularly with gynecologic laparoscopic operations. The reason for the higher risk with laparoscopy may be explained by the lack of tactile sensation, decreased mobility, reduced vision, especially depth perception and panoramic view, reluctance of the gynecologist to open into the retroperitoneal space, suboptimal knowledge of pelvic anatomy and reliance on hemostatic devices which increase the risk for urinary tract injury.

Prevention of injury and recognition of injury are sentinel pillars for high quality medical practice standards. Varying opinions have been reported relative to ureteral catheter placement or stenting for the prevention of injury during major surgery, particularly relating to laparoscopic surgery. Tactile sensation is not given in laparoscopic surgery.

Late Complications

Late complications occurring in the postoperative period are also called secondary lesions and occur in 0.5% of cases, e.g. secondary bowel lesions associated with peritonitis and massive intra-abdominal infection. Small vascular lesions are often not recognized until a hematoma appears and ureter lesions are sometimes only recognized after the development of an urinoma. This may occur many days after surgery. All patients have to be counseled to immediately report adverse symptoms or conditions whether they are still in the hospital or already discharged.

FUTURE PERSPECTIVE

No matter what kind of entry technique is used, it is essential that the operating surgeon is well trained in his preferred technique. Beyond that, all surgeons should be familiar with alternative entry sites and techniques to be able to solve any kind of obstacle or complication.

Laparoscopic surgeons of all disciplines tend to divide laparoscopic surgery into different pillars, one of which is laparoscopic entry. During the training of young surgeons, it is important that more focus is given to laparoscopic entry alongside the more popular pillars of endoscopic preparation and suturing. There are plenty of dry and wet laboratories for the training of surgical skills and safe surgical practice; however, it is more complicated to train the safety steps which demand a high learning curve and are difficult or impossible to train in a virtual setting. Laparoscopic entry is associated with more than half of all complications during laparoscopic surgery. A major problem remains the feasibility of establishing training programs that focus on this domain with the highest risk for complications as this kind of training is difficult to implement in a training program. Nevertheless, the intention is that laparoscopic surgeons have appropriate training, supervision and thereby gain stepwise experience corresponding to the operational requirements. It is essential that surgeons undertaking laparoscopic surgery are well-acquainted with the equipment, instrumentation and energy sources used. There also exists an obligation to ensure that the nursing staff and surgical assistants are appropriately trained. An awareness of the complications which can be encountered, early detection and professional treatment are prerequisites for a high quality operating unit.[1]

All operational procedures including port placement, even under direct vision, carry an inborn risk. For the prevention of complications we doctors can never be careful enough and require God's protection.

ACKNOWLEDGMENTS

We thank Mathias Podlovics for all graphic designs.

We also thank Dawn Rüther for editing the manuscript and Thoralf Schollmeyer for his valuable contributions to the manuscript.

REFERENCES

1. Gynaecologists RCoOa. Preventing entry-related gynaecological laparoscopic injuries. RCOG Green-top Guideline. 2008;49:1-10.
2. Levine R. Instrumentation and equipment. In: Pasic R, Levine R, (Eds). A Practical Manual of Laparoscopy: A Clinical Cookbook. Abingdon, UK: Informa Healthcare; 2007. pp. 19-38.
3. Pasic R. Creation of pneumoperitoneum and trocar insertion techniques. In: Pasic R, Levine R, (Eds). A Practical Manual of Laparoscopy: A Clinical Cookbook. Abingdon, UK: Informa Healthcare; 2007. pp. 57-74.
4. Cogliandolo A, Manganaro T, Saitta FP, et al. Blind versus open approach to laparoscopic cholecystectomy: A randomized study. Surg Laparosc Endosc. 1998;8(5):353-5.
5. Hasson HM. Open laparoscopy: A report of 150 cases. J Reprod Med. 1974;12(6):234-8.
6. Hasson HM, Rotman C, Rana N, et al. Open laparoscopy: 29-year experience. Obstet Gynecol. 2000;96(5 Pt 1):763-6.
7. Ballem RV, Rudomanski J. Techniques of pneumoperitoneum. Surg Laparosc Endosc. 1993;3(1):42-3.
8. Gunenc MZ, Yesildaglar N, Bingol B, et al. The safety and efficacy of direct trocar insertion with elevation of the rectus sheath instead of the skin for pneumoperitoneum. Surg Laparosc Endosc Percutan Tech. 2005;15(2):80-1.
9. Jansen FW, Kolkman W, Bakkum EA, et al. Complications of laparoscopy: an inquiry about closed- versus open-entry technique. Am J Obstet Gynecol. 2004;190(3):634-8.
10. Magrina JF. Complications of laparoscopic surgery. Clin Obstet Gynecol. 2002;45(2):469-80.
11. Semm K. Cutting versus conical tip designs. Endosc Surg Allied Technol. 1995;3(1):39-47.
12. Vilos GA, Ternamian A, The Society of Gynaecologists of Canada, et al. Laparoscopic entry: a review of techniques, technologies, and complications. J Obstet Gynaecol Can. 2007;29(5):433-65.
13. Bemelman WA, Dunker MS, Busch OR, et al. Efficacy of establishment of pneumoperitoneum with the Veress needle, Hasson trocar, and modified blunt trocar (TrocDoc): A randomized study. J Laparoendosc Adv Surg Tech A. 2000;10(6):325-30.

14. Berch BR, Torquati A, Lutfi RE, et al. Experience with the optical access trocar for safe and rapid entry in the performance of laparoscopic gastric bypass. Surg Endosc. 2006;20(8):1238-41.

15. Garry R. Laparoscopic surgery. Best Pract Res Clin Obstet Gynaecol. 2006;20(1):89-104.

16. Veress J. Neues Instrument zur Ausführung von Brust- und Bauchpunktionen und Pneumothoraxbehandlung. Deutsche medizinische Wochenschrift. 1938;64:1480-1.

17. Vilos GA, Vilos AG. Safe laparoscopic entry guided by Veress needle CO_2 insufflation pressure. J Am Assoc Gynecol Laparosc. 2003;10(3):415-20.

18. Teoh B, Sen R, Abbott J. An evaluation of four tests used to ascertain Veress needle placement at closed laparoscopy. J Minim Invasive Gynecol. 2005;12(2):153-8.

19. Vilos GA, Vilos AG, Abu-Rafea B, et al. Three simple steps during closed laparoscopic entry may minimize major injuries. Surg Endosc. 2009;23(4):758-64.

20. Sammour T, Kahokehr A, Hill AG. Meta-analysis of the effect of warm humidified insufflation on pain after laparoscopy. Br J Surg. 2008;95(8):950-6.

21. Peng Y, Zheng M, Ye Q, et al. Heated and humidified CO_2 prevents hypothermia, peritoneal injury, and intra-abdominal adhesions during prolonged laparoscopic insufflations. J Surg Res. 2009;151(1):40-7.

22. Ott DE. Laparoscopy and tribology: the effect of laparoscopic gas on peritoneal fluid. J Am Assoc Gynecol Laparosc. 2001;8(1):117-23.

23. Ternamian AM. Laparoscopy without trocars. Surg Endosc. 1997;11(8):815-8.

24. Ternamian AM, Vilos GA, Vilos AG, et al. Laparoscopic peritoneal entry with the reusable threaded visual cannula. J Minim Invasive Gynecol. 2010;17(4):461-7.

25. Ternamian AM, Deitel M. Endoscopic threaded imaging port (EndoTIP) for laparoscopy: Experience with different body weights. Obes Surg. 1999;9(1):44-7.

26. Granata M, Tsimpanakos I, Moeity F, et al. Are we underutilizing Palmer's point entry in gynecologic laparoscopy? Fertil Steril. 2010;94(7):2716-9.

27. Malik E, Stoz F, Moebus V, et al. Subkostaler Einstich in der Medioklavikularlinie zur primären Insufflation und Inspektion im Rahmen der gynäkologischen Laparoskopie. Geburtshilfe und Frauenheilkunde. 1997;57:388-90.

28. Palmer R. Safety in laparoscopy. J Reprod Med. 1974;13(1):1-5.

29. Nezhat F, Brill AI, Nezhat CH, et al. Laparoscopic appraisal of the anatomic relationship of the umbilicus to the aortic bifurcation. J Am Assoc Gynecol Laparosc. 1998;5(2):135-40.

30. Hurd WW, Bude RO, DeLancey JO, et al. The relationship of the umbilicus to the aortic bifurcation: implications for laparoscopic technique. Obstet Gynecol. 1992;80(1):48-51.

31. Hurd WH, Bude RO, DeLancey JO, et al. Abdominal wall characterization with magnetic resonance imaging and computed tomography. The effect of obesity on the laparoscopic approach. J Reprod Med. 1991;36(7):473-6.

32. Semm K. New methods of pelviscopy (gynecologic laparoscopy) for myomectomy, ovariectomy, tubectomy and adnectomy. Endoscopy. 1979;11(2):85-93.

33. Semm K. Visible control of peritoneal perforation in surgical pelviscopy. Geburtshilfe Frauenheilkd. 1988;48(6):436-9.

34. Semm K. Morcellement and suturing using pelviscopy- not a problem any more. Geburtshilfe Frauenheilkd. 1991;51(10):843-6.

Section 2
THE LEARNING CURVE

- Gray's Anatomy of Female Pelvis as seen through the Laparoscope
- Principle and Use of Electrosurgery in Laparoscopy
- Laparoscopic Suturing
- Tissue Retrieval
- Anesthesia in Laparoscopy

"True knowledge exists in knowing that you know nothing."

Socrates

CHAPTER 4

Gray's Anatomy of Female Pelvis as Seen through the Laparoscope

Shailesh Puntambekar

■ INTRODUCTION

The pelvic anatomy is fairly constant with very few variations. Therefore, it easy to understand and master the anatomy. The knowledge of anatomy is more relevant when one has a limited view as in laparoscopy. Better understanding will lead to better surgery. This anatomy is beneficial to surgeons, gynecologist, urologist and any other surgeon who wishes to do pelvic surgery.

The book has described the following structures:
❏ Organs in the pelvis
❏ Attachments and ligaments
❏ Bones and muscles in the pelvis
❏ Vascular anatomy
❏ Spaces in the pelvis
❏ Ureteric anatomy
❏ Nerves in the pelvis
❏ Lymphatic drainage.

The description is as per the anatomy and its applications in the surgery.

■ PELVIS BOUNDARIES

The pelvic cavity starts at the level of sacral promontory and is bounded by bony structures laterally. The caudal limit is the pelvic floor. The structures included are the uterus with adnexa, ureters, urinary bladder, rectum and prostate in males. The anatomy defers in males and females only in the region of the prostate. The pelvic organs are the uterus, bladder and the prostate. The rectum and ureters enter the pelvis from the upper abdomen. With the exception of the ovaries, the blood supply of the organs entering the pelvis arises from above the pelvis. The blood supply of the pelvic organs comes from the lateral side traversing quite a distance from their origin before reaching the organ. This understanding is important.

Relevance: Thus, there is enough length of the vessels available for ligation.

■ ORGANS IN THE PELVIS

❏ Uterus
❏ Ovaries
❏ Tubes
❏ Bladder
❏ Rectum.

■ LIGAMENTS/SUPPORTS OF THE UTERUS

The uterosacrals, the cardinal ligaments and the paracolpos form a continuous fan-shaped structure. Medially is the rectum, laterally is the internal iliac artery and caudally is the levator ani muscle. The ligaments go from the uterus to the sacrum traversing pararectal and paravesical spaces. The ureter lies on the ligaments and hence has to be retracted laterally to go to the insertion of the ligament into the pelvic wall. The lymphatics and the veins traverse through these ligaments while the uterine artery traverses above the ureter and does not lie in the ligaments.

■ BONES AND MUSCLES

The psoas muscle is the lateral most structure in the pelvis. The external iliac artery rests on the muscle. The levator ani and the obturator internus muscle form the base of the pararectal space; they are covered by the endopelvic fascia.

❑ This is a tough fascia. This fascia forms an important landmark for all pelvic floor repairs
❑ The pubic bone is exposed as the lateral most boundary during the ileo-obturator lymphadenectomy
❑ The circumflex iliac vein is in close proximity to this bone. This vein forms the distal limit of the lymphadenectomy
❑ Anteriorly the pubic symphysis is visualized during the exenteration and pelvic floor repairs.

Thus, the bony boundaries of the pelvic cavity are:

❑ Superiorly sacral promontory
❑ Laterally the ala of the pelvic bone
❑ Posteriorly sacrum
❑ Inferiorly pubic symphysis.

■ VASCULAR ANATOMY

The vascular anatomy has been described from the bifurcation of the aorta. *The bifurcation of the common iliac is at the level of sacral promontory.*[1,2] This is an important anatomical landmark. The line of small bowel mesentery crosses at the level of sacral promontory on its way to the right sacroiliac joint. Thus, the pelvic organs can be separated at this level from the upper abdominal organs. There are no vessels (branches) arising from the major vessels at this level anteriorly. *Thus, the organs anterior to the bifurcation can be easily separated from the great vessels.* It is important to recognize these fascial planes. Unless there is inflammation, the loose areolar planes can be easily dissected. In the presence of any branches of aorta or vena cava, this would not have been possible. These planes are essential in the surgeries of the rectum and the vault suspension in females.

The bifurcation of aorta is always at the level of sacral promontory, and it can be considered as the upper boundary of the pelvis.

The only structure of importance is the hypogastric plexus, which is formed at this level. This has been described in details later.

The aorta divides into the common iliac vessels on either side. The division of inferior vena cava is at the lower level and to the left of the aorta.[3]

The veins are in close proximity to the arteries, posteriorly, and hence, the lymphatic clearance anterior to the arteries can be easily achieved without the fear of damaging the veins. *The common iliac, external and internal iliac arteries and veins have no branches or tributaries on the anterior or lateral region. This is important to understand, as this is the reason the lymph node dissection can be done by sweeping all the fibro-fatty tissues. Any branch would have prevented this from happening. These fibro-fatty tissues are outside the fascial covering of the vessels. Knowledge of this plane is important for the lymph nodal dissection.*

The ureter crosses the common iliac artery from the lateral to the medial side at this level.[4,5] The ureter thus continues to be medial to the artery in the pelvis. This should take out the misconception that the ureter has segmental supply, as there is no direct branch of internal iliac supplying the ureter. *This also ensures that the ureter can be completely separated from the major vascular structures thus enabling major cancer surgery to be performed.*

The common iliac then divides into the external and internal iliac arteries.[6,7]

The external iliac artery travels along the iliopsoas muscle on its way to the lower limbs. The external iliac vein lies posteromedial to the artery.[8] Both the external iliac artery and vein are devoid of any branches till they reach the inguinal ligament. At this level, the inferior epigastric artery arises from the anteromedial aspect of the external iliac artery.[9] This artery then ascends on the posterior aspect of the transversalis fascia extraperitoneally and goes cranially to supply the lower abdominal muscles. The origin of inferior epigastric artery is the distal limit of ileo-obturator nodal dissection.

Important Aspects of Inferior Epigastric Artery and Vein

The inferior epigastric vein also drains into the external iliac vein on the anteromedial aspect. Both the vein and artery are closely approximated and are on the medial side of internal inguinal ring. *The inferior epigastric artery is close to the position of inferior ports and has to be visualized before the port insertion, as it is likely to be damaged.* These vessels are the dividing line of direct and indirect inguinal hernias.

❑ They are extraperitoneal
❑ They are the only branches of external iliac artery and vein in the pelvis
❑ They lie on the medial aspect of deep inguinal ring and form the boundaries for classifying hernias either into direct or indirect hernias.

The only tributary of external iliac vein is the deep circumflex iliac vein and it hugs the pelvic bone.

Arteries

Internal Iliac Artery

The internal iliac artery arises from the common iliac artery at the level of sacral promontory.[10] It courses downward and medially and divides into two divisions: The anterior and the posterior. This division takes place about 2–3 cm distal to the division of common iliac. The posterior division dips into the presacral fascia to supply the gluteal vessels.[11] *The anterior division of internal iliac artery should be ligated distal to the posterior division otherwise, there is claudication in the gluteal region.*[12]

The anterior division continues downward toward the iliac bone and is the main source of supply to the pelvic organs. The first branch arises about 5–6 cm distal to the division of common iliac artery. Thus, enough length of internal iliac is available for ligation before it gives its first branch. This is the most important anatomical landmark. *The internal iliac vein closely hugs the artery posteriorly, and hence, care should be taken while ligating the artery as during emergency situations; the vein can be damaged.*

The first branch of the anterior division of internal iliac is the uterine artery in females and the superior vesicle artery in males. Both, the uterine as well as superior vesicle traverse a long distance through the pararectal space before they supply the organs. Both the vessels cross the ureter anteriorly and supply the ureter through a small branch. *Thus, there is enough length of these vessels available for the surgeon from its origin to its insertion.*[13] *In case of bleeding from the organ, one can go laterally and be sure that there is enough length of artery available for ligation. Also, one has to differentiate between the arterial and venous bleeding. If it is arterial bleeding then one should depress the ureter posteriorly and go lateral to the ureter, while if it venous bleeding, one should retract the ureter upward and go lateral because the vein comes from below the ureter.*

Lateral vascular control can be easily achieved once this anatomy is understood. The easiest way of achieving this lateral control is to open the peritoneum at the level of sacral promontory and identify the ureter as it crosses the common iliac from lateral to medial and then open the plane parallel to the ureter in the direction from cranial to caudal.[14] This opens the pararectal space and the first structure, which crosses transversally, is the artery that can be ligated. *The main trick is remaining lateral and parallel to the ureter.*[15]

After giving the first branch, the anterior division continues caudally and gives two branches in females and one branch in males and then continues as obliterated hypogastric artery and ends by entering into the bladder at the level of the urethra. The two branches in females are superior and inferior vesicle while in males, it is the inferior vesicle. Since the bladder lies anterior to the uterus, the superior vesicle also arises at a plane higher than the uterine artery. *This allows the preservation of superior vesicle during radical surgeries of the uterus.*

The middle rectal artery, which is considered as a branch of anterior division of the internal iliac is absent in 30% of patients. *Thus, during the rectal surgery for cancer, this artery may not be visualized.* The area lateral to the obliterated artery is vascular and harbors the lymph nodes. *Thus, if one stays medial to the artery, the risk of damaging the obturator nerve or external vessels is minimal.*

Salient points of surgical anatomy of internal iliac artery:

❏ There is 6 cm length of internal iliac artery available for ligation before it gives its first branch
❏ The uterine artery and the superior vesicle traverse a long distance before they enter the organs
❏ Obliterated hypogastric artery divides the vascular and avascular spaces
❏ The internal iliac artery forms the lateral boundary of paravesical and pararectal spaces. The only structures that cross these spaces transversally are the arteries on their entrance to the organs
❏ The internal iliac vein is closely hugging the artery posteriorly
❏ The middle rectal artery is inconsistent.

Uterine Artery

The artery originates as the first branch of anterior division of internal iliac artery. It is tortuous and traverses a long distance transversely in the pararectal space to reach the uterus. This course allows it to be accommodated in during the enlargement of uterus.

The artery crosses the ureter anteriorly on its way to uterus. It gives a branch to the ureter. This branch needs to be separated to free the ureter. During surgery, the artery needs to be cut with scissors as any energy source will cause thermal damage to the ureter.

The artery enters the uterus at the level of internal os. It then divides into ascending and descending branches. The descending branch is called as cervical branch and supplies the cervix and upper vagina. The ascending branch runs paracervically upward for some distance before entering the uterus. This allows the surgeon to clamp the uterine in the parcervical region easily. The descending cervical can be avoided by staying medial to the uterine artery after cutting.

The main supply to the uterus comes from the ascending branch and hence all the fibroids grow in the upward direction. The arterial supply thus comes from below. This allows the entire separation of the myoma till the base. Had there been supply coming from all around the myoma, separation would not have been possible. Also, the blood supply coming from the base, the depth of the cavity needs to be closed carefully to avoid secondary hemorrhage.

In a radical hysterectomy, the stump of the uterine has to be carefully reflected medially to lateralize the ureter.

Superior Vesicle Artery

The superior vesical artery is the first branch of anterior division of internal iliac artery in males. It crosses the ureter anteriorly to reach the bladder.

In females, it is the second branch and arises at an anterior plane than the uterine artery (due to the fact that the bladder is anterior to the uterus). It, therefore, does not cross the ureter. Thus, it can be avoided when opening the pararectal space.

Obliterated Hypogastric Artery

The anterior division of the internal iliac artery ends as the obliterated hypogastric artery. This forms the medial umbilical ligament on the either side of the bladder. It ends by entering the bladder at the level of urethra. The paravesical space lies medial to it. The obturator fossa lies lateral to it. To avoid damage to the obturator vessels and nerves, the dissection should remain medial to the artery.

Obturator Artery

The obturator is the only medial branch of the internal iliac artery. It runs parallel and posterior to the obturator nerve in the obturator fossa. Thus, it can be damaged during lymph node dissection. The plane of dissection should always be superficial and parallel to the nerve and artery.

Inferior Epigastric Artery

This is already described in the text.

Veins

Common Iliac Vein

The common iliac vein divides into the internal and external vein at caudal to the division of common iliac artery. The veins essentially lie medial or posterior to the main arteries as surrounded by some free space. This is due the reason that the veins have to adjust the diameter as per the venous blood while the arteries can accommodate the increased volume without increasing the diameter.

There are no tributaries of common iliac vein. It is closely approximated to the presacral fascia, and thus rarely damaged during surgery.

Internal Iliac Vein

This is closely applied to the anterior branch of internal iliac artery and is posterior to it. It drains the veins of pelvic organs. This can be damaged during the artery if care is not taken. The presacral veins also drain into this. Hence, damage to the presacral veins is difficult to control as the tributaries retract. The parasympathetic fibers arise medial to the vein on their way to the pelvic organs.

External Iliac Vein

The external iliac vein runs medial to the artery and continues as femoral vein. The only tributaries are inferior epigastric and circumflex iliac.

Uterine Vein

The uterine vein is either single or double as it enters the internal iliac vein. It passes underneath the ureter. At its origin, it is closely in association with the parasympathetic fibers. Thus, it is an important landmark in nerve sparing radical hysterectomy. The veins should be ligated medial to the hypogastric nerve so as to preserve the inferior hypogastric plexus.

If there is venous bleeding during surgery one should lift up the ureter anteriorly to visualize and control the bleeding

■ THE SPACES

Pouch of Douglas or the Rectovaginal Space

The pouch of Douglas is bounded by cardinal and uterosacral ligaments on either side, the uterus anteriorly and rectum posteriorly.

There are two layers of Denonvilliers' fascia. One layer covers the rectum completely while the other lies on the posterior vaginal wall.

Pararectal Space

This is the most important space for the pelvic surgeon. It is a potential space lateral to the ureter. It needs to be exposed surgically, and this can be achieved by opening the peritoneum at the level of sacral promontory. The boundaries of pararectal space are ureter medially, and internal iliac artery. It is a pyramidal space, the apex of which is at the level at which the ureter crosses the common iliac and the base is formed by the levator ani muscle, with its covering endopelvic fascia. The space is traversed by the uterine vessels and superior vesicle vessels in females and males, respectively. The parasympathetic nerves from S2, S3 and S4 also traverse this space on their way to the pelvic organs. All the supports of uterus and bladder also traverse this space. The space is opened by remaining parallel and lateral to the ureter. This space dissection helps to expose the entire vascular anatomy. The uterosacral ligament and the hypogastric nerves lie on the medial side of the ureter while the deeper (dorsal) part, Mackenrodt, goes underneath the ureter and carries the uterine vein and the lymphatics. Thus to achieve a good oncological clearance one has to cut the Mackenrodt as lateral as possible.

Paravesical Space

The paravesical space lies lateral to the urinary bladder, and the boundaries are: laterally—the obliterated hypogastric artery, medially—the urinary bladder, inferiorly—pubic bone and superiorly—the pararectal space. Both these spaces are connected to each other and hence the entire vascular structures can be separated from the solid organs. During the radical surgeries, this space needs to be opened to reach the lateral side wall and achieve an optimum oncological clearance. The obliterated hypogastric artery is also called as the lateral umbilical ligament (Hernia surgery—transperitoneal).

Prevesical Space

The prevesical space lies anterior to the urinary bladder and is bounded by pubic symphysis anteriorly and bladder neck and urethra posteriorly. It is continuous space that communicates with the paravesical spaces on the either side. The base is formed by the levator ani muscles.

This space is important during the extraperitoneal as well as transperitoneal hernia surgery. The opening of this space ensures the safety of bladder and the mesh is placed in this space.

This space is also opened selectively in Burch repair and radical prostatectomy. The space can be opened by taking a peritoneal on the urachus and then dissecting the space bluntly as this space is completely avascular.

■ URETERIC ANATOMY

The ureteric anatomy is probably the most important consideration in pelvic surgery. The ureter crosses the common iliac at the level of sacral promontory from lateral to medial side. The ureter travels in its own endopelvic fascia. It travels in between the fork of the uterine artery and the uterine vein. It then turns medially and anteriorly to pass on the anterolateral aspect of the upper third of the vagina toward the bladder in its own "tunnel" of the endopelvic fascia. This commonly known as the ureteric tunnel is actually the uterovesical ligament. This ligament consistently contains two veins. The ureters enter the bladder at the corners of the trigone approximately 2.5 cm apart.

Blood Supply

The blood supply of the ureter is divided into upper third, middle third and lower third.
- ❑ The upper segment is supplied by branches of the renal, gonadal or adrenal arteries
- ❑ The middle portion receives small peritoneal twigs and branches from the arteries of the posterior abdominal wall
- ❑ The lower segment is the pelvic ureter, which is supplied by branches of common iliac artery or internal iliac artery and its branches.

All these vessels run up and down the ureter to form an anastomotic plexus in the adventitial coat of the ureter.

This anastomosis is deficient in some individuals, hence excessive mobilization of the ureter can lead to necrosis.

Remember: The blood supply of the ureter is parallel to its course. This can be seen as a separate mesentery. This ureteric mobilization when done, should be done along with its mesentery. This avoids the ureteric denudation and avascular fistula at a later date. The presence of mesentery also allows the complete ureteric mobilization from the sacral promontory up to the uterovesical junction, thus, allowing type III radical hysterectomy to be performed.

The ureter seems to be attached to the paracolpos by small fibrous bands, which have to be cut to reach the uterovesical junction.

The ureter is vulnerable for injury at the entry into the bladder, which is the narrowest part of the ureter, and at the point where the uterine artery crosses the ureter.

■ NERVES

There are four nerves in the pelvic area.

Genitofemoral Nerve

It lies lateral to the external iliac artery on the psoas muscle. The nerve should be protected during pelvic lymphadenectomy. It runs parallel till it dips down into the muscle.

Obturator Nerve

It lies in the bifurcation between the iliac arteries. The obturator artery and the veins run parallel to the nerve. The vein drains directly into the presacral veins. Thus, the plane of dissection during obturator lymphadenectomy should be superficial to the nerve.

Hypogastric Nerve

It arises from the superior hypogastric plexus, which lies at the bifurcation of the aorta. They carry the postganglionic sympathetic fibers from L1–3. The hypogastric nerves then traverse posterolaterally on the either side of the rectum on their way to the bladder and the pelvic floor. At the level of the uterine vein, this is joined by pelvic splanchnic nerves S2–4. These carry the parasympathetic supply. The hypogastric nerve is identified medial to the ureter at the level of the uterosacral. It lies in the space between the ureter and the uterosacral. The branches of these nerves, which arise medially, supply the rectum, uterus and part of cervix. These branches have to be sacrificed to achieve a nerve sparing radical hysterectomy.

Pelvic Splanchnic Nerve

They arise from S2–4 sacral nerves; they run parallel to the uterine vein on their way to join the hypogastric nerve from the lateral side. Thus, the distal part of the uterine vein becomes an important landmark to identify and preserve these nerves.

Lymphatics

The lymphatics from the uterus travel along the infundibulopelvic ligament and drain into the para-aortic group of nodes. Lymphatics from cervix and upper vagina go along the paracolpos and cardinal ligament, and drain into the ileo-obturator nodes. The obturator node is the first echelon of spread from the cervical cancers.

The ileo-obturator nodal region is defined from the obliterated hypogastric artery medially, to the fascia of obturator internus muscle laterally, and from the external iliac vein above to the obturator nerve below. The contents of this space are the obturator nerve, which is covered with the endopelvic fascia and fatty areolar tissue. During dissection, the nerve is easily exposed by gently sweeping away the areolar tissue over it.

Ten Commandments/"Mantras"

1. The uterine artery arises 6 inches beyond the bifurcation of the common iliac artery. Six inches of internal iliac artery is available for ligation.
2. The uterine artery and vein cross the pararectal space. The ureter lies in the fork between the artery and vein.
3. The pararectal and paravesical spaces are potential spaces that can be dissected easily.
4. The Denonvilliers' fascia consists of two layers, one layer over the cervix and vagina, and the second layer over the rectum.
5. The uterosacral ligaments, the cardinal ligaments and the paracolpos form a continuous fan-shaped structure.
6. The ureteric tunnel is a condensation of pelvic fascia and is vascular. Strands of endopelvic fascia fix the ureter to the vagina.
7. The vesicouterine ligament always has two veins.
8. The hypogastric nerves are medial to the ureter and lateral to the uterosacral ligament.
9. The uterine vein is an anatomical landmark for identification of the pelvic splanchnic nerves.
10. The anatomical variations of the vascular structures and the nerves of the pelvis are uncommon in females.

CHAPTER 5

Principle and Use of Electrosurgery in Laparoscopy

Helder Ferreira, Carlos Ferreira

"Surgeons do not know what they do not know about the safe use of energy in surgery."

■ INTRODUCTION

For many centuries heat started to be used to perform hemostasis. The discovery of the principle of heat production by passing electrical current through tissue (electrosurgery) resulted in the progressive development of electrosurgical devices, which are now crucial in surgeon´s armamentarium. Also called diathermy, electrosurgery consists in cutting and coagulation of body tissue with a high frequency current.[1] This technique is used in almost all kinds of surgeries to reduce blood loss and surgical time. In the last decades, researchers have developed many technological advances to minimize adverse events while refining its execution both in open or endoscopic surgeries. Despite widespread usage, awareness about electrosurgical principles and its potential complications is scanty among its users[2] and gynecologists are no exception.[3] All surgeons should be absolutely familiar with all equipment and inherent technology in the operating room.

■ HISTORY

The effect of intense heat on tissues is well known since the antiquity. The use of cautery (from Greek 'kaien' – burn) dates back as far as prehistoric times, when heated stones or hot iron were used to obtain hemostasis. An aphorism counseled to Hippocrates counseled the following: "Those diseases which medicines do not cure, iron cures; those which iron cannot cure, fire cures; and those which fire cannot cure, are to be reckoned wholly incurable."[4] Hot iron cauteries were used until the end of Modern Age to treat disease by lightly touching the skin as a counterirritant to dry up infected ulcers and gangrenous tissues, to destroy tumors, and perhaps to coagulate bleeding vessels.

In the 18th century, many scientific discoveries about electricity coincided with the beginning of its application in medicine. In 1786, Luigi Galvani´s demonstrated that electricity was the medium by which nerve cells passed signals to the muscles. His discovery and subsequent experiments led to the birth of electrophysiology.[5] The first applications of electricity in human tissues began in the early 19th century when Becquerel, a French physicist, first used electrocautery. He passed direct current though a wire, thereby heating it and effectively cauterizing tissue upon contact.[1] Also Eugène Sèrè, heated the blade of the first "electric scalpel" with a galvanic battery in 1863. The temperatures used were variable but very high. Tissues were coagulated at 600°C and cut at 1,500°C. Between this values—by varying the length of the blade—cutting and coagulation could be graded.[6]

Between 1880 and 1890, an important development in electrosurgery occurred with the discovery of alternating and high-frequency currents. D'Arsonval pioneered the use of an alternating electrical current in biological tissues. This French biophysicist discovered that high-frequency (over 10,000 Hz) alternating electrical currents could pass through the body safely. Rather than causing muscle stimulation, electrical current at a frequency of 200 kHz or higher generated heat in tissue.[7] From this accumulative work, Doyen developed an electrocoagulation machine[8] and Nagelschmidt first introduced the concept of "surgical diathermy" to explain how high frequency electrical current created heat in the body through the agitation of cellular ions and molecules.[9]

William T Bovie, seen as the father of modern electrosurgery for many surgeons, basing his electrosurgical unit on the work and discoveries of his predecessors, constructed a diathermy unit that produced high-frequency current delivered by a "cutting-loop" to be used for cutting, coagulation, and desiccation. The first use of this apparatus in a patient was at the Peter Bent Brigham Hospital in Boston, on October 1, 1926, when Dr Harvey Cushing solicited Bovie help for a second attempt to remove an enlarging, vascular myeloma from the head of a 64-year-old man. The initial success of this operation led to Cushing and Bovie´s further collaboration in other difficult cases as the first was not altogether comfortable with the hazards of the new approach. Over the course of the next year, Cushing's operative mortality increased significantly, reflecting the increased use of the Bovie's apparatus to perform more complex procedures he had not attempted without electrosurgical technology.[10] This electrosurgical unit model was used until 1968. Until this date, electrosurgical generators were "ground referenced", in other words, the flow of energy was in relation to earth ground. In this situation, anytime the patient came in contact with a potential path to ground, the current would choose the path of least resistance. This could potentially result in current flow through an electrocardiogram pad or through an intravenous pole in contact with the patient. If the current density were high enough at the point of contact, there was the possibility for a patient burn. This potential hazard was eliminated with the introduction of generators that were isolated from the ground confining the current flow to the circuit between the electrode and the patient return electrode, which offers a low-resistance pathway for current to return to the generator from the patient[11] (Fig. 1).

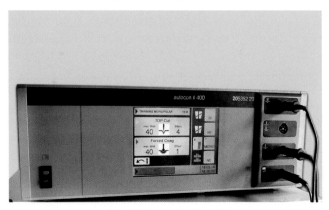

Fig. 1: Electrosurgical unit

NOMENCLATURE

The terms *electrosurgery, electrocautery, radiosurgery, diathermy and radiofrequency heating*, have all been used to refer to tissue application of radiofrequency electricity to obtain a desired effect. This overlapping of definitions can easily confuse those who use these products daily.

Electrocautery, in its classic meaning, is defined as the use of electricity to heat an object, which is then touched to the tissue to single vessels. This corresponds to the "hot iron" cautery referred before which differs from *electrosurgery*. *Electrosurgery or diathermy* uses radiofrequency electricity to generate heat in the tissue itself rather than applying heat from an outside source. The term *radiofrequency* is purely descriptive. The frequency of an electrical signal, in simple terms, is the rate at which the signal´s voltage rises and falls. Frequency is measured in cycles per second, and the unit of measurement is Hertz. Electrosurgical devices deliver electricity with high frequencies (0.1 MHz and 4 MHz) falling within the radio wave spectrum (0.01 to 300 MHz), that is why it is called radiofrequency electricity.

BIOPHYSICAL PRINCIPLES

Electrical current is created by the movement of electrons in a closed circuit. Voltage is the force that causes this movement. For example, the application of a voltage across human tissue results in a simple electrical circuit being formed between the voltage source and the tissue.

There are two types of electrical current: Direct current (DC), where electrons move in the same direction (e.g. our computer battery), and alternating current (AC), where the current changes direction periodically (e.g. our house current). In surgeries, alternating current is used to avoid electrolysis effects and with high frequencies (over 300 kHz) to avoid the Faraday effect on nerves and muscles stimulation associated with AC with a low frequency (under 10,000 Hz).[12] Electrosurgical units used in operating rooms convert electrical frequencies from the wall outlet, which are 50–60 Hz, to much higher frequencies, 500,000–3,000,000 Hz. The generated electrical current passes through the tissue, which acts as a resistor within this circuit. This resistance converts the electrical energy into thermal energy and is dependent on tissues' water content. This heat production rises body tissue temperature causing its destruction or damage.

Every electrical circuit obeys to Ohm´s Law: $V = R \times I$ [V: voltage in Volts (V), R: resistance of the tissue in Ohms (ω), I: current in Amperes (Amp)]. In cases of alternating current, the concept of impedance (Z) appears instead of resistance because there are two additional impeding mechanisms to be taken into account besides the normal resistance of direct current circuits: The induction of voltages in conductors self-induced by the magnetic fields of currents (inductance), and the electrostatic storage of charge induced by voltages between conductors (capacitance). Therefore, to achieve the same current flow, a greater voltage is needed as the resistance (or impedance) increases.

Resistance to current is inherent within all human tissues and electrical current flows through less resistant medias. In other words, electrons, when acted on by an electric field created by an electrosurgical unit, will be set in motion, forming a current that always seeks to travel the path of least resistance. This notion is fundamental on monopolar electrosurgery in which, high-frequency current passes through the patient from the active electrode, generally a forceps or probe, to the return electrode connected to the generator.

The power generated (in Watts) is the product of the voltage and current flow ($P = I \times V = I^2 \times R$). As $I = V/R$, the power generated is $V \times V /R$ equals V^2/R. Therefore, the larger voltage applied, the greater destructive effect. The transformation of electrical energy into heat occurs in accordance with Joules law and can be expressed by the following formula: Energy (joules) $= P \times t = I^2 \times R \times t$. So the amount of thermal energy delivered and the time rate of delivery will dictate the observed tissue effects. Moreover heat produced is inversely proportional to the surface area of the electrode [$E = (\text{Current/cross-sectional area})^2 \times R \times t$]. On the one hand, the smaller the surface area, the more localized heating energy produced; on the other hand, larger electrodes require longer periods of current application to achieve the same heat production.

ELECTROSURGERY: MONOPOLAR OR BIPOLAR MODALITY

There are two modalities of delivering current flow through tissue—monopolar or bipolar. The main difference between these two methods is that in monopolar surgery, the current passes through the patient to complete the current cycle, while in bipolar surgery, the current only passes through the tissue between the two electrodes of the instrument.

Monopolar electrosurgery is the most commonly used mode in open surgery. The monopolar delivery of energy to tissue requires that the current from the generator passes from the active electrode (with little surface) through body tissues and out of the patient through a dispersive or neutral electrode pad connected to the generator to form a closed circuit. At the tip of the active electrode, a high current density is produced with a resultant thermal effect and localized tissue destruction. This density of electrons diminishes rapidly as the distance from the electrode increases. Where body tissue resists current flows and chooses the least resistant paths. A return electrode is necessary to complete the circuit and disperse the electrical current. The large surface area of the dispersion pad results in low current density at the attachment site, thus minimizing the risk of skin burns. To reduce the length of the circuit, it is recommended to attach the dispersive pad as close as possible to the surgical field. Conditions such as surgical scars, metal implants, hairiness, bubbles increase impedance and can result in burns. To avoid these risks, the pad should be applied to well-perfused, dry, hairless skin over a large muscle and away from metallic bone implants. The modern electrogenerators have sensors that measure pad-to-skin contact and current density and block its function in case of any contact failure.

In a bipolar modality, the current flow is confined to the tissue grasped between the two electrodes. In other words, in a bipolar circuit, the surgeon uses forceps that have one tine connected to one pole of the generator (active electrode) and the other connected to the opposite pole (return electrode). The electrodes can also be blades of scissors, or graspers. Since the return electrode is included in the circuit at the site of surgery, the dispersive patient return electrode pad is unnecessary and patient body does not make part of the electrosurgical circuit. The current density on tissues is almost constant and because the pathway between tissues is shorter, the system is considered safer with little current dispersion and with minimal thermal damage to surrounding tissues. A disadvantage of bipolar systems is that for a fixed power output, the impedance load is lower and the tissue effects may be less than that for a monopolar generator resulting in longer times for coagulation, charring and adherence to tissue with incidental tearing of adjacent blood vessels.

TISSUE EFFECTS

Electrical current is a flux of electrons that collides with molecules of substances, particularly water molecules containing intracellular fluid. These collisions cause molecular agitation or motion increasing the temperature of the fluid. To understand the surgical applications of electrosurgery, it is necessary to know the effects of temperature on cells and tissues. The mean of human body temperature is 37°C. If we have a systemic infection, our cells can experience temperature elevations up to 40°C or so without damage to its integrity. As tissue temperature exceeds 45°C, the proteins in the tissue become denatured, losing their structural integrity. Heating body tissues in a progressive way over 60°C results in proteins denaturation of intracellular components before the water boils. The cells retract and the tissue turns white (white coagulation) and slowly desiccates. This effect is similar to heating the albumin of an egg. If the cells' temperature rises fast to 100°C or more, an explosive vaporization of intracellular water occurs, causing a rupture of cells membranes and its separation. Over 200°C or more, the organic molecules are broken down in a process called carbonization (black coagulation).[13]

The specific tissue effects of electrical current depend on the shape and size of electrode, time and speed of use, natural resistance of the tissue, frequency, waveform and peak voltage of current flow. As expected, the greater the current that passes through an area, the greater the effect will be on tissue. Also, the greater the amount of heat that is produced by this current, the greater the thermal damage on tissue. This thermal effect is a function of current density (current per cross-sectional area). Consequently, the heat produced is inversely proportional to the surface area of the electrode whereby, the smaller the surface area, the more localized heating is produced. On contrary, larger electrodes require longer periods of current application to achieve the same heat production.

The activation of the probe for long periods will produce wider and deeper tissue damage. In opposition, shorter lengths of time of activation result in an absence of the desired tissue effect. Besides that, faster movements will result in less coagulation and thermal spread.

Various tissue types have a different electrical resistance, which affects the rate of heating. Adipose tissue and bones have high resistance and are poor conductors of electricity; whereas, muscle and skin are good conductors of electricity and have low resistance.

The electrosurgical generators have different heating modalities with distinct tissue effects. These effects can be achieved by electric wave modulation in two ways: The voltage can be altered to drive more or less current through the tissues, or the waveform can be modified which influences the tissue effect. A variation in waveform mediates corresponding changes in tissue effects. Sinusoidal current waves with relative low voltages provided in a continuous way produce a rapid and intense heating. Higher voltages with sinusoidal current waves but functioning in an interrupted way (cycles), result in a progressive and moderate heating. In electrosurgery, the basic types of current waveform used are: Cutting, coagulation and blended current (Fig. 2).

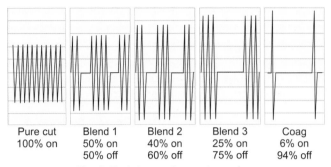

| Pure cut 100% on | Blend 1 50% on 50% off | Blend 2 40% on 60% off | Blend 3 25% on 75% off | Coag 6% on 94% off |

Fig. 2: Basic types of current waveform

Cutting Current

The cutting current waveform is sinusoidal and continuous with a high current but relatively low voltage (up to 300 Volts). A discharge arc from the probe is created at a specific location causing a sudden rise in temperature (over 100°C), vaporizing intracellular fluid leading to the rupture of the cell membranes and cleavage of the tissue with minimal coagulation effect. The continuous current does not allow for tissue cooling. To be effective, a cutting current power setting must be between 50 Watt and 80 Watt. Ideally, a monopolar instrument with a narrow, pointed or blade-shaped electrode is held near but not in contact with the tissue to create a spark gap through which the current arcs to the tissue. This spark results from the active ionization of the air gap between the active electrode and the target tissue. A precise incision is created in biological tissues with minimal hemostasis (coagulation) without extensive thermal damage (Fig. 3).

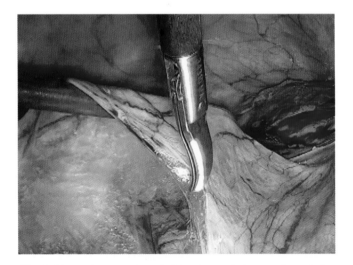

Fig. 3: Monopolar current applied to scissors tip to open the anterior leaflet of broad ligament

Coagulation Current

The aim of coagulation is to denature tissue or to constrict vessels to an extent where bleeding stops. The coagulation current is characterized by high voltage (over 400 Volts) intermittent bursts of dampened sine waves. The electrical activation time represents 6% of the duty cycle. In between bursts of current, the heat dissipates into the tissues reducing the cutting effect whilst enhancing the coagulation during the 94% off cycle. Unlike the case for vaporization, the cellular proteins are altered but not destroyed. When temperature is maintained between 60°C and 95°C, protein denaturation and dehydration occurs. This culminates in coagulum formation. The coagulation current is operated with the power setting between 30 Watt and 50 Watt. Effective coagulation for the purposes of sealing vessels or other lumen-containing structures like Fallopian tubes requires contact of the electrode with tissue.

Desiccation (from Latin: *dessicare*, to dry out) is used to define a very special form of application of coagulation rather than specific form of current. In this case, a needle-shaped electrode is pricked into the tissue and the electrical energy is totally converted into heat within the tissue, not seen with other current waveforms. It uses low current density, produced by low current and high voltage, applied over a broad area resulting in loss of water from the tissue cells but no significant protein damage. The end result is deeper necrosis and greater thermal spread. Desiccation is used in tumors or metastasis treatment, to reach tissue volumes as large as possible.

Fulguration or spray coagulation is a noncontact form of coagulation, producing a spark gap and electric discharge arc to mediate the ionization of air between the electrode and the tissue. Very high pulsed and extremely strongly modulated output voltages of several thousands volts (up to 8 kV) are used elevating the temperature beyond 100°C, reaching levels of 200°C or more. When fulgurating, the electrode is hold at some distance (3 to 4 mm) away of the tissue. Unlike the case of low-voltage continuous current (cutting current), the interrupted high-voltage discharges identify variable paths to the tissue and manifest in what appears to be a spraying effect onto an area of tissue that is much larger than the electrode itself and coagulating it, hence the term spraying coagulation. When a current pulse impacts a focal area of tissue, intracellular temperature increases, but then reduce again because of the lack of sustained current in that focal area. This results in a superficial coagulation, typically to a depth of approximately 0.5 mm. This type of coagulation is most preferred for the arrest of capillary or small arteriolar bleeding over a large surface area.

Blended Current

A blended waveform is a modification of the cutting waveform and is used when hemostasis is needed while cutting.[14] This waveform type consists of a combination of both cutting and coagulation waveforms. Higher blend settings translate into more time between bursts of current and greater coagulation, as seen in the following examples: Blend 1 (80% cut, 20% coagulation); Blend 2 (60% cut, 40% coagulation); and Blend 3 (50% cut, 50% coagulation). Although the total energy remains the same, the ratio of voltage and current is modified to increase hemostasis during dissection.

To conclude this point, the authors underline that the most important factor in achieving the desired surgical effect with electrosurgery lies in the surgeon's manipulation of the electrode. Allowing arcing of current by holding the electrode in close proximity to the tissue or activating the electrode while in direct contact allows the surgeon to achieve a wide variety of effects at a given generator power output and mode.

There is an evidence that the use of electrosurgery may lead to inadvertent damage to nearby structures through the lateral spread of thermal energy.[15] This collateral effect can cause tissue necrosis at the site of application leading to wound progressive damage at early stages of healing after thermal injury.[16] Thermal spread can also cause injury to adjacent organs (ureter, bladder, or bowel). The degree of thermal spread depends on the type of instrument, the power settings used and the duration of application.

Lateral thermal spread with bipolar instruments seem to be reduced when compared monopolar instruments. The traditional bipolar device produces an expected thermal spread of 2–22 mm.

■ BIPOLAR INSTRUMENTS

Although the introduction of bipolar devices started at the beginning of 20th century, its use was only to coagulate or to seal small blood vessels with a maximum diameter of 2–3 mm. However, in the end of the last century, bipolar vessel sealing instruments appeared as the most recent advance in electrosurgery with growing acceptance in open and laparoscopic surgeries. Vessels up to 7 mm in diameter and large tissue bundles can now be surgically ligated. The main principle of these new advances is the thermofusion of parietal collagen of vessels creating a mechanical resistance able to occlude permanently vessels lumen. Specifically, high current and low voltage are delivered to the targeted tissue and denature the collagen and elastin in the vessel wall. This advanced electrical current is combined with optimal mechanical pressure delivery by the instruments to fuse vessel walls and create a seal allowing the denatured protein to form a coagulum. To ensure that sufficient energy and pressure can be delivered into the tissue for adequate sealing, these bipolar devices rely on tissue response electrogenerators. In other words, this process is controlled and automatically stopped only after the intended sealing level has been reached. Additionally, thermal spread appears to be reduced compared to traditional bipolar electrosurgical systems.

There are three innovative bipolar devices that use low constant voltage and impedance feedback along paired ligating—cutting devices: the LigaSure˚ Vessel Sealing Device, the Enseal˚ Laparoscopic Vessel Fusion System and the Plasmakinetics˚ Cutting Forceps. These vessel sealing devices are also associated with lateral thermal spread effects.[17]

Although ultrasonic instruments are not electrosurgical, they are mentioned here as an alternate energy source of cutting and coagulation to clear up the confusion often encountered when defining this technology. The work principle of ultrasonic devices is based on the vibration of piezoelectric crystals at frequencies above 1 MHz that generate sound waves that travel through the tissues. This mechanical energy transmitted to tissues and the heat that is generated causes protein denaturation and formation of a coagulum that seals small vessels. The Harmonic˚ Scalpel, an ultrasonic cutting and coagulation device seem to be the safest instrument in terms of lateral thermal spread (< 0–3 mm), but is dependent upon application time and setting. The reduced risk of collateral tissue damage makes harmonic scalpels ideal for use close to vital structures such as bowel or ureter.

CURRENT USES OF ELECTROSURGERY IN MINIMALLY INVASIVE PROCEDURES IN GYNECOLOGY

The use of electrosurgery in operating rooms to perform surgical procedures is very common. In minimally invasive gynecological surgery, electrosurgery is used to cut or coagulate, and in a monopolar or bipolar way. The biophysical principles and effects on tissues of these endoscopic devices are very similar to laparotomic surgery. That is why, all gynecologists should be aware about all the theoretical concepts surrounding these new versatile and powerful electrosurgical instruments.

As the active electrodes in laparoscopy have a small surface area, the output power needed is low. The majority of modern generators have specific programs designed to

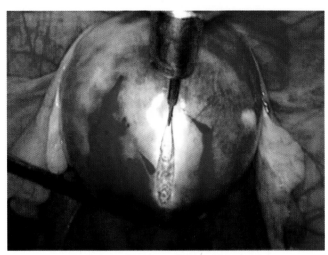

Fig. 4: Monopolar needle during a myomectomy

perform different laparoscopic procedures. The surgical instruments in laparoscopy need to be long and thin to pass through a trocar that can be made of plastic, metal or both. These characteristics impose constraints of insulation of all these materials to avoid injuries to adjacent structures.

Various electrosurgical devices to perform minimally invasive procedures have been introduced in recent years to achieve a safe and faster hemostasis. The preference for one electrosurgical tool over another is based on surgeon´s preference, availability and cost.[18] Total laparoscopic hysterectomy can be performed with bipolar forceps or vessel sealing devices with no differences in intraoperative blood loss.[19]

The example of a laparoscopic myomectomy, the uterine incision should be made with a monopolar needle with pure cutting current in order to avoid lateral thermal damage that may cause future uterine dehiscence (Fig. 4).

For the myoma traction is helpful to use the bipolar grasper to coagulate the myoma's pedicle.

In laparoscopic hysterectomy, the bipolar forceps (such as RobiKelly®) is very efficient most of the times to coagulate the uterine and cervicovaginal arteries (Figs 5A and B).

UNDESIRABLE EFFECTS OR ACCIDENTS AND ITS PREVENTION

The incidence of electrosurgical complications is 1–5 recognized injuries per 1,000 cases.[20] Although basic and advanced energy-based devices are commonly used, there is no well-defined requirement to demonstrate competency in the skills and knowledge required to use them.[21,22] Electrosurgical injuries may result from the following situations: Direct coupling and/or insulation

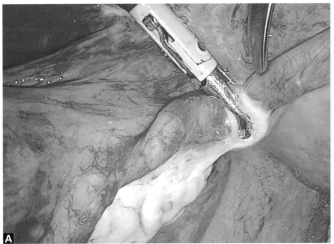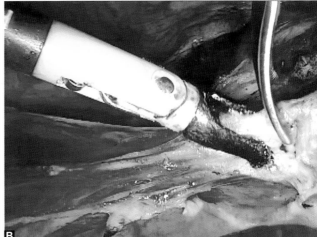

Figs 5A and B: RobiKelly® bipolar forceps

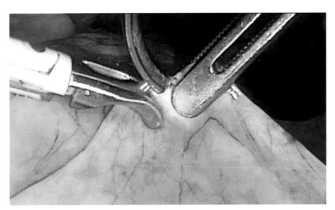

Fig. 6: Direct coupling when applying monopolar current at the scissors tip

failure, capacitive coupling, return electrode and alternate site burns.

Direct coupling results from inadvertent contact activation of the generator while the active electrode is in close proximity to another metallic instrument (such as a metallic trocar or a metallic grasper) (Fig. 6). Electrical current flows from the primary to the secondary instrument (path with least resistance), which acts as a second conductor. The former can injury adjacent structures or organs in contact with this secondary instrument out of surgeon´s visual field. Consequently, some injuries, such as burns to the bowel, may not be recognized immediately.

Insulation defects are not rare in laparoscopic instruments, particularly in reusable ones more exposed to damage of the material covering the active electrode. Also, the exposition of these long instruments to high-voltage currents of coagulation can create "blow holes" and break their insulation sheath. These defects can create an alternate route for the current to flow with capacity to cause iatrogenic burns.

Electrophysics defines a capacitor as two nearby conductors separated by a nonconducting medium. Capacitive coupling is not specific of laparoscopy, but the risk is higher with the utilization of different conductive and insulating materials, specially the trocars. The current flow can accumulate in an insulator and form a stored energy. This capacitor creates an electrostatic field between the two conductors such that current through one conductor is transmitted to the second conductor once the net charge exceeds the insulator´s capacity. This results in capacitive coupling able to cause visceral injuries away from surgeon´s visual field. The best way to reduce this effect is using trocars exclusively made of plastic or metal. The use of an active electrode monitoring system and limiting the amount of time that a high voltage setting is used can also eliminate concerns about capacitive coupling.[9]

In monopolar mode, the most common site of injury is at the patient return electrode. To avoid possible burns, the dispersive electrode pad must be of low resistance with a large enough surface area to decrease current density and heat producing on the smaller area of skin. If the patient´s return electrode is not wet or is not completely in contact with the patient´s skin, then the current exiting the body can have a high enough density to produce an unintended burn. Surface area impedance or in other words, the quality of contact between the return electrode and the patient´s skin can be compromised by excessive hair, adipose tissue, bony prominences, fluid invasion, adhesive failure, scar tissue and many other variables.[9] The best pad site location is on well vascularized muscle tissue.

In an effort to avoid this type of injury, contact quality monitoring systems were introduced in 1981. This system inactivates tne generator before an injury can occur if it detects a dangerously high level of impedance at the patient/pad interface.

Alternate site burns are another possible complication. This type of injury is a result of improper grounding. Prior to the development of the isolated generator systems, the patient was not properly grounded and many accidents occurred in the past. Originally, the generator systems were ground referenced where the electrical current passed through the patient´s body and returned to ground. Electrical currents seek to travel down choosing the pathways of least resistance. Therefore, the stray current could exit the patient through any conductive grounding object, which is in contact with the patient as a method of ground return: such as ECG electrodes or tables and operating staff. This increases the possibility of creating alternate site burns on the patients at alternate grounding sites where the high frequency current has exited the patient.

Recommendations for avoiding electrosurgical accidents during laparoscopic surgeries:

- Train the hand-eye coordination sequentially: didactic phase, laboratory experience, observation and/or assistance and preceptorship
- Learn the biophysical principles of electrosurgery
- Choose the proper current waveform mode
- Use all-metal or all-plastic cannula system
- In monopolar fashion:
  - Use the lowest possible power setting
  - Use low voltage waveform (cut)
  - Use brief, intermittent activation
  - Do not activate the electrode in the air when not in use (risk of capacitive current effect)
  - Do not activate the electrode in close proximity or direct contact with another instrument
- In bipolar fashion:
  - Terminate current at the end of vapor phase
  - Apply current in pulsatile fashion
  - Pay attention to the tip´s metallic part
- Use electrosurgical accessory safety equipment
  - Use a return electrode monitoring system
  - Use active electrode monitoring to detect stray energy generated by insulation failure or capacitive coupling
- Smoke evacuation can significantly improve visualization in the operation field
- Organize a laparoscopic team (biomedical engineer, perioperative nurses)
- Promote extended education activities and participation in medical conferences

Key Points
- Despite widespread usage, awareness about electrosurgical principles and its potential complications are scanty among its users and gynecologists are no exception.

■ REFERENCES

1. Massarweh N, Cosgriff N, Slakey D. Electrosurgery: history principles and current and future uses. J Am Coll Surg. 2006;202(3):520-30.
2. Feldman LS, Fuchshuber P, Jones DB, et al. FUSE (Fundamental Use of Surgical Energy™) Task Force. "Surgeons don't know what they don't know about the safe use of energy in surgery". Surg Endosc. 2012;26:2735-39.
3. Mayooran Z1, Pearce S, Tsaltas J, et al. Ignorance of electrosurgery among obstetricians and gynaecologists. BJOG. 2004;111(12):1413-8.
4. Cruse JM. History of medicine: The metamorphosis of scientific medicine in the ever-present past. Am J Med Sci. 1999;318:171-80.
5. Picollino M. Luigi Galvani and animal electricity: two centuries after the foundation of electrophysiology. Trends Neuroscience. 1997;20:443-78.
6. Ségal A, Ferrandis JJ. Le premier bistouri électrique. Pour la science. 1999;265.
7. Laquerrière A. Le professeur d'Arsonval. Journal de radiologie. 1941;24:3-4.
8. Doyen, Eugène-Louis. Surgical therapeutics and operative technique. London: Baillière, Tindall and Cox. 1917;1:439-52.
9. Wang K, Advincula AP. "Current thoughts" in electrosurgery. Int J Gynaecol Obstet. 2007;97 (3):245-50.
10. Carter PL. The life and legacy of William T. Bovie. Am J Surg. 2013;205(5):488-91.
11. Moak E. Electrosurgical unit safety. The role of the perioperative nurse. AORN J. 1991;53(3):744-6.
12. Doucet BM, Lam A, Griffin L. Neuromuscular electrical stimulation for skeletal muscle function Yale J Biol Med. 2012;85:201-15.
13. Munro MG, Fundamentals of Electrosurgery Part I: Principles of Radiofrequency Energy for Surgery, The SAGES Manual on the Fundamental Use of Surgical Energy (FUSE). 2012;2:15-59.
14. Alkatout I, Schollmeyer T, Hawaldar NA, et al. Principles and safety measures of electrosurgery in laparoscopy. JSLS. 2012;16(1):130-9.
15. Sutton PA, Awad S, Perkins AC, et al. Comparison of lateral thermal spread using monopolar and bipolar diathermy, the Harmonic Scalpel and the Ligasure. Br J Surg. 2010;97(3):428-33.
16. Lu S, Xiang J, Qing C, et al. Effect of necrotic tissue on progressive injury in deep partial thickness burn wounds. Chin Med J (Engl). 2002;115(3):323-5.
17. Abstracts of the Global Congress of Minimally Invasive Gynecology, 34th Annual Meeting of the American Association of Gynecologic Laparoscopists, Chicago, Illinois, USA, November 9-12, 2005, J Minim Invasive Gynecol. 2005;12(5 Suppl):S1-124.

18. Law KS1, Lyons SD. Comparative studies of energy sources in gynecologic laparoscopy, J Minim Invasive Gynecol. 2013;20(3):308-18.

19. Janssen PF, Brölmann HA, van Kesteren PJ, et al. Perioperative outcomes using LigaSure compared with conventional bipolar instruments in laparoscopic hysterectomy: a randomised controlled trial. BJOG. 2011;118(13):1568-75.

20. Hulka JF, Levy BS, Parker WH, et al. Laparoscopic-assisted vaginal hysterectomy: American Association of Gynecologic Laparoscopists' 1995 membership survey. J Am Assoc Gynecol Laparosc. 1997;4(2):167-71.

21. Feldman LS1, Brunt LM, Fuchshuber P, et al. Rationale for the fundamental use of surgical Energy™ (FUSE) curriculum assessment: focus on safety. Surg Endosc. 2013;27(11):4054-9.

22. Wu MP, Ou CS, Chen SL, et al.. Complications and recommended practices for electrosurgery in laparoscopy, Am J Surg. 2000;179 (1):67-73.

CHAPTER 6

Laparoscopic Suturing

Meenu Agarwal

"We are what we repeatedly do. Excellence, then, is not an act, but a habit."

Aristotle

■ INTRODUCTION

The historic Japanese shrine Izumo-taisha is built entirely of wood without the use of a single nail. It is an example of approximation at its best. This is how a good tissue approximation should appear after suturing.

The skill of laparoscopic suturing is crucial for a laparoscopic surgeon not only to perform surgeries which involve suturing but also for dealing with the intraoperative complications. It is rather ironic that we do not begin with laparotomies without the suturing skills but could start with laparoscopic surgeries without the know-how of laparoscopic suturing. It was because, in the past, the suturing in laparoscopy seemed to be difficult as we did not have the correct methodology of suturing. A correct systematic approach to suturing needs to be followed, backed up with a good training and practice on pelvic trainers and simulators. It may be cerebrally intensive in the initial learning phase but over a period of time, suturing becomes a habit just like in open surgery. Suturing skills can be mastered easily with practice even by an average surgeon.

■ METHODOLOGY

❏ Equipment
❏ Knots
❏ Suturing techniques
❏ Ergonomics and port placement.

■ EQUIPMENT

The equipment needed for laparoscopic suturing:
❏ Needle holder
❏ Needle
❏ Suture material.

Needle Holder

A good set of needle holders is a good investment. One should avoid changing the needle holders for a sustained efficiency. The needle holders must always be deployed as a pair (we recommend using two needle holders instead of one grasper as they give better needle handling and also the ability to suture with both hands).

Practical Hints

❏ A surgeon should chose one pair of needle holders and be thoroughly familiar with its usage which would increase his efficiency. After repeated usage of the same instruments, they get incorporated into the reflexes so well that they almost become an extension of his hands.

For right-handed surgeons, the active instrument should be in the right hand and the control button to open the jaws would be on the side of thumb with the movable upper jaw and a fixed lower blade and this would be opposite in the left-handed instrument which will used as a passive instrument to lift up the tissue for countertraction and to take out the needle from the tissue. An ambidextrous surgeon can also use identical straight needle holders in both the hands and can interchange the function of the instrument by just reversing the role of active hand to the passive hand and vice versa.

A good way to practice hand-eye coordination for suturing is to put inside the pelvic trainer, a loosely knotted Vicryl, and then try to open the knot with two needle holders.

The tip of the needle holder should be of multiutility type, i.e.

- Handle the tissue gently
- Handle the suture
- Hold the needle firmly but should not deform it.

Jaw

The jaw can be:

- *Curved vs straight*: We have a preference for curved jaws as they have more stability.
- *Universal vs self-rightening*: We prefer universal as self-rightening auto-adjusts the needle and we cannot change the direction of needle in cases where we need to take a stitch at an odd angle (many surgeons prefer self-rightening needle holders).
- *Surface*: The surface should hold the needle but not needle deforming.
- *Micro vs macro*: Depending on the type of surgery, e.g. for tubotubal anastomosis, you should have 4 mm microsurgical needle holders to take the stitches with 5/0 or 6/0 suture material.

The additional feature of the jaw is that the edges of the jaw should be rounded and should not have a rough joint, which might catch the suture when you wrap the suture around it.

Shaft

The shaft should have glare reduction.

Handle

The handle can be curved or straight and with a rachet. The holding and releasing mechanism of the rachet is the key. It should be smooth and easy.

The grasper used by the assistant to maintain tension on the suture during continuous suturing should be atraumatic with smooth nonslip jaws to prevent fraying of the suture.

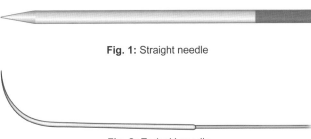

Fig. 1: Straight needle

Fig. 2: Endoski needle

Needles

- *Straight needle*: The straight needle was used by the initial pioneers of laparoscopy. It was mainly because the control over the needle to drive through the tissues was better. The needle could be introduced through the small port. Over a period of time we have realized that the straight needle is not ideal for atraumatic suturing, especially in cases of thick tissues as it does not have a curved path. Another main disadvantage of straight needles is that it is difficult to suture pedicles (Fig. 1).
- *Endoski needle*: It is curved at the tip and straight at the base so it combines the good feature of both straight and curved needle. It has the ease of passing through small ports and also has the curve to negotiate the depth of the tissues while suturing (Fig. 2). The distal end is tapered half circle and proximal shaft of the needle is straight. The shaft of the needle is 1.5 times the length of curved portion of Endoski needle.
- *Curved needle*: You can rotate the needle and also get the depth for suturing. The curved needle is by far the most superior for suturing as it replicates the pronating movement of the wrist same as in laparotomy. It can be ¼ circle, ½ circle, 3/8 circle, 5/8 circle (Figs 3A to C). Most commonly used is ½ circle.
- *CT needle*: A majority of surgeons use CT needles as these are bigger and strong curved needles for vault suturing and myomectomy suturing.

> **Points to Remember**
> - The needle should always be held with the tip of needle holder
> - The needle should be held close to the tail end so as to have an adequate effective length which is important especially in cases of deep bites
> - The distance between the two sutures should be approximately equal to the visible width of the tied suture
> - The tissues should be tightened down just enough to achieve an edge-to-edge anastomosis

Passage of Needle

- Either a one stage pass or a two stage pass can be used depending on the thickness of the bite required to be taken. In a single stage pass, the entire length of the needle is passed through both the edges of the tissue in

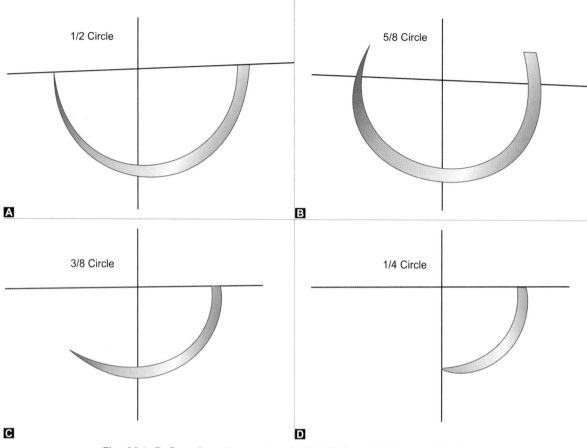

Figs 3A to D: Curved needle. (A) 1/2 circle; (B) 5/8 circle; (C) 3/8 circle; (D) 1/4 circle

one go and in a double stage pass, the needle is taken out from one edge and again reintroduced into the second edge. Two stage pass is better where the gap is big and a precise approximation is required and also the safety margin is more as the exact route of the needle is under vision.

❑ The tip of the needle must always approach the tissue at right angles and the direction of the driving force must be perpendicular to the cut surface so that the needle goes head on against the resistance of the tissue. If the direction of the force is not correct, the needle will deflect.

❑ The extraction of the needle should be in 12 O'clock direction by the passive needle holder after having released the needle from the active needle holder.

Points to Remember

- In a two stage pass after the needle is taken out from one edge advances the suture length just enough to regrasp the needle for the next bite
- Do not try to pull the suture till you have taken out the second bite as that can sometimes cause entangling of the thread and unnecessary confusion and wastage of time

Suture Material

There has been evidence in archaeology of the use of horse hair as the suture material applied to human wounds in the ancient times.

Today, we have many types of suture materials which are broadly classified as:

❑ Permanent
  ❖ Used in Burch colposuspension, sacrocolpopexy, etc.
  ❖ We use GORE-TEX suture in these cases. Prolene can be used for tubotubal anastomosis.

❑ Delayed absorbable
  ❖ The purpose is to maintain the approximation of the tissue until the approximation is attained naturally by the healing process.
  ❖ Vicryl: It is the work horse suture material used in most of the surgeries, e.g. myomectomy, hysterectomy, etc.

Introduction of a Suture in the Peritoneal Cavity

We use the back loading technique. We withdraw the lower accessory port cannula out, put the needle holder through the cannula and hold the thread 2 cm from the needle and then needle holder is introduced into the accessory port site with a little push under visual control along with the thread. The thread is pulled in by the assistant grasper till the needle and the entire suture material is pulled in and then the cannula is slipped over the needle holder (Figs 4 and 5).

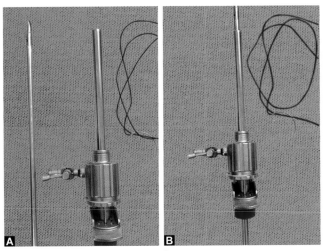

Figs 4A and B: (A) Withdraw the lower port from the abdomen; (B) Insert the needle holder through the cannula

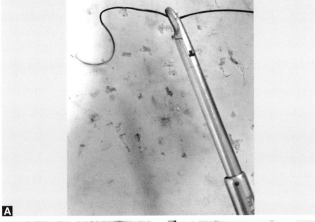

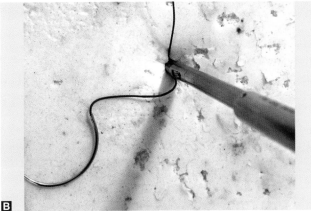

Figs 5A and B: (A) Hold the thread 2 cm away from needle; (B) Introduce the needle holder through the lower accessory port with the thread, pull the needle in with the opposite side grasper, slide the cannula over it

Transferring a Suture Ligature into the Peritoneal Cavity through a Cannula

❑ The other technique is that you withdraw the lower port out of the abdomen and then push the grasper from the opposite port into the lower port site to come out, hold the thread 2 cm away from the needle and pull it inside the abdominal cavity (Figs 6 to 10).

❑ Since the length available is always long, the suture length needs to be cut approximately 10–15 cm from the needle end. Although the suturing becomes a bit easier if only the required length is taken, sometimes a longer suture is taken to save on the cost which should be avoided to facilitate a hassle-free suturing.

❑ It is very important to hold and grasp only the suture and not the needle. The needle is only held during suturing and transferring of the needle.

❑ The loading of the needle into the needle holder can be done in many ways:

❖ The needle is placed on any serosal surface and the active needle holder approaches the needle at right angles with its jaws open since its inferior jaw is fixed that can be gently pressed on the mucosal surface for a perfect alignment of the needle before the jaws are closed to pick up the needle.

❖ The suture is held by the passive needle holder about 3–4 cm from the needle and is dangled with its tip touching the tissue. Wait till the needle stops moving and then the active needle holder approaches the needle and the passive needle holder slowly rotates the needle into a favorable position till the active needle holder grasps it at the correct angle.

❖ The needle is held with the passive needle holder and then transferred to the active needle holder to and fro till the correct angle of holding the needle is achieved making sure that these movements are happening away from the tissue.

▮ KNOTS

After the needle is passed through the tissue, the suture is pulled out leaving 2–3 cm of the suture tail and the knot is tied by wrapping the suture around it with the assistant needle holder or grasper.

Types of Knots

Different types of knots are:

❑ Overhand or half knot: This is an incomplete basic knot and can be untied easily. We need to pull both the ends of the thread in opposite directions with uniform

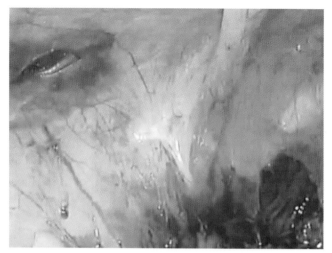

Fig. 6: Withdraw the lower port cannula

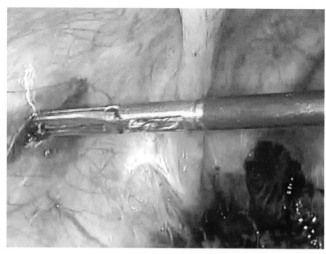

Fig. 7: Insert the grasper from the opposite site into the lower port site (make sure that there is no gas leakage by gentle pressure with a gauze at the skin end)

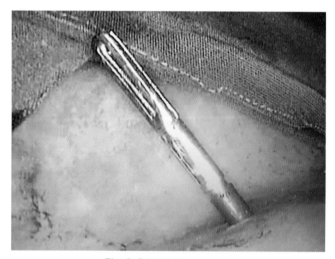

Fig. 8: Bring the grasper out

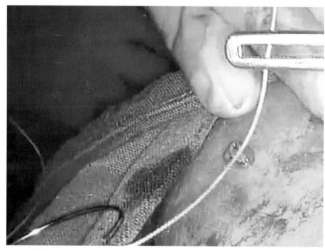

Fig. 9: Hold the thread about 4 cm from the needle end

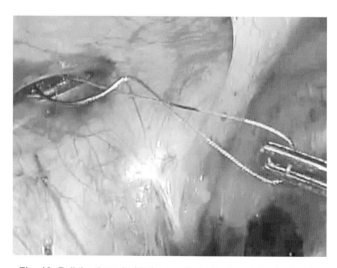

Fig. 10: Pull the thread with the needle inside the abdominal cavity

tension. Ideally, both the halves should be of the same length but to save the length of the suture material we can keep one end small and hold the other end in such a way that the knot forms the hypothetical midpoint (Figs 11A and B).

❑ The square or reef knot: It consists of two opposite half knots. This is a safe knot for securing small blood vessels but the first half knot needs to be stepped on to hold before the second knot is put (Fig. 12).

❑ Ligature knot: It consists of an initial double half knot followed by a single half knot. It is more secure than the classic reef knot. However, it does not capsize as easily as the square knot. This is important as a capsized knot converts into a sliding configuration and the tissue tension and edge approximation can be adjusted in such a knot (Fig. 13).

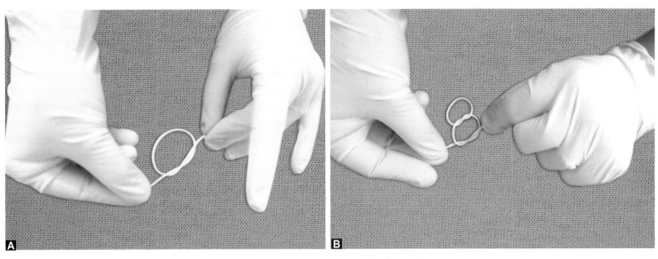

Figs 11A and B: (A) Half knot; (B) Square knot

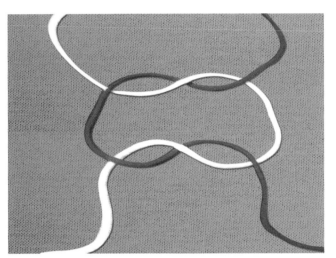

Fig. 12: The square or reef knot

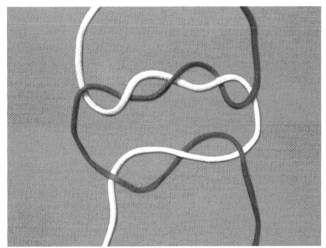

Fig. 13: Ligature knot

❏ Double knot: It consists of two double half knots (Fig. 14).
❏ Mayo knot: The Mayo knot consists of two identical half knots forming a granny knot followed by a third and opposite half knot which locks the completed knot. The second and third half knots will form a square knot as a unit. We can do fine adjustment of tissue tension and approximation before taking the third knot (Fig. 15).
❏ Granny knot: Two identical half knots form a granny's knot, but it is not advisable as they can lock prematurely or may sometimes slide making it an unstable knot (Fig. 16).
❏ Surgeons knot: It is favored for interrupted suturing. It consists of a double half knot and then two opposite half knots (forming a square knot). If a surgeon has to get familiar with only one type of knotting, this surgical knot is the one (Fig. 17).

❏ Double knot: Two double half knots would form a double knot. It is a very secure knot (Fig 18).
❏ Multiple knots: These are used when slippery suture material with a memory is used such as Prolene (Fig. 19).

▊ SUTURING TECHNIQUE

The different types of suturing techniques are:
❏ Loop ligatures
❏ Extracorporeal
❏ Intracorporeal
❏ Automated systems
❏ Robotics.

Loop Ligatures

Endoloops are available as preformed slipping loops. The pusher mechanism used is a plastic push rod.

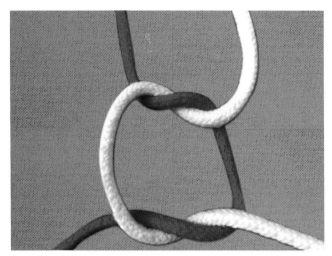

Fig. 14: Double knot

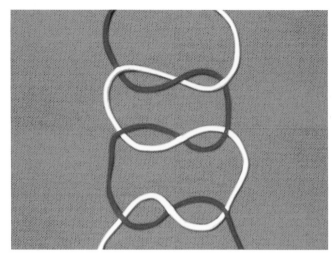

Fig. 15: Mayo knot

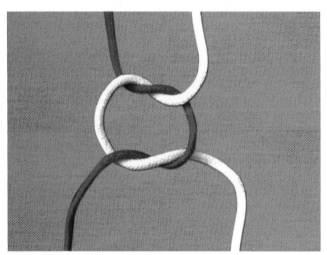

Fig. 16: Granny knot

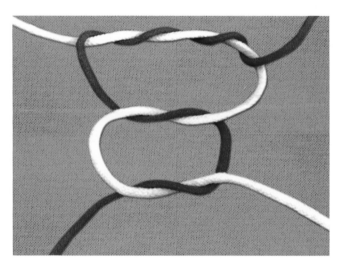

Fig. 17: Surgeon's knot

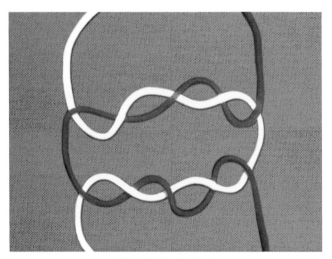

Fig. 18: Double knot

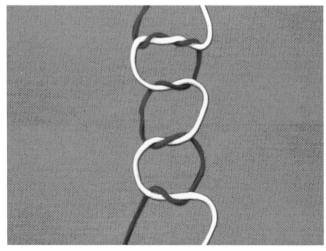

Fig. 19: Multiple knots

Use of Slipping Endoloops

❏ Ligature of small tubular structures
❏ Ligature of small blood vessels
❏ To ligate the base, e.g. of a subserous fibroid.

Technique of Inserting Slipping Endoloops

The site of insertion through a 5.5 mm port must be near the intended target. Ideally, the loop is inserted at an angle of 60–90° from the port where the grasper is inserted to hold the structure to be ligated. Once the loop is inside, put the grasper through the loop to hold the structure to be ligated then push the loop over it till it reaches the base of the structure to be ligated and then tighten the loop. We, many a times, use it for subserous fibroids to ligate them at the base and then cut with a monopolar hook or harmonic little above the loop. It is very quick and saves time.

Intracorporeal

In this, the knot is tied inside the peritoneal cavity using two needle holders which are an extension of your hands or we can also use one needle holder and one grasper.

Extracorporeal

In this technique, loose knot is fashioned outside suture, outside the abdominal cavity and then pushed inside with the help of a knot pusher and then tightened. Some knots are partially tied extracorporeally and completed intracorporeally.

There are various types of extracorporeal loops, e.g. Roeder's knot.

One should know at least one type of extracorporeal knot and use it when required.

Roeder's Knot

Technique: The needle is introduced in the peritoneal cavity and is passed through the tissue to be sutured. The needle is then taken out keeping the other end inside which is supported by the assistant's grasper. The needle is cut off and then we start assembling the extracorporeal knot.

First, it is performed a single flat knot (or half knot) then the free tail of the suture wraps three times around the top of a suture loop and locks it with a single throw through the proximal suture leg of the loop. Once the knot is tightened, the free end of the suture is cut to approximately 3 mm.

Steps:

❏ Initial half knot

❏ The free tail of the suture is wrapped around the top of the suture loop by the surgeon keeping the initial half loop between his thumb and middle finger
❏ Three and a half coils are wrapped around the suture loop
❏ The free tail of the suture is tied around the proximal leg of the loop, from the anterior to posterior, forming a half knot
❏ The free tail of the suture is pulled back between the second and the last coil
❏ The tail is held taut and the final configuration of Roeder's knot is achieved by pressing the turns between two half knots. This is then pushed down into the cavity until tightened over the suture line (Figs 20A to D).

Auotomated Systems

The sewing machines do not have the depth and the versatility and hence are not so popular.

Robotics

❏ Hugely expensive sewing machine
❏ It definitely has a lower learning curve and the suturing versatility is immense but is very expensive. It may not be a cost-effective option in a primarily gynecological set-up.

EROGONOMICS AND PORT PLACEMENT

❏ Contralateral
❏ Ipsilateral
❏ Triangular
❏ *Contralateral:* In the contralateral suturing, both the ports are on the either side of the primary port. It gives a good angle for suturing in the pelvis. The distance between the instruments is adequate but ergonomically it is not a good port placement as you have to crossover to the other side to suture and can be a cause for the shoulder pain for the surgeon.
❏ *Ipsilateral:* In the ipsilateral suturing, both the ports are on the same side of patient. We use the lower port 2 cm medial to the anterior superior iliac spine which is always lateral to the inferior epigastric artery. The second port is at the same level as the primary port in the straight line from the lower port. The movements are same as contralateral suturing so if you have been trained for contralateral suturing, it is not difficult to get adapted to ipsilateral suturing. The tremors are much less and the arms are relaxed and just next to your body, so ergonomically it is the correct position. The down

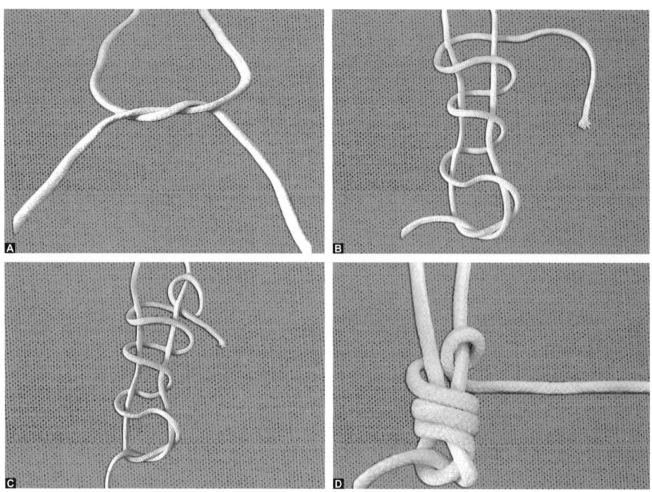

Figs 20A to D: Roeder's knot. (A) The initial half knot; (B) Three and a half turns around the two loops behind the half knot; (C) A second half knot between the tail and one limb of standing part; (D) The tail is pulled back to stack the turns between the first and second half knot

side is that the ports may be very close to each other, especially in small built patients and the angulation between the instruments may not be optimal.

❏ *Triangular*: The triangular suturing used mainly by general surgeons where they can rotate their port placement depending on what they want to suture.

▊ SUTURING IN A VERTICAL ZONE

It is an ipsilateral suturing with both the ports on the same side of the patient, lower left lateral and a paraumbilical port. So, in this technique surgeon uses two hands on the same side just like in open surgery. The needle holders are parallel to the suture line. This technological innovation of vertical zone described by Prof Charles Koh is the biggest breakthrough in the history of laparoscopic suturing (Fig. 21).

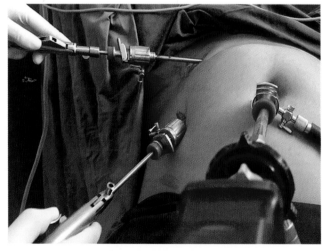

Fig. 21: Suturing in a vertical zone

Change is the only constant so even if a laparoscopic surgeon is trained for contralateral suturing, it is not difficult for him to adapt to the ipsilateral suturing in the vertical zone which is much more natural to a surgeon as he is already trained for ipsilateral suturing in open surgery.

Key Points

- The proficiency in laparoscopic suturing reduces the complication rates and the conversion to laparotomies
- Ipsilateral suturing in the vertical zone increases the efficiency of a laparoscopic surgeon
- The training, practice and the correct methodology is the key

CHAPTER 7

Tissue Retrieval

Namita Joshi

■ INTRODUCTION

Today almost every conventional gynecological surgery that performed open earlier can be done laparoscopically.

It is very important to get a pathological specimen for correct diagnosis and further management of the case.

Surgeons have improvised ways to retrieve tissue from abdominal cavity after a laparoscopic surgery. The larger the specimen, the difficult and time consuming is the retrieval.

Sometimes the surgery does not take as long as the retrieval of specimen.

In this chapter, we have discussed various methods of tissue retrieval used and described over the period.

■ TISSUE RETRIEVAL THROUGH 5 MM PORT

Soft and small tissues like tubes, ovarian cysts can be retrieved through 5 mm port site. Remove the port, insert a long artery forceps, increase the inner diameter of the port site by opening the artery forceps perpendicular to the skin incision, hold the specimen in long artery forceps and pull it out under vision. The port site can be closed in the usual way using Ethilon No 3. The left lower quadrant port is used for retrieval (Figs 1 to 4).

■ REPLACING 5 MM PORT BY 10 MM PORT

Small and soft structures like tube after salpingectomy, appendix, ovarian cyst wall can be removed through a 10 mm port. Again, the left lower quadrant port is converted to 10 mm port. Debulking of specimen can be done by making spiral cuts in the specimen so as to enhance the extraction. We have cut a 3–4 cm fibroid into 2–3 pieces after enucleating it, but while it is still attached to the uterus by using monopolar current. This way it was extracted through 10 mm port site. Allis Grasper Forceps give a good hold for removing the specimen (Figs 5 to 7).

■ ENDOBAGS FOR TISSUE RETRIEVAL

Some surgical specimen warrant retrieval without spillage of its content. They include dermoid cysts, endometriotic cyst, chronic ectopic, malignant ovarian cyst, infected TO masses.[1-4] In all these cases, it is ideal to use endobags. Use of endobag needs a port size of 10–12 mm. Endobags are available in various sizes. The commercial endobags are costly. To reduce the surgical cost, surgeons have used gloves (Fig. 8), plastic bags and converted them in a bag by placing purse string suture using No. 2 silk. Though cheap, their strength can, sometimes, be compromised. The endobag is placed in the abdominal cavity either through the umbilical port or through the left lower quadrant port. After removal, the specimen is placed in the endobag. If it contains fluid, it is drained inside the endobag. The bag is then closed by tightening the purse string suture or tightening the clasp of the commercially available endobags. The bag can then be removed through the 10 mm port site or through CCL vaginal extractor.

■ MORCELLATION FOR TISSUE EXTRACTION

Electromechanical morcellation using a hand instrument was first described in 1993.[5,6] There are various morcellators available depending on weight, blade size, diameter, cutting

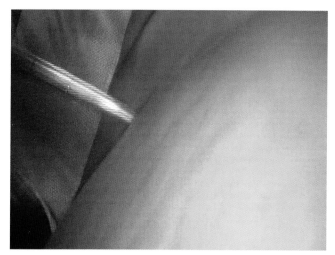

Fig. 1: Long artery forceps being inserted through left lower quadrant port

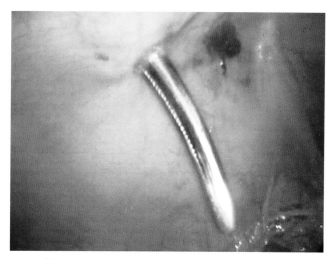

Fig. 2: Long artery forceps inside the abdominal cavity

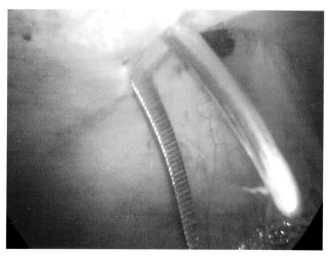

Fig. 3: Long artery forceps opened to increase the inner diameter

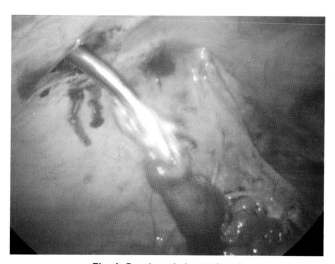

Fig. 4: Specimen being retrieved

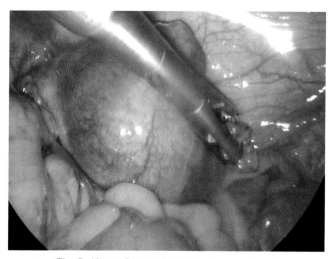

Fig. 5: 10 mm Grasper in use for tissue retrieval

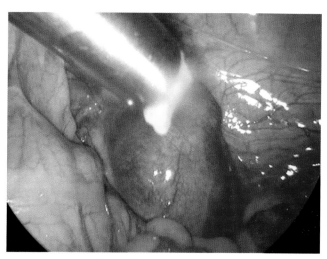

Fig. 6: 10 mm Grasper in use

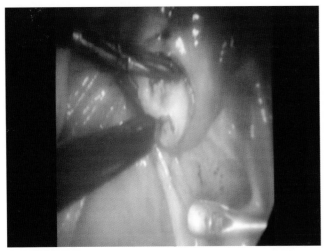

Fig. 7: Monopolar cautery in use for debulking of fibroid

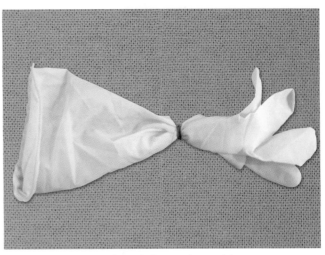

Fig. 8: Glove being used as endobag

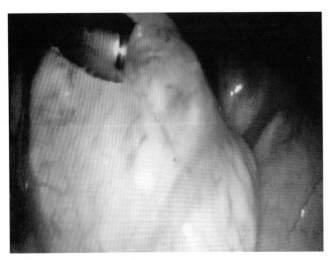

Fig. 9: Morcellator in use

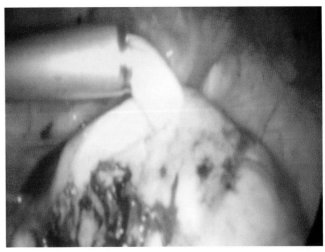

Fig. 10: Tissue morcellated in strips

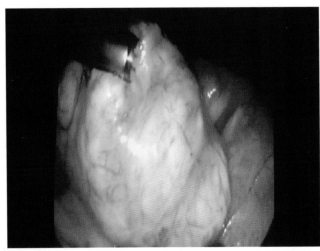

Fig. 11: Morcellation in progress

speed, etc. Commonly available morcellators need a 12–15 mm port for entry. Because of its motor peeling feature, these morcellators have faster morcellation capability. Karl Storz has introduced SAWALHE II SuperCut Morcellator, it has a handle with a pistol grip and motor once introduced in the handle is locked in place. The obturator is conical with atraumatic spirals that allow its entry by dilatation and deflection mechanism. The knife is secure in a sheath and should be activated only once the position is correct and safe. This is important to avoid injuries during morcellation.[7] The Company recommends the use of motor at 650 rpm.

While morcellating, the tissue should be pulled toward the blade and the blade should be in vision at all times. Tissue is removed in long strips (Figs 9 to 11).

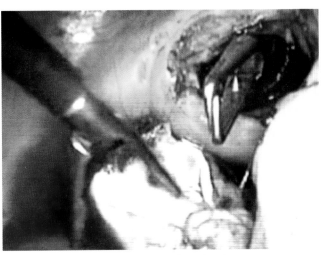

Fig. 12: Tissue removal through colpotomy

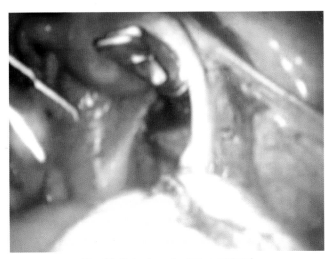

Fig. 13: Colpotomy for tissue retrieval

There are some concerns over spread of malignancy when used in case of unsuspected borderline malignancies and fibroids with sarcomatous changes and some guidelines have been issued by Food and Drug Administration.[8,9]

❑ Food and Drug Administration does not recommend use of morcellation in a case of surgery for fibroid.

❑ Its use should be avoided in a case of suspected malignancy.

❑ All treatment options should be discussed with women for treatment of fibroids.

❑ If morcellation is to be used, the possibility of spread of an unsuspecting malignancy should be discussed with the patient.

The American Association of Gynecologic Laparoscopists also recommends following these precautions.

ENDOSCOPIC KNIFE FOR TISSUE MORCELLATION

De Grandi P et al.[10] have developed a knife that can be used to morcellate a myoma and uterus that are later retrieved using a CCL vaginal extractor. The knife is introduced through a 10 mm port. While introducing the knife, the blade is protected in a sheath. The specimen should be cut from posterior to anterior side so as to reduce the injury to bowel and vessels. Morcellated tissue is removed through a colpotomy.

COLPOTOMY

When the tissue to be removed is larger than the conventional 10–12 mm port site then it is advisable to remove it through posterior colpotomy route (Figs 12 and 13).

Almost every tissue can be retrieved through this route. The problem with this route is loss of pneumoperitoneum. The CCL vaginal extractor overcomes this problem. It has a trocar fitted with a ball-shaped head at one end. Some surgeons have used sponge on a holder in place of CCL vaginal extractor to guide the incision between two uterosacral ligaments. Monopolar cautery or scissors can be used to open the posterior fornix laparoscopically. CCL vaginal extractor is better as the pneumoperitoneum is maintained. Now the specimen to be removed is held in a grasper inserted through the vaginal port and is brought out. If the specimen is still larger, it can be kept in an endobag; the bag's mouth is delivered out vaginally, the specimen is then morcellated inside the bag and retrieved later. The colpotomy incision can be closed either using endosuturing through laparoscope or by the conventional vaginal route. The technique is much better than removing the specimen by enlarging abdominal incision, as there are chances of hernia. Some surgeons have modified the vaginal extraction of a large myoma by placing the extracted myoma in pouch of Douglas and making an incision directly over the myoma[11] as it is held with an Allis Grasper laparoscopically. The myoma prevents the loss of pneumoperitoneum. Once the posterior pouch is opened the myoma is held with a tenaculum and is pulled out vaginally or morcellated manually using a knife and retrieved. Tissue retrieval through colpotomy gives less postoperative pain as compared to abdominal retrieval after enlarging the incision.

ACKNOWLEDGMENTS

I would like to thank Dr Meenu Agarwal for motivating and guiding me while writing this chapter.

∎ REFERENCES

1. Amso NN, Broadbent JAM, Hill NCW, et al. Laparoscopic oophorectomy–in-a-bag for removal of ovarian tumour of uncertain origin. Gynecol Endo. 1992;2:59-63.

2. Volz J, Koster S, Potempa D, et al. Pelviscopic ovarian surgery: A new methods of safe organ preserving surgery. Geburt shilfe and Frauenhelkunde. 1993;53:132-4.

3. Davies A, Mohamed H, Richardson RE, et al. Laparoscopic ovarian cystectomy; inside a bag: a new technique for dermoid cysts. J Gynaecol Surg. 1997;13:35-8.

4. Russel JB. Laparoscopic oophorectomy. Current Opinions in Obstet Gynaecol. 1995;7:295-8.

5. Steiner RA, Wight E, Tadir Y, et al. Electrical cutting device for laparoscopic removal of tissue from the abdominal cavity. Obstet Gynecol. 1993;81:471-4.

6. Carter JE, Mc Carus SD. Laparoscopic myomectomy. Time and cost analysis of power vs. manual morcellation. J Reprod Med. 1997;42:383-8.

7. AAGL Advancing Minimally Invasive Gynecology Worldwide. AAGL position statement: route of hysterectomy to treat benign uterine disease. J Minim Invasive Gynecol. 2011;18(1):1-3.

8. US Food and Drug Administration. Laparoscopic uterine power morcellation in hysterectomy and myomectomy: FDA safety communication. Available at: http://www.fda.gov/MedicalDevices/Safety/Alertsand Notices/ucm 393576.htm. [Accessed on January 2015].

9. Magdy P, Milad MD, Sokol E. Laparoscopic Morcellator-Related Injuries. J Am Assoc Gynaecol Laparoscop. 2003;10(3):383-5.

10. De Grandi P, Chardonnens E, Gerber S. The morcellator knife. A new laparoscopic instrument for supracervical hysterectomy and morcellation. Obstet Gynecol. 2000;95:777-8.

11. Jain N. State of the Art Atlas of Endoscopic Surgery in Infertility and Gynecology. New Delhi: Jaypee Brothers Medical Publishers; 2004.

CHAPTER 8

Anesthesia in Laparoscopy

Manisha Bijlani

■ INTRODUCTION

Surgical and anesthetic procedures and also equipment are undergoing continuous and rapid evolution, and many procedures are being performed through laparoscopy. A number of endoscopic procedures are faced by the anesthesiologist. Although they are visually "minimally invasive" to the patient, the intraoperative requirements of laparoscopic surgery produce significant physiological changes, some of which are unique to these procedures. Therefore, it is essential that the surgeon and the anesthesiologist thoroughly understand the pathophysiology and management of the potential problems and complications associated with laparoscopic surgery.

The anesthesiologist has to be alert at every step of the surgery.

■ TROCAR INSERTION

The first step is the establishment of pneumoperitoneum by placing a cannula intra-abdominally. A Veress needle is usually introduced blindly into the peritoneal cavity periumbilically. Visceral and vascular perforations are reported complications by this technique. Injury to the urinary bladder and stomach can be avoided by decompressing them using urinary catheter and nasogastric tube respectively.[1]

Safer technique to avoid such injuries is the "Hasson" minilapratomy technique (Fig. 1).[2] The pneumoperitoneum is established with the patient in a slight Trendelenburg position.[1]

■ INSUFFLATION

Once the cannula is intra-abdominal, the insufflator is put on with a set pressure of 15 mm Hg. If the cannula is displaced accidently, subcutaneous emphysema or retroperitoneal emphysema can occur.

Extraperitoneal insufflation of CO_2 is a common complication of laparoscopy (this may be desirable in cases of inguinal hernia repair).[2] The anesthesiologist should be alert to the possibility of vagally mediated reflexes (excessive stretching of the peritoneum). Bronchospasm, brady-arrhythmias and even sinus arrest have been reported during insufflations. Cardiovascular collapse and gas emboli have been reported when CO_2 has been inadvertently insufflated directly into a blood vessel.[1]

CO_2 is instilled at a low flow initially at 1–1.5 L/min and once adequate pneumoperitoneum has been established, a higher flow rate is used to avoid above complications.[1]

Pressure limiters are used to decrease the deleterious effects of raised intra-abdominal pressure. Intra-abdominal pressure of 40 mm Hg and higher, causes circulatory impairment, respiratory embarrassment, increased risk of CO_2 embolism and peritoneal and subcutaneous emphysema. Today's equipment limits the intra-abdominal pressure to 15 mm Hg.[1]

■ CHANGES DUE TO CARBON DIOXIDE (CO_2)

Carbon dioxide is the standard gas for insufflation because of its valuable properties like:[3]

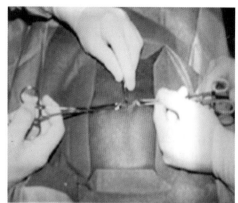
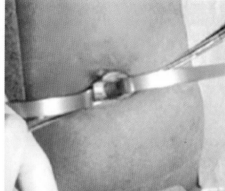
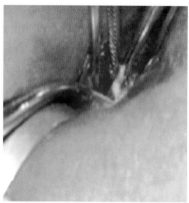

Safe entry

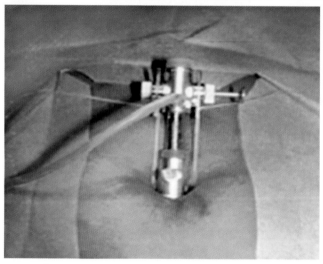

Fig. 1: Hasson's minilapratomy technique

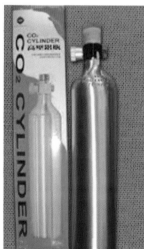
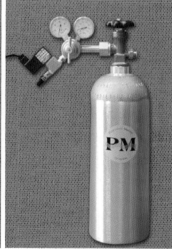

Fig. 2: CO₂ cylinders

❏ It is noninflammable and does not support combustion
❏ Readily diffuses across membranes and is rapidly removed from the lungs

❏ Risk of CO₂ embolism is small as compared to air embolism
❏ Increasing ventilation can augment elimination of CO₂. As long as oxygen requirements are met, a high concentration of blood CO₂ can be tolerated
❏ Medical grade CO₂ is readily available and is inexpensive
❏ It is more soluble in blood than either air, oxygen or nitrous oxide[4]
❏ Lethal dose of embolized CO₂ is approximately five times more than that of air.

Various Complications due to CO₂

CO₂ Embolism

Although rare, the most dreaded and dangerous complication of laparoscopic surgery is CO₂ embolism.[4] If a pressure gradient exists between the peritoneal cavity and the venous system, the insufflated gas may enter an open vein resulting in a gas embolism.[2] This develops principally during the induction of pneumoperitoneum.

Therefore, peritoneal insufflation must be started as slowly as 1 L/min. High insufflating pressures greater than 15 mm Hg in the presence of open venous channels (surgical dissection and trauma) and CO_2 under pressure may gain intravascular access.[1]

The clinical effects depend on the volume of gas entrained, the rate of entrainment, the type of gas used for insufflation and the patients' intravascular volume status.[2] Small amounts of CO_2 are not harmful because they are quickly absorbed and excreted by the lungs. A large bolus of CO_2 when gaining access to the circulation causes hemodynamic collapse.[1]

Early signs of CO_2 embolism:

❑ Decrease end tidal CO_2[2]
❑ Fall in systolic blood pressure, tachycardia, increase in central venous pressure, cardiac arrhythmias and development of a mill wheel murmur[4]
❑ Cyanosis and desaturation evident on pulse oximetry[1]
❑ Pulmonary edema[4]
❑ Electrocardiographic changes of right heart strain.[4]

Treatment of CO_2 embolism:

❑ Administer 100% O_2[2]
❑ Release of pneumoperitoneum[2]
❑ Steep head low position with left lateral decubitus (Durant position)[4]
❑ Raising the central venous pressur (CVP) by IV fluids administration[2]
❑ Inotropic support and hyperventilation[2]
❑ Aspiration of gas via a central venous line, if embolus is large[2]
❑ Cardiopulmonary resuscitation, if necessary[4]
❑ External cardiac massage may be helpful in fragmenting CO_2 emboli into smaller bubbles[4]
❑ Hyperbaric oxygen treatment should be considered if cerebral gas embolism is suspected.[4]

Effects of CO_2 embolism:

❑ CO_2 is not inert and causes direct peritoneal irritation and pain due to formation of carbonic acid when it comes in contact with moist peritoneum.[3] It remains intraperitoneally after laparoscopy causing referred shoulder pain when it is insoluble in the absence of red blood cells.[3]
❑ Hypercarbia and respiratory acidosis can occur and may manifest as hypertension, tachycardia when buffering capacity of blood exceeds temporarily.[3]
❑ Severe hypercarbia exerts a negative inotropic effect on the heart and reduces left ventricular function.[5]

VENTILATORY AND RESPIRATORY CHANGES AND COMPLICATIONS[4,5]

The introduction of several liters of gas into the abdominal cavity results in an increased intra-abdominal pressure.[5] This causes various changes in ventilation and respiration as follows:

❑ Reduction in thoracopulmonary compliance by 25–30%, decrease in tidal volume and minute ventilation[4]
❑ Reduction in functional residual capacity due to elevation of diaphragm and increased intra-abdominal pressure[4]
❑ Increase in airway pressure and risk of barotrauma during intermittent positive pressure ventilation[5]
❑ Ventilation perfusion mismatch can occur due to position of the patient and uneven distribution of ventilation to the nondependent parts of the lungs[5]
❑ During controlled ventilation in the Trendelenburg position, an intra-abdominal pressure of 15 mm Hg raises the $PaCO_2$ by 10 mm Hg and the $PaCO_2$ by 4 mm Hg and decreases the total lung compliance by 25%[1,5]
❑ Prolonged surgical time, along with underlying pulmonary disease, results in diminished respiratory capacity for CO_2 elimination leading to detectable hypercapnia and serum acidosis. The $PaCO_2$ usually correlates well with the end tidal CO_2 except in patients with cardiopulmonary compromise and associated ventilation perfusion mismatch. A direct estimation of $PaCO_2$ may be necessary in such patients by blood gas analysis.[5]

Causes of Increased $PaCO_2$[4]

❑ Absorption of CO_2 from the peritoneal cavity
❑ Impairment of pulmonary ventilation and perfusion by:
  ❖ Abdominal distension
  ❖ Patient position (steep tilt)
  ❖ Volume controlled mechanical ventilation
  ❖ Respiratory depression due to premedication and anesthetic agents in spontaneously breathing patients.

These mechanisms are accentuated in obese, American Society of Anesthesiologists (ASA) II, III and above.

❑ Increased metabolism (insufficient plane of anesthesia)
❑ Accidental events:
  ❖ CO_2 emphysema (subcutaneous or body cavities)
  ❖ Capnothorax
  ❖ CO_2 embolism
  ❖ Selective bronchial intubation.

Monitoring end tidal CO_2 and other respiratory parameters will help identify the problem so that measures can be taken to avoid them.

PNEUMOTHORAX, PNEUMOMEDIASTINUM AND PNEUMOPERICARDIUM[4]

These are rare complications of pneumoperitoneum. Movement of gas during the creation of a pneumoperitoneum can produce pneumomediastinum, unilateral and bilateral pneumothorax and pneumopericadium.[4] Embryonic remnants constitute potential channels of communication between the peritoneal cavity and the pleural or pericardial sacs which can open when intraperitoneal pressure increases.[4] These defects or weak points occur at the:

❑ Foramen of Bochdalek (the lumbocostal triangle) the outer crus or the esophageal hiatus.[2]
❑ Defects of the diaphragm (patent pleuroperitoneal canal)[5, 6]
❑ Diaphragmatic hiatus for esophagus and aorta.[2,5]

Excessively high intra-abdominal pressures during CO_2 insufflation may cause the gas to pass into the mediastinum.[2] Pneumothorax may develop during a laparoscopic procedure due to a ruptured bleb or bulla following increased alveolar inflation secondary to increase minute ventilation (independent of pneumoperitoneum), usually occurring on the right side.[4,5]

These complications are potentially serious and may lead to respiratory and hemodynamic disturbances.[4]

Pneumothorax should be suspected when there is:[2]

❑ Subcutaneous emphysema

❑ Increased airway pressure
❑ Hemodynamic compromise
   ❖ Oxygen desaturation
❑ Unexplained hypoxemia or hypercarbia.
   Auscultation and X-ray chest will confirm the diagnosis.[2]
   The following guidelines are provided if pneumothorax develops during laparoscopy:[4]
❑ Stop N_2O administration
❑ Adjust ventilator settings to correct hypoxemia
❑ Apply positive end-expiratory pressure (PEEP)
❑ Reduce intra-abdominal pressure as much as possible
❑ Avoid thoracocentesis unless necessary as it will spontaneously resolve after exsufflation.
❑ In case of pneumothorax secondary to rupture of preexisting bullae, PEEP must not be applied and thoracocentesis is mandatory.

If the pneumothorax occurs at the beginning of procedure:[2]

❑ Deflate the abdomen
❑ Correct hypoxemia
❑ Keep the chest drain
❑ Apply PEEP.

Procedure is continued if patient is stable, and if it is detected towards the end of the procedure, surgery can be completed without intervention.[6] Once the abdomen is deflated, the CO_2 in the pleural cavity will be quickly reabsorbed, thereby obviating the need for a chest drain.[2]

In presence of tension pneumothorax, standard therapeutic treatment should be instituted including needle thoracotomy deflation of abdomen and insertion of chest drain. PEEP must not be applied.[2,4]

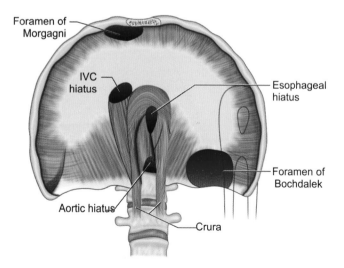

Fig. 3: Foramen of Bochdalek

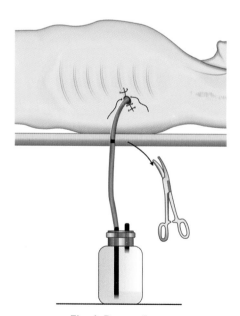

Fig. 4: Pneumothorax

HEMODYNAMIC AND CARDIOVASCULAR CHANGES AND COMPLICATIONS

Hemodynamic alterations occur only when $PaCO_2$ is increased by 30% above the normal levels. Hypercapnia causes sympathetic stimulation, which results in tachycardia, increased systemic vascular resistance, systemic arterial pressure, central venous pressure and cardiac output. This shortens the pre-ejection period and the left ventricular ejection time and shortens the diastolic filling phase of the coronary arteries, resulting in coronary ischemia. Patients with ischemic heart disease thus are at a higher risk if not properly managed.[5]

Intra-abdominal pressure greater than 10 mm Hg induces significant alterations of hemodynamics:

❑ Elevation of arterial pressure
❑ Increase of systemic and pulmonary vascular resistance
❑ Heart rate either remains unchanged or increases only slightly
❑ Decreased cardiac output is proportional to the increased intra-abdominal pressure. The mechanism of decreased cardiac output is multifactorial:[4]
  ❖ Decrease in venous return with increased intra-abdominal pressure
  ❖ The increased intra-abdominal pressure results in caval compression leading to pooling of blood in the legs and increase in venous resistance
❑ Increase in systemic vascular resistance can cause a deleterious effect in patients with cardiac diseases and may lead to further decrease in the cardiac output[4]
❑ Increase in systemic vascular resistance is considered to be because of mechanical and neurohumoral factors. It is affected by patient position, Trendelenburg position attenuates this and head-up position aggravates it. Catecholamines, the renin-angiotensin system and especially vasopressin are all released during pneumoperitoneum and may contribute to increasing afterload
❑ The increase in systemic vascular resistance can be corrected by administration of vasodilating anesthetic agents (isoflurane), nitroglycerin or nicardipine[4]
❑ The increased $PaCO_2$ results in hemodynamic alterations by causing vasodilatation directly and by stimulating the sympathetic nervous system. Hypercapnia can result in cardiac arrhythmias and pulmonary vasoconstriction leading to right ventricular failure[4]
❑ Cardiac arrhythmias: Arrhythmias are common during laparoscopy and usually occur during or shortly after CO_2 insufflation[4]

Bradyarrhythmias are the most common because of reflex increase of vagal tone from sudden stretching of the peritoneum[5] (Vagal stimulation will be accentuated in lighter planes of anesthesia and if the patient is on β-blocking drugs)

Gas embolism can also result in cardiac arrhythmias.[4] These events are quickly reversible. Treatment consists of interruption of insufflation, atropine administration and deepening of anesthesia after recovery of heart rate.[4]

❑ In patients with mild to severe cardiac disease, the pattern of change in mean arterial pressure, cardiac output and systemic vascular resistance is quite similar to that in healthy patients. Increased afterload is a major contributor to the altered hemodynamics seen during pneumoperitoneum in cardiac patients. Nitroglycerine and nicardipine are the drugs of choice in such patients[4]
❑ Acute hypotension, hypoxemia and cardiovascular collapse described during laparoscopy may be due to:[5]
  ❖ Hypercarbia due to hypoventilation and CO_2 absorption which may cause arrhythmias more in the presence of halothane[2]
  ❖ Compression of the vena cava causing decrease in cardiac output[2]
  ❖ Hemorrhage[2]
  ❖ Venous gas embolism[2]
  ❖ Severe hypercarbia exerts a negative inotropic effect on the heart and reduces left ventricular function.[2]

OTHER SYSTEMIC CHANGES

Acid Aspiration

High intra-abdominal pressure due to pneumoperitoneum during laparoscopy may increase the likelihood of an intraoperative reflux of gastric contents causing acid aspiration syndrome. Insertion of orogastric or nasogastric tube to decompress the stomach decreases the risk.[1] The problem of reflux is significant during regional anesthesia with sedation or if mask ventilation is chosen. Antacids and gastric propellants help to increase the gastric pH and decrease gastric volume and increase the lower esophageal tone.[1]

Renal Function

Increased intra-abdominal pressure affects renal hemodynamics by alterations in cardiac output and by a direct effect on renal blood flow. Mechanical obstruction of renal venous blood flow along with increased sympathetic activity, elevation of plasma antidiuretic hormone (ADH) and raised plasma renin-angiotensin activity increase the renal vascular resistance leading to a fall in filtration pressure and urine output.[5]

Intracranial Pressure and Intraocular Pressure

The raised intra-abdominal pressure compresses the inferior vena cava and increases the lumbar spinal pressure by reducing drainage from lumbar plexus, thus increasing the intracranial pressure and the intraocular pressure. Hypercarbia produces reflex vasodilatation in the central nervous system and also contributes to the increase in intracranial pressure.[5]

Thromboembolism

An intra-abdominal pressure above 14 mm Hg, reverse Trendelenburg position, obesity, pelvic surgery and surgery of long duration reduce venous flow in the lower extremities, increasing the chance of thromboembolism.[5] Compression stockings or pneumatic calf compression may counteract this effect.

Temperature Variations

During laparoscopy, the continuous flow of dry gases over the peritoneal surfaces under pressure can lead to a fall in the body temperature because of the Joule-Thomson effect (sudden expansion of gases), higher flow rates, especially during prolonged surgery and leakage through the ports because of various reasons (leakage during changing of cannulae, aspiration of gases and during lavage). There is a 0.3°C decrease in core temperature per 50 L volume flow of CO_2 pneumoperitoneum.[5]

Neurohumoral Stress Response

Levels of adrenocorticotropic hormone (ACTH), cortisol, insulin and glucagon rise during laparoscopy. Pain and discomfort secondary to peritoneal stretching, hemodynamic disturbances and ventilatory changes induced by pneumoperitoneum might contribute to the stress response of laparoscopy.[4] Thus, it is concluded that laparoscopy is as stressful as conventional surgery.[5]

Positioning of the Patient

Apart from cardiovascular and respiratory changes occurring during the Trendelenburg and the reverse Trendelenburg positions, other problems faced during these positions are:

❑ Shift of the diaphragm upward during pneumo-peritoneum and prolonged Trendelenburg position results in cephalad movement of carina potentially leading to endobronchial intubation. This complication results in a decrease in SpO_2 associated with increase airway pressure.[4,5]

❑ Deep vein thrombosis: A step head-up position causes venous stasis in the legs predisposing these patients to deep vein thrombosis, particularly in procedures of long duration. Pneumoperitoneum further increases blood pooling in the legs.[4]

❑ Nerve injury: Nerve compression is a potential problem during the head-down position. Over extension of arm must be avoided. Shoulder braces must be used with great caution and must not impinge on the brachial plexus.[4]

Lower extremity neuropathies have been reported after laparoscopy.[4]

Common peroneal nerve is particularly vulnerable and must be protected when the patient is placed in the lithotomy position.[4]

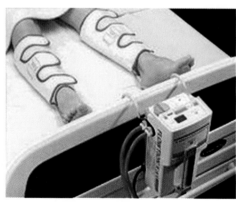

Fig. 5: Calf compressions

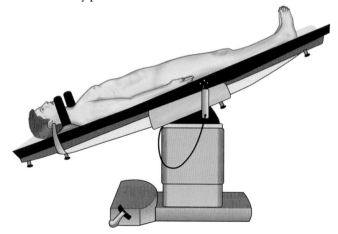

Fig. 6: Trendelenburg position

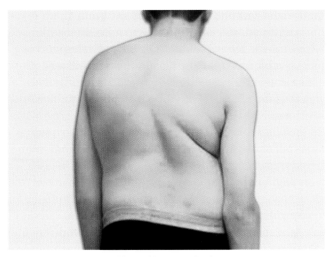

Fig. 7: Kyphoscoliosis

Lower extremity compartment syndrome can occur in prolonged lithotomy position.[4]

❏ Intracranial and intraocular pressure: The Trendelenburg position may also affect cerebral circulation resulting in an elevation of the intracranial and intraocular pressure.[5]

❏ The lithotomy position used for hysteroscopy and urological procedures does not cause any hemodynamic or respiratory alterations except in obese patients. But the irrigation solution can pass into the intravascular space or abdominal cavity if urinary bladder or uterus respectively is perforated.[7]

❏ The risk of air embolism is very high if the irrigating solution gets over suddenly and the air enters the uterine cavity with open blood vessels during hysteroscopy.

❏ The central venous pressure increases by an average 8 mm Hg at an intra-abdominal pressure of 15 mm Hg. in the supine position. It increases by an additional 6 mm Hg at similar intra-abdominal pressure in the Trenedelenburg position.[5]

▌ANESTHETIC MANAGEMENT

A well-planned and executed general anesthesia, which not only provides a complete anesthetic effect but also enables cardiovascular and respiratory stability, should be used for laparoscopy.[1] Recovery from anesthesia should be rapid with minimal side-effects.[5] The fact that any laparoscopic surgery can be converted into open surgery should be kept in mind.[1]

Preoperative or Preanesthetic Assessment

Apart from the detailed history physical examination, the cardiac and pulmonary status of all patients should be carefully assessed on priority and optimized preoperatively. In some patients, pneumoperitoneum may be risky or undesirable. These include:

❏ Elderly patients, i.e. age above 70 years: These patients already have a compromised cardiopulmonary function which may worsen during laparoscopy under general anesthesia.

❏ Patients with kyphoscoliosis: It is not only difficult to anesthetize such patients but the pulmonary function can worsen with the condition. In such cases, regional anesthesia or total intravenous anesthesia with propofol is desirable.

❏ In patients with morbid obesity, there are multiple problems including difficult intubations. Trendelenburg position along with pneumoperitoneum will cause excessive pressure on the diaphragm and ventilation perfusion mismatch. Increase in $PaCO_2$ due to retention in lipid tissue will delay recovery from anesthesia. Difficulty in trocar insertion and barotraumas can occur. Such patients have to be properly assessed before extubation.[3]

❏ Patients with ventilatory problems, like asthmatic patients with history of breathlessness or wheeze, decreased exercise tolerance and smokers, have poor pulmonary functions. Need for bronchodilators, antibiotics and antisialogogues should be assessed. Forced expiratory volume less than 70% in pulmonary function test is undesirable for laparoscopy.

❏ Patients with heart disease, especially failure and terminal valvular insufficiency, are more prone to develop cardiac complications. Recent history of myocardial infarction is again a high-risk for laparoscopy. Halothane has to be totally avoided in patients with arrhythmias. A record of input/output has to be maintained in patients with renal failure and concomitant use of nephrotoxic drugs should be avoided.[4]

❏ Patients with increased intracranial pressure due to space occupying lesions have to be treated with caution.[4] Correction of shock in hypovolemic patients before induction of anesthesia is a must.[4]

❏ The ventriculoperitoneal and peritonojugular shunts should be clamped before insufflation.[4] Sickle cell crisis may be precipitated in patients with sickle cell disease due to acidosis.

❏ Hemodynamic changes induced by pneumoperitoneum are similar in pregnant and nonpregnant patients. The following recommendations are for safe laparoscopy in pregnant patients:[7]

❖ The surgery must be performed during second trimester, ideally before the 23rd week of pregnancy, to minimize the risk of preterm labor and to maintain adequate intra-abdominal working room.

❖ Open laparoscopy technique should be used for abdominal access to avoid damage to the uterus.
❖ Use of tocolytics to arrest preterm labor is debatable.
❖ Fetal monitoring can be performed using transvaginal ultrasonography.
❖ Mechanical ventilation must be adjusted to maintain physiological maternal alkalosis.

An inexperienced surgeon is good contraindication for laparoscopy.[8] Most of the contraindications of laparoscopic techniques become relative with increasing experience and skilled surgeons.

Preoperative Investigations

Apart from the routine investigations, i.e. basic tests some additional tests have to be done for laparoscopy.
❑ Blood urea and serum creatinine and baseline electrolytes are necessary for renal functions.[2]
❑ 2-D echocardiography to assess the ventricular functions in patients with cardiac problems.[2]
❑ A baseline X-ray chest to compare if any acute change, like mediastinal or subcutaneous emphysema, pneumothorax or pulmonary edema has occurred.[9,10]
❑ Pulmonary function tests, arterial blood gas analysis, oxygen saturation while breathing room air should be done in patients with chronic obstructive airway disease and in chronic smokers. Abnormal values may suggest the need for antibiotics and bronchodilators and delay in surgery until pulmonary function is optimal.[9,10]

Preoperative Preparation

❑ The patients should be on clear liquids the day before surgery and nil by mouth 6–8 hours before surgery. A complete bowel preparation is necessary.[9,10]
❑ Preoperative antibiotic as per surgeon's choice should be started. An antacid or antiemetic combination, which decreases acid formation and gastric volume and increases the tone of the esophageal sphincter, is to be given preoperatively to prevent gastric reflux during induction of pneumoperitoneum.[5]
❑ Anxiety can be controlled with alprazolam the night before surgery.[5]
❑ Written consent, which should include consent that the laparoscopic surgery can be converted into an open surgery.[9,10]

Premedication

Premedication is adapted according to the duration of surgery and necessity of quick recovery.

❑ An antacid or antiemetic combination to be given intravenously if not given orally to prevent postoperative nausea and vomiting.[9,10]
❑ A vagolytic should be given intramuscularly either half an hour before surgery or should be kept at hand because increase in vagal tone is known with pneumoperitoneum.[9,10]
❑ Narcotic medication can be used to supplement analgesia only if controlled ventilation is planned. Morphine and other narcotics are to be avoided in patients with pulmonary dysfunction.
❑ Deep vein thrombosis prophylaxis is recommended for long duration procedures.[9,10]
❑ An antisialogogue, like glycopyrrolate, reduces oral secretions.[9,10]

Intraoperative Management

❑ Intraoperative management starts with securing an IV line with 18G or 20G intravenous cannula.
❑ A nasogastric tube and urinary catheter are inserted after the patient is asleep to decompress the stomach and bladder to prevent perforation by trochars.[2,10] An arterial and central venous line is recommended whenever laparoscopic procedure is either complex or long or when patient has significant cardiopulmonary disease.
❑ Special precautions have to be taken to prevent hypothermia like warm intravenous fluids and irrigating bottles, cover the patients with plastic covers or blanket and use of CO_2 gas warmers.

Monitoring

Monitoring begins before induction of anesthesia to know the baseline reading. The recommendations for routine patient monitoring include:[4]

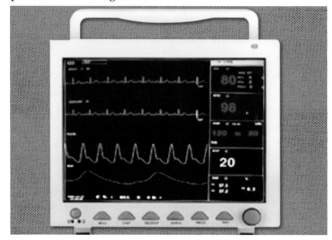

Fig. 8: Multipara monitor

❏ Pulse rate
❏ Continuous ECG
❏ Intermittent noninvasive blood pressure (NIBP)
❏ Pulse oximetry (SpO_2)
❏ Capnography end tidal CO_2
❏ Temperature
❏ Intra-abdominal pressure
❏ Pulmonary airway pressure.

Optional monitoring includes:[5]

❏ Esophageal stethoscope to detect mill-wheel murmur of CO_2 embolism
❏ Precordial Doppler
❏ Transesophageal echocardiography is recommended in patients with severe cardiac disease with ejection fraction of less than 30%.
❏ Invasive monitoring is required in severely deranged patients.
❏ Intra-arterial blood pressure and $PaCO_2$ are helpful in patients with cardiopulmonary disease as end tidal CO_2 may not be the correct indication of hypercarbia in such patients.
❏ Venous oxygen saturation is a better indicator of hypoxemia in case of gas embolism as it can be first detected in venous blood.
❏ Pulmonary artery catheterization helps in detection of pulmonary artery wedge pressure, pulmonary hypertension and aspiration of blood in case of CO_2 embolism.

Observations regarding the position of endotracheal tube, the color of the skin, the feel of upper chest wall for subcutaneous emphysema, and the extent of corneal and conjunctival edema are carried out periodically.[9] It is extremely important to maintain a record of the volume of fluids infused and the patient's hourly urine output along with observation of its color and concentration.[9]

Choice of Anesthesia Technique

The choice of anesthesia depends on the type and duration of surgery. The procedure may be conducted under regional, general or local anesthesia.

Regional Anesthesia

Regional anesthesia including epidural or subarachnoid block is used for pelvic and short procedures without major impairment of ventilation.[4] Our experience with regional anesthesia for short procedures, like tubal banding for sterilization, diagnostic laparoscopies have been excellent. Extensive sensory block T_2-T_4 is necessary for good muscle relaxation. Administration of opiates helps to provide adequate analgesia and attenuates the shoulder pain caused by diaphragmatic irritation. Spraying of local anesthetic such as bupivacaine also helps to relieve the shoulder pain and for postoperative analgesia. Patient cooperation, skilled laparoscopic surgeon, low intra-abdominal pressure and low degrees of patients tilt guarantee the success of regional anesthesia. Continuous epidural technique using a syringe pump can be used depending on the type of surgery for prolonged cases. Similarly, combined spinal or epidural can be used in some cases.

Advantages of regional anesthesia:[5]

❏ Simple and economical technique
❏ Excellent relaxation
❏ An awake patient helps in early detection of complications.
❏ Induced vasodilatation and absence of positive pressure ventilation may reduce the cardiovascular changes seen during pneumoperitoneum.
❏ Reduces the need for sedatives and narcotics
❏ Sympathetic blockade decreases bowel distension, which gives clear exposure to surgical field.
❏ It provides excellent postoperative analgesia with lower incidence of postoperative nausea and vomiting.[5]

Disadvantages of regional anesthesia:

❏ Sympathetic block may exaggerate development of vagal reflexes, hypotension and decreased cardiac output.[6]
❏ Combined effect of pneumoperitoneum and sedation can lead to hypoventilation and arterial oxygen desaturation.[6]
❏ Shoulder tip pain has to be taken care of with analgesics and by maintaining low intra-abdominal pressure that is disliked by the surgeon.
❏ High level of sensory block is required that may cause dyspnea in Trendelenburg position.[6]
❏ Procedures requiring only extraperitoneal hernia repair may be successfully conducted under regional anesthesia.[5]
❏ A nasogastric tube may not be tolerated by the patient.[6]

General Anesthesia

Almost any combination that provides amnesia, good analgesia, good muscle relaxation, ability to control hypercarbia and protects aspiration of gastric contents can be used for laparoscopic surgery. A wide variety of anesthetic drugs have been used for laparoscopies but since most of these procedures are being conducted on an outpatient basis, the choice is shifting toward short-acting drugs. Halothane is the only anesthetic that should probably be avoided because it can cause arrhythmias in the presence of hypercarbia.[11]

General anesthesia with spontaneous ventilation is best suited to lower abdominal surgeries, laparoscopy of short duration, using low intra-abdominal pressure and small degrees of tilt with close monitoring by an experienced anesthesiologist.[1,4] The use of laryngeal mask airway (LMA) might improve the safety of anesthesia in such patients but does not protect the airway from aspiration of gastric contents. General anesthesia can be performed without intubation safely and effectively with LMA ProSeal in nonobese patients.[12] Legal binding may restrict the use of such a technique. Total intravenous anesthesia with propofol and fentanyl is a popular technique for outpatient laparoscopic procedures.

Adequate abdominal and diaphragmatic relaxation is essential for easy laparoscopic maneuvers.[5] Controlled ventilation is the best choice for laparoscopies. There is apparently no clinical advantage to omitting nitrous oxide, and any benefit from its elimination must be balanced against greater risk of awareness.[12]

Maintenance of anesthesia with nitrous oxide during laparoscopic surgery is controversial because of concerns about its ability to produce bowel distension during surgery and increased incidence of postoperative nausea or vomiting.[5]

Maintenance of anesthesia with inhalation agents like sevoflurane or isoflurane ensures rapid recovery with minimal postoperative nausea, vomiting and shows least sensitivity to arrhythmias in the presence of increased catecholamines due to hypercapnia.[5]

In addition to the usual criteria for extubation, prolonged laparoscopic procedures in Trendelenburg position require other considerations.

Extubation should be delayed if patient has conjunctival edema or lid edema, venous congestion, duskiness of head and neck and increased end tidal CO_2. The patient kept in head-up position should be kept intubated until normal ventilation, blood pressure, oxygen saturation and normal end tidal CO_2 are achieved.

Monitoring of the vitals should be continued in the recovery room as the hemodynamic changes induced by pneumoperitoneum outlast the release of pneumoperitoneum.[4]

All patients should be administered O_2 postoperatively since slow release of CO_2 from the tissues may result in hypoxia.[4] Whereas no anesthetic technique has proved to be clinically superior to any other, general anesthesia with controlled ventilation seems to be the safest technique for operative laparoscopy.[4]

Advantages of general anesthesia:
❑ Good for anxious patients and for long duration surgery.

❑ Respiratory compromise, which occurs during regional anesthesia due to hypercarbia and sedation, is well managed during general anesthesia.
❑ Good muscle relaxation.

Disadvantages of general anesthesia:
❑ Postoperative respiratory complications with general anesthesia are more
❑ Increased incidence of postoperative nausea and vomiting which is already more because of peritoneal insufflation, bowel manipulation and pelvic surgery.
❑ High risk in elderly patients, obese patients and patients with cardiopulmonary disease.

Postoperative Analgesia

The pain is often intense, though short, and up to 80% of patients will require opioid analgesia. Wound infiltration with local anesthetic is useful and reduces postoperative analgesic requirement. Intraperitoneal or spraying over the diaphragm of bupivacaine reduces postoperative pain and opioid requirement.

Postoperative Nausea and Vomiting

The use of ondansetron and an antacid preoperatively decreases the incidence of postoperative nausea and vomiting.

Combined Regional and General Anesthesia

This technique is the best in our opinion. Spinal or epidural anesthesia is given along with general anesthesia with controlled ventilation.

There are many advantages when you combine regional and general anesthesia:
❑ Good hemodynamic stability can be maintained
❑ Requirement of anesthetic agent is reduced
❑ Quick recovery and good postoperative analgesia
❑ Good muscle relaxation, less bowel motility and distension
❑ Anesthesia can be titrated because full view of the surgery is available.

Local Anesthesia

Laparoscopy under local anesthesia is uncommon due to the peritoneal irritation that occurs with CO_2. N_2O may be a better option because of its decreased systemic absorption and minimal irritation of the peritoneal cavity. "Microlaparoscopy" office procedures may be conducted under local anesthesia with or without sedation.

■ REFERENCES

1. Black TE. Anaesthesia for laparoscopic assisted surgery. In: Healey, Cohen OJ (eds). Wylie Churchill-Davidson; Practice of Anesthesia, 6th edn. pp.1391-6.
2. Cunningham AJ, Kelly DJ. Laparoscopic surgery. In: Morgan M, Hall GM (Eds). Short Practice of Anaesthesia. London: Chapman and Hall; 1997. pp. 493-501.
3. Fishburne JI. Anesthesia for laparoscopy: considerations, complications and techniques. J Reprod Med. 1978;21(1):37-40.
4. Miller RD. Anaesthesia for laparoscopic surgery. Anaesthesia, 5th edition. Philadelphia: Churchill Livingstone Sec III; 2000. pp. 2003-23.
5. Jayashree S, Kumar VP. Indian journal of surgery. 2003;65(3):232-40.
6. Wiengram J. Laparoscopic and laser surgery. In: Malhotra V (Ed.) Anesthesia for Renal and Genitourinary Surgery. New York: Mc Graw-Hill; 1996.
7. Maria F.martin_Cancho, Celdran D, Lima JR, Maria S. Carrasco_Jimenez, Francisco M, Sanchez_Margallo, Jesus Uson_Gargallo. Anaesthetic Considerations during Laparoscopic Surgery. 2011. Spain: Jesús Usón Minimally Invasive Surgery Centre.
8. Gunningham AJ, Schlanger M. Intraoperative hypoxemia complicating laparoscopic cholecystectomy in a patient with sickle hemoglobin apathy. Aneasth Analg. 1992;75:838-43.
9. Brull SJ. Anaesthetic considerations for laparoscopic procedures. ASA Refresher Courses in Anaesthesiology. 1995;23:15-28,
10. Chui PT, Gin T, Oh TE. Anaesthesia for laparoscopic general surgery. Anaesthesia and Intensive Care. 1993;21:163-71.
11. Seed RF, Shakespeare TF, Muldoon MJ. Carbon dioxide homeostasis during anaesthesia for laparoscopy. Anaesthesia. 1970;25(2):223-31.
12. Nguyen JH, Tanaka PP. Anaesthesia for lap. surgery. Prevention and Management of Laparoscopic Surgical Complications. 3rd edition.

Section 3

LAPAROSCOPY

- Diagnosis and Treatment of Ectopic Pregnancy
- Laparoscopic Hysterectomy
- Laparoscopic Myomectomy
- Adenomyosis—Management and Laparoscopic Surgery
- Laparoscopic Management of Endometriosis
- Laparoscopic Colposuspension

"Science is not only a disciple of reason but, also, one of romance and passion."

Stephen Hawking

CHAPTER 9

Diagnosis and Treatment of Ectopic Pregnancy

Ibrahim Alkatout, Ulrich Honemeyer, Liselotte Mettler

■ INTRODUCTION

After fertilization in the ampullary part of the fallopian tubes, the growing morula moves in a circular fashion for 4–5 days through the tube towards the uterine cavity while differentiating into the embryoblast and trophoblast.[1] Today, 2% of early pregnancies implant in extrauterine sites. They can be removed safely by laparoscopic surgery. The histological examination (Fig. 1) is always required. The prevalence of ectopic pregnancy in all women presenting with first-trimester bleeding, lower abdominal pain or a combination of the two to an emergency department is between 6% and 16%.[2]

The tubal diameter increases from the tubouterine junction to the fimbria, but remains a narrow pathway. This may be the reason why 97% of all ectopic pregnancies are located in the fallopian tube. Furthermore, the ampullary region is the most distal place where ascending infections can cause phymosis and occlusion. Three percent of ectopic pregnancies are located in the rudimental uterine horn, ovary, abdominal cavity, broad ligament, cervix and vagina or are simultaneously in the uterine cavity and tubes (Fig. 2 and Table 1).[3]

Today, the mortality rate of ectopic pregnancies worldwide is estimated to be 3.8 per 1,000 ectopics. Early diagnosis before the occurrence of hemoperitoneum and/or hypovolemic shock leads to a striking decrease of mortality and to a better recognition at the initial medical assessment.[2-5] Owing to the advances made in transvaginal ultrasound and radio immunoassays for serum β-hCG levels and an increased vigilance by clinicians with more experience of diagnostic laparoscopy, more than 80% of ectopic pregnancies are now diagnosed intact and offer an opportunity for conservative nonmedical or medical nonsurgical treatment.[6,7]

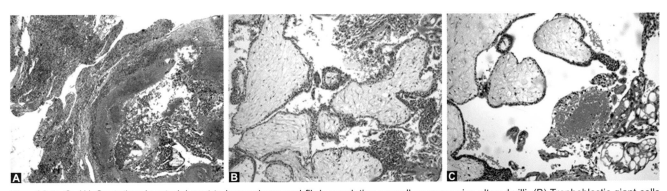

Figs 1A to C: (A) Gestational material next to hemorrhage and fibrin exudation as well as regressive altered villi; (B) Trophoblastic giant cells next to regressive altered villous stroma, trophoblast, and decidual stroma; (C) Regressive altered villous stroma, trophoblast, hemorrhage and fibrino trophoblastic giant cells

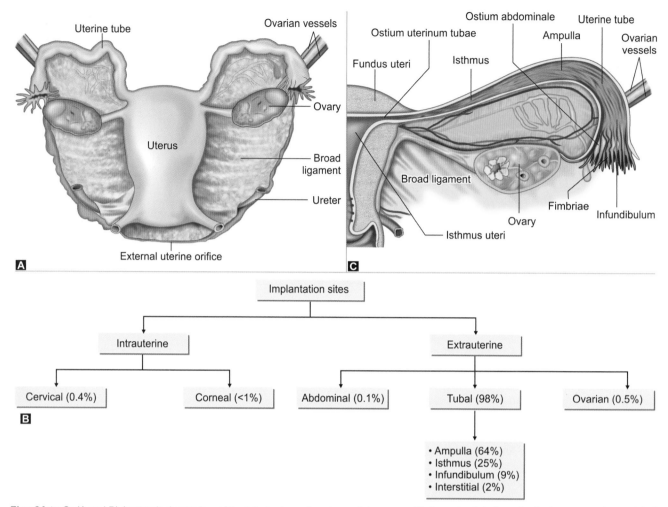

Figs 2A to C: (A and B) Anatomical overview of the interior inner female genital organs with the potential sites of ectopic pregnancies and their percentage distribution; (C) Schematic drawing of the expected ultrasound layer. Ovary, Fallopian tube and the transition to the uterus are clear beside the surrounding meso

Table 1: Different localizations of ectopic pregnancies and the associated percentages	
Localizations of ectopic pregnancy	
Fallopian tube	97%
Rudimental uterine horn	
Ovary	
Abdominal	
Intraligamental gravidity	3%
Cervical gravidity	
Vaginal gravidity	
Simultaneous intra- and extrauterine	

THE IMPLANTATION WINDOW

Any impedance of the conceptus migration to the uterine cavity may precipitate an ectopic gestation (Table 2). Previous surgeries or infections, anatomic defects in the tubal epithelium, hormonal factors that interfere with normal transport of the conceptus and pathologic conditions that affect normal tubal function may arise. Estrogens and gestagens show different hormonal effects on the growth and movement of the epithelial tubal cilia. The influence of smoking also has to be considered.[5,8,9]

DIAGNOSTICS—PRETREATMENT ASSESSMENT OF ECTOPIC PREGNANCIES

Additional unspecific parameters after a positive β-hCG are a slightly enlarged uterus, vaginal bleeding or spotting, pelvic pain and a palpable adnexal mass. Apart from mimicking the symptoms of other gynecological and even non-gynecological diseases, ectopic pregnancies appear in many variations often causing no pain at vaginal

Table 2: Potential sites of ectopic pregnancy implantation and their percentage distribution					
Implantation sites of ectopic pregnancy					
Intrauterine			Extrauterine		
Cervical (0.4%)	Corneal (<1%)	Abdominal (0.1%)	Tubal (98%)	Ovarian (0.5%)	
			Ampulla (64%)		
			Isthmus (25%)		
			Infundibulum (9%)		
			Interstitial (2%)		

examination. Severe pain can also be experienced in a normal pregnancy.[8]

Breakthrough bleedings appear as spotting because these ectopic pregnancies show only small hCG levels which do not support the continuous decidual transformation of the endometrium. The earliest appearance of symptoms occurs in the 6th week after the last period.[5]

Serum Level of β-hCG

Human chorionic gonadotropin starts with secretion on day 5 to day 8. A serum array detects levels as low as 5 mIU/mL while the detection limit in urine is 20–50 mIU/mL. The β-hCG levels double every 1.5 days in the first 5 weeks of a regular gestation and every 3.5 days after 7 weeks.

Normal hCG levels for the time of pregnancy are only found in 30% of ectopics and the daily doubling increase of β-hCG is lacking. An abnormal β-hCG pattern is highly suspicious for an ectopic gestation or a no longer intact gestation.[9-12]

Imaging Signs in Ultrasound Scan

At a gestational age of about 5 weeks, a normally developing gestational sac can be visualized showing an ovoid collection of fluid clinging to the endometrium as well as a yolk sac of 8 mm or more in diameter. However, a pseudo-gestational sac can mimic a gestational sac at an early stage. The pseudo-gestational sac is often situated in the center of the uterine cavity. Its margin is homogenous and round but it is difficult to define its boundary to the outside tissue. By contrast, a physiologic gestational sac is asymmetric and contains two concentric rings, separated by a thin echogenic layer. At a gestational age of 6–6.5 weeks the embryonic structures measure 4–5 mm and cardiac activity might already be detected.

At a serum β-hCG level of 1,500 mIU/mL, an intrauterine chorionic sac can be detected. The "Comet sign" of intervillous flow in power Doppler (PD) assessment of the decidua around the double echogenic ring and visualization of a yolk sac at 5 weeks plus, confirm the impression of an intrauterine implantation. Color-coded flow signals of the ectopic pregnancy are clearly separated from ovarian tissue and corpus luteum. The extent of vascularity reflects trophoblastic vitality and invasiveness (neoangiogenesis), enhanced by vasodilatation of the fallopian vessels under the influence of maternal progesterone.[13]

In 85% of all ectopic pregnancies the corpus luteum is found ipsilateral. Luteal color or PD flow may be used as a guide while searching for an ectopic pregnancy, and could be called the "light house-effect" of corpus luteum which directs the investigator to the color Doppler signals of the ectopic pregnancy (Fig. 3).[14,15]

The combination of transvaginal ultrasonography and serial quantitative β-hCG serum levels detects, with a sensitivity of 96% and a specificity of 97%, an ectopic pregnancy and remains the gold standard as well as the most cost-effective strategy for diagnosing ectopic pregnancy. A positive fetal heart beat is often absent because extrauterine pregnancies seldom develop vitally and only display an agglomeration of trophoblast tissue and a surrounding hematoma.[16-18]

Progesterone Levels

The progesterone serum level has a sensitivity of 15% to detect pregnancy failure. As a stable marker in the first trimester, a serum level above 22 ng/mL speaks for a viable intrauterine pregnancy whereas levels under 5 ng/mL are indicative of a nonviable pregnancy.[3,18,19]

Uterine diagnostic curettage as well as the puncture of the pouch of Douglas have become obsolete as diagnostic procedures.[18]

This straightforward diagnosis of ectopic pregnancy is therefore based on three pillars: Symptoms, clinical features, laboratory (Fig. 4).

■ DIFFERENTIAL DIAGNOSIS

For possible differential diagnosis of ectopic pregnancy see Table 3.[20]

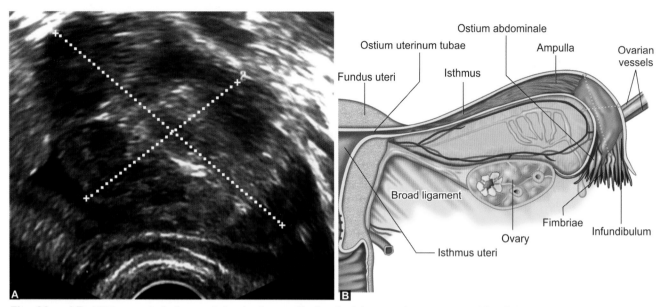

Figs 3A and B: (A) Transvaginal ultrasound showing in magnification the inhomogenic structures and free fluid in the pouch of Douglas. The capsule and the boundary of the fallopian tube are respected and visual. (B) The ectopic pregnancy detected by ultrasound is visualized in a schematic drawing of the ultrasound layer

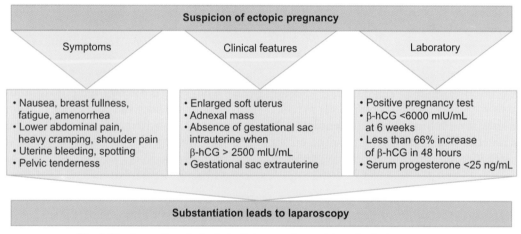

Fig. 4: The three pillars that substantiate an early suspicion of ectopic pregnancy

TREATMENT OF ECTOPIC PREGNANCIES

The treatment decision includes operative and medical management as well as the option not to treat and follow-up with observation and clinical and laboratory tests. It is known that many early ectopic pregnancies result in spontaneous abortion and reabsorption and this might make aggressive treatment unnecessary. Medical treatment with MTX is restricted to a few limited indications.

Expectant Treatment

Ectopic pregnancies might have a natural tendency to terminate in tubal abortion or complete resorption.

Modern monitoring might be sufficient and enhance the preservation of tubal function and fertility. We consider the following prognostic parameters: lack of clinical symptoms, a sonographic adnexal tumor below 4 cm with a decreasing tendency, less than 50 mL of free fluid and an initial β-hCG level of below 2,000 mU/mL with a decreasing tendency after a 48-hour interval. However, more than 90% of all affected women with ectopic pregnancies develop increasing and endangering symptoms that lead to an operative intervention.[5,7,21-25]

Medical Treatment

Today MTX as well as actinomycin D, potassium chloride, prostaglandins and mifepristone (RU 486) are applied. In

Table 3: Major contributing factors for ectopic pregnancy
Risk factors for ectopic pregnancy
❖ Previous tubal surgery
❖ History of ectopic pregnancy
❖ Sexually transmitted disease
❖ Pelvic inflammatory disease
❖ In utero diethylstilbestrol exposure
❖ History of infertility
❖ Anatomical uterine/tubal abnormality
❖ Previous tubal ligation
❖ Previous or current intrauterine device use
❖ Assisted reproductive technologies
❖ Current smoking
❖ Nonwhite (all races other than white)
❖ Age between 35 and 44 years (compared to those from 15 to 24 years)
❖ Induced abortion
❖ T-shaped uterus
❖ Myomata
❖ Progestin-only contraceptives

view of the uncertainty of treatment success and possible adverse side effects, the indication for a conservative treatment has to be weighed up carefully.

Methotrexate can disrupt the rapidly-dividing trophoblastic cells. The expected time to resolution of the ectopic pregnancy is 3–7 weeks after MTX application. The selective use of MTX can be as effective as surgery although adverse side effects are possible, such as bone marrow suppression, elevated liver enzymes, rash, alopecia, stomatitis, nausea, diarrhea, and to a lower extent pleuritis, dermatitis, conjunctivitis, gastritis and enteritis. The success rate of MTX is up to 94%. Nevertheless, this depends on the β-hCG level. The lower the serum level at the beginning of the therapy, the higher the success rate is.

The use of MTX to destroy an ectopic pregnancy has been advocated for women with an atypical localization in the cervix, interstitially, cornually or in the abdominal cavity, an incomplete resolution of a surgically treated ectopic gestation, residual trophoblast tissue or persisting low β-hCG levels after curettage with no evidence of trophoblast material in the histological examination. Furthermore, patients with a high operative risk and contraindications to anesthesia, e.g. after induced ovarian hyperstimulation syndrome and patients who are expected to have extensive intraperitoneal abdominal adhesions might be optimal candidates for a preliminary medical treatment if they are hemodynamically stable.[20]

Methotrexate can be given locally or systemically by intramuscular injection of 1 mg/kg or 50 mg/m^2. Patients with a hematocrit below 35% should take 325 mg ferrous sulfate twice daily as they may bleed within the laparoscopic removal and afterwards. If the β-hCG levels do not decrease by at least 15% after 7 days, a second dose of MTX has to be given.[20]

Surgical Treatment General Beginning

In most cases of ectopic pregnancy surgical treatment is without doubt necessary.

Diagnostic Laparoscopy—Evacuation of the Hemoperitoneum—followed by Operative Laparoscopic Treatment in the Same Session

A diagnostic laparoscopy visualizes the location, size and nature of the ectopic pregnancy. A hemoperitoneum (Figs 5A and B) can complicate the whole operation. Depending on the degree of bleeding, a primarily inserted grasper localizes the ruptured tube and tamponades the bleeding site. After safe compression or preferably suture of the bleeding source, blood and blood clots can be removed by suction and irrigation.[3-5,26-28]

The following specific techniques can be applied dependent on the individual case.[9]

Surgical Treatment of Tubal Pregnancy

Milking of Tubal Pregnancy through the Fimbrial End
If the product of conception is located at the outer region of the fallopian tube or the fimbrial end, it can be removed by grasping the tubal segment and stepwise milking the gestational product out of the fimbriae of the tube (Fig. 6). The product of conception is gently pushed until it is extruded. The stepwise movements begin in the proximal part and gently push the product into the abdominal cavity. Although this type of operation is gentle and organ-saving, it has a higher rate of incomplete removal and, therefore, a higher risk of recurrence and of trophoblast residuals.[5]

Salpingostomy

The majority of ectopic pregnancies located in the infundibulum (Figs 5C and D) have to be operated either by salpingostomy or by segmental tubectomy and secondary reanastomosis after a certain interval.[4,5] However, approximately 8% of patients have persistent ectopic pregnancy after salpingostomy. This has to be kept in mind and be part of the preoperational discussion.[2]

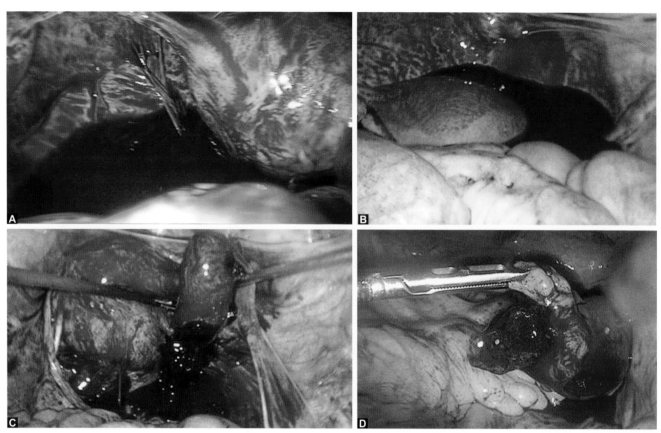

Figs 5A to D: (A) Severe hemoperitoneum with the volume of 1200 mL blood in the pouch of Douglas. (B) Hemoperitoneum of a ruptured tubal pregnancy. Site after insertion of the optic trocar. (C) Tubal pregnancy already protruding from the fimbrial end into the abdominal cavity. (D) Ectopic pregnancy protruding from the fimbrial end with the option of extirpation without incising the tube

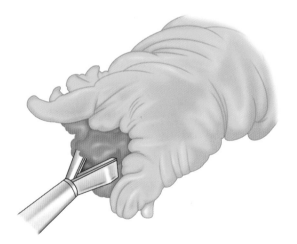

Fig. 6: Schematic drawing of the ectopic pregnancy protruding out of the fimbrial end with the option of extirpation without incising the tube; however, this operation technique is only feasible if total extraction of the ectopic pregnancy is assured

Before opening the tube, vasopressin, 20 IU diluted in 100 mL of normal saline, is injected into the mesosalpinx over the mesenteric surface of the tubal segment containing the gestational products. As the trophoblast has a high cell division, its metabolic rate is equivalently high.[4,9]

Evacuation by Aquadissection or Aspiration, Luxation and Preparation

A 1–2 cm longitudinal incision is made on the most distended part of the antimesenteric tubal wall, which is often of bluish discoloration. Usually it is possible to identify the different tubal wall layers: serosa, muscularis externa and interna and the mucosa. Once the lumen is open, the friable gestational sac bulges out of the wound and can be evacuated by aspiration. If the product of conception is surrounded by blood clots, it must be extracted through the tubal incision with alternating pressurized suction and irrigation or with the aid of a grasping or biopsy forceps. The site of implantation is then irrigated extensively. The irrigation fluid must drain from both sites, the salpingotomy and the fimbrial end. Minimal bleeding from the tubal bed is normal and ceases in most cases spontaneously.[3,4]

The decision to suture after salpingotomy is taken by the surgeon. Usually the incision does not require suturing.

Suturing can be recommended if bleeding occurs and requires extensive coagulation. If the defect has to be closed, a continuous suture or single knots approximating the edges with single 4-0 resorbable sutures are made. Nevertheless, the follow-up and prognosis for recurrent extrauterine pregnancies is not improved after suturing.[3,4,28]

Partial Salpingectomy

If salpingostomy cannot resolve the problem, a partial salpingectomy can be tried before salpingectomy is performed. Indications for a partial salpingectomy are tubal rupture, a pregnancy located in the isthmus or a recurrent tubal pregnancy. In most cases of isthmic pregnancy a linear salpingostomy is unsuccessful as these gestations grow through the lumen of the tube and into the tunica muscularis; therefore, segmental resection is recommended.

Coagulation of the tubal part is done by bipolar forceps on both ends of the affected part including the corresponding mesosalpinx. After resecting the affected part of the tube the mesosalpinx is cauterized stepwise. The partial salpingectomy can be completed by reanastomosis.

Salpingectomy

The indications for salpingectomy include no desire for future pregnancies, recurrent tubal pregnancies and the occurrence of extrauterine pregnancy after a failed sterilization or a previously reconstructed tube. Other indications for salpingectomy are made intraoperatively, e.g. severe adhesions, hydrosalpinx, tubal rupture, persistent bleeding after a safe tubal procedure or if the tubal pregnancy is over 5 cm in diameter.

It is of utmost importance to resect the tube right within the utero-tubal junction to avoid cornual pregnancies after IVF if further pregnancy is desired.[28]

An ectopic pregnancy is defined as extraluminal when the gestational product is situated between the muscularis externa and the serosa. Incision with the monopolar needle or hook over the point of maximum distention results in the product of conception slipping out without need of a long incision.

Surgical Technique for Nontubal Ectopic Pregnancy

Ovarian Pregnancy

The unusual site and rarity of ovarian pregnancies leads to a more complex clinical course. The difficulty in making an early and accurate diagnosis can lead to an inconsistent therapeutic approach with an unpredictable outcome and a life-threatening status if the ovary ruptures.

❑ *Superficial pattern:* The implantation takes place in an ovarian focus of endometriosis
❑ *Intrafollicular pattern (90% of ovarian pregnancies):*
   ❖ *Primary*—insemination of an ovum that has not yet ovulated.
   ❖ *Secondary*—after regular ovulation implantation of the inseminated ovum in the follicle or corpus luteum.

Tubal pregnancy, hemorrhagic ovarian cyst, endometrioma and other pelvic diseases have the same clinical findings as ovarian pregnancies. Therefore, the diagnosis is quite difficult.

The traditional operative treatment for ovarian pregnancies has been oophorectomy. However, the desire to maintain reproductive capability and improvements in laparoscopy has more recently led to the ovarian-preserving operational technique. By enucleating the gestational sac bluntly from the ovary, the surrounding ovarian tissue is protected to the greatest possible extent (Figs 7A and B, and 8A to F).

Abdominal Pregnancy

Abdominal pregnancy can be either primary or secondary in case of rupture of a tubal pregnancy and abdominal implantation. This rare localization occurs in only about 1% of all ectopic pregnancies. Nevertheless, it has a high morbidity and mortality rate and makes detection by ultrasound or MRI necessary.

Due to comparatively few symptoms the abdominal gravidity is often recognized very late. The treatment of an advanced abdominal pregnancy is associated with an enormous risk for life-threatening maternal bleeding. The removal of the placenta is dependent on its localization as it can be implanted on any organ in the abdominal cavity. Sometimes the placenta is better left intra-abdominally to be calcified and reabsorbed or embolized by an interventional radiologist prior to removal at a second intervention. Its management is strictly by laparotomy (Figs 9A to D).[5]

Interstitial or Cornual Pregnancy/Rudimental Uterine Horn

If a pregnancy implants in the interstitial area of the fallopian tube, we speak of an interstitial or cornual ectopic pregnancy (incidence 1–3% of extrauterine pregnancies. The interstitial line has been described as an echogenic line extending from the cornual side of the endometrium

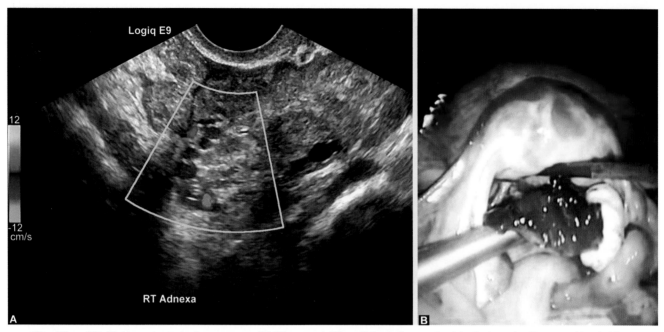

Figs 7A and B: Right ovarian ectopic pregnancy. (A) Ultrasound differentiates between physiological ovarian tissue and trophoblast; (B) Intraoperative situs with extraction of trophoblast of the right ovary

into the cornual region, reaching the ectopic gestational sac, and is said to be a highly specific sign for interstitial pregnancy. Its mortality rate is about 2%. This is due to the high vascularity of this area where the uterine and ovarian vessels join together. The classical treatment methods are laparotomy, uterine horn resection or even hysterectomy (Figs 10A to F).[29]

The cornual pregnancy, implants in the same anatomical area of the tube, but opens to the uterine cavity. Therefore, the operative method of choice can be hysteroscopy. To avoid uterine perforation, larger pregnancies can be removed by curettage under laparoscopic guidance.

Cesarean Scar Ectopic Pregnancy

Deficient uterine scars are a frequent finding in women with a history of previous cesarean section. The risk of scar deficiency is increased in women with a retroflexed uterus and in those who have undergone multiple cesarean sections.

Early diagnosis can offer treatment options to avoid uterine rupture and hemorrhage. Available data suggest that termination of pregnancy is the treatment of choice in the first trimester soon after the diagnosis. Expectant treatment in these cases is not indicated.[30] Laparoscopy enables the successful treatment of an unruptured ectopic

pregnancy in a previous cesarean scar and makes it possible to preserve the patient's reproductive capability. Figures 11A to D clearly demonstrate the striking diagnosis with a Doppler ultrasound.

Viable cesarean scar pregnancies have been treated safely by selective transarterial embolization in combination with subsequent dilatation and curettage and local or systemic injections of MTX. Hysteroscopic management has also been reported.

Intraligamental Gravidity

For intraligamental development (1 in 250 ectopic pregnancies) the gestational sac must split the oviduct precisely between the leaves of the broad ligament. With an intact amnion, the embryo develops in its extraperitoneal sac. Rupture occurs early enough so that the villi are capable of expanding their areas of nidation.

Cervical and Vaginal Pregnancy

The criteria for a cervical pregnancy have been described by Rubin in 1911:

❑ Cervical glands must be present opposite the placental attachment
❑ The attachment of the placenta to the cervix must be intimate

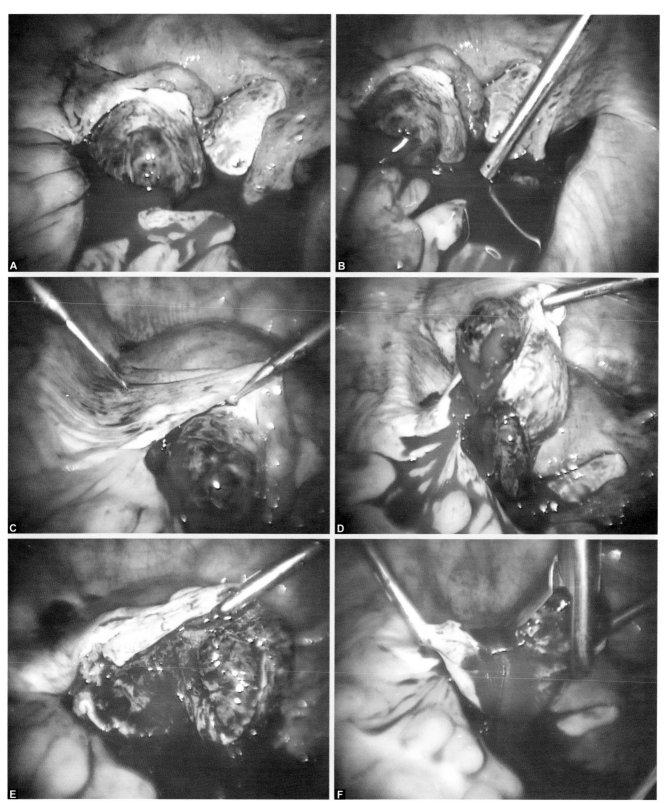

Figs 8A to F: (A) Overview after creating a pneumoperitoneum for diagnostic laparoscopy. Bleeding from the ruptured ectopic pregnancy of the left ovary. In the background, the slightly enlarged uterus and the right ovary with the corpus luteum cyst. (B) Suction of the blood out of the cul-de-sac. (C) Preparation of the left ovary and injection of ornipressin into the infundibulo pelvic ligament. (D) Blunt preparation and enucleation of the gestational sac from the orthotopic ovarian tissue. Removal of the product of conception by (E) enucleation. Healthy ovarian tissue can be seen on the left. (F) Removal after complete separation of the trophoblast from the ovary[26]

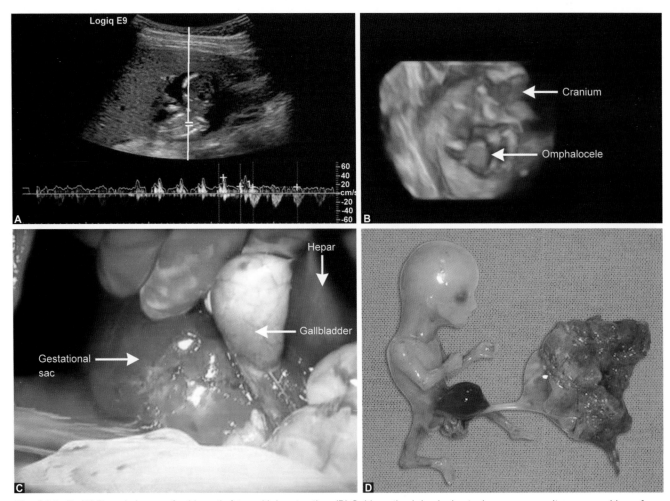

Figs 9A to D: (A) B-mode image of subhepatic fetus with heart action; (B) Subhepatic abdominal ectopic pregnancy: ultrasonographic surface-rendered image of the fetus; (C) Intraoperative image with subhepatic gestational sac; (D) Intraoperative image of the fetus after rupture of membranes

❑ The placenta must be below the peritoneal reflection of the anterior and posterior surfaces of the uterus
❑ Fetal elements must not be within the uterine cavity.

Cervical and vaginal pregnancies are threatening localizations for the patient. Due to their anatomic closeness to the uterine artery they connect early to the corresponding drainage. Diagnostic detection of a cervical pregnancy should implicate a local or systemic medical treatment with MTX. The medical treatment can be accompanied by selective uterine artery embolization. It is therefore essential to know the sonomorphology of cervical ectopic pregnancy: homogene decidual reaction, closed inner cervical os and round gestational sac (Figs 12A and B).

An isthmic localization is associated with a severe risk for uncontrollable intraoperative bleeding; however, this can be handled well by laparoscopy. Rarely is a laparotomy necessary.

Simultaneous Intra-and Extrauterine Pregnancy

Simultaneous intra- and extrauterine pregnancy has increased with the wide application of assisted reproductive technologies (ART).

In the majority of the cases the simultaneous pregnancy is an incidental finding. Persistent abdominal pain or other clinical features alongside an irregular rise in the β-hCG level can lead to this infrequent diagnosis. Once a simultaneous pregnancy has been discovered, the operative method of choice is laparoscopic salpingectomy.[5]

Bilateral tubal pregnancy is diagnosed and treated during single laparoscopy following clinical and sonographic diagnosis of tubal ectopic pregnancy of mostly only one side. Before the undetected second ectopic pregnancy becomes clinically obvious, persisting β-hCG levels after the initial surgery raise suspicion.

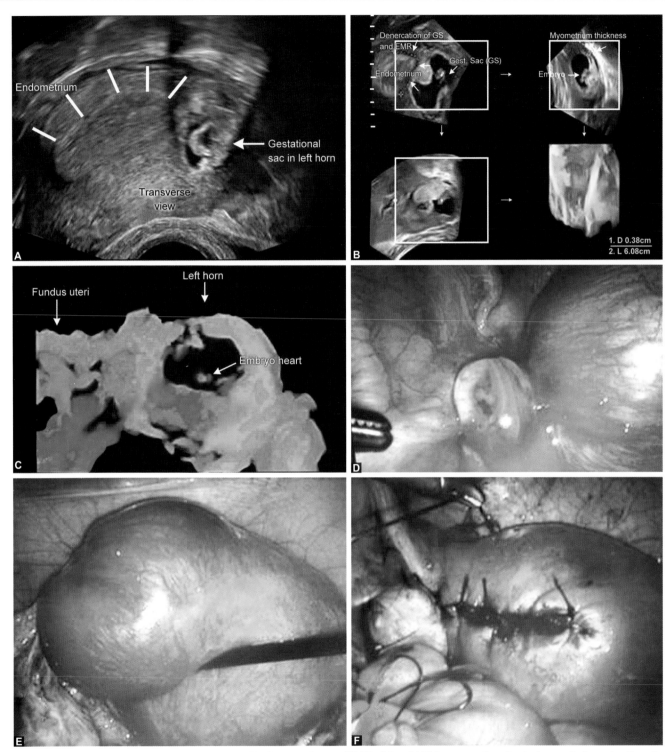

Figs 10A to F: Ectopic cornual pregnancy (A and B) Ultrasound scan; (C) 3D vision; (D-F) Intraoperative situs before and after extraction of the trophoblast and uterus wall reconstruction

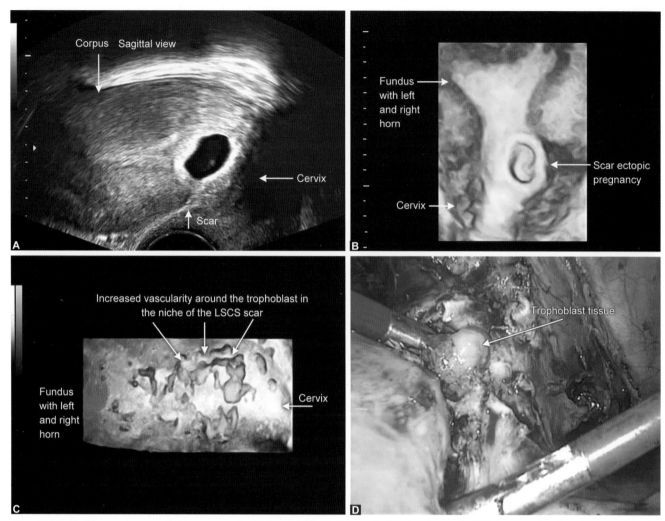

Figs 11A to D: Cesarean scar ectopic pregnancy in (A) 2D and (B) 3D vision with (C) Doppler mode (D) Intraoperative situs demonstrates the trophoblast in the uterus scar

▌COMPLICATIONS

Precedent bleedings are caused by the invasion of trophoblast tissue into the local vascular system leading to intraluminal hematoma and bleeding of the fimbrial end. If the stretching capacity of the tube is exceeded, this results in tubal rupture.

It should be emphasized that the possibility of leaving behind products of conception is the same after laparoscopy as after laparotomy (5–15%). Attention should be focused at surgery on the medial portion of the tube as this is the preferential site where trophoblastic tissue can outlast and be responsible for elevated serum β-hCG levels.

At times the differential diagnosis of ectopic pregnancies is difficult. They can be of gynecological origin (e.g. early stage of normal pregnancy, miscarriage, intrauterine abortion, torsion of ovary or fallopian tube, ovarian cyst, ruptured corpus luteum cyst or follicle, necrotic myoma, pelvic inflammatory disease and tubo-ovarian abscess) or of non-gynecological origin (e.g. acute appendicitis; cystitis; pyelonephritis; nephrolithiasis; perforation of hollow organs, such as stomach, bowel or gallbladder; obstruction of hollow organs; intraabdominal inflammation; rupture of parenchymatous organs, such as liver, spleen or kidney; vascular ischemic disease and vascular hemorrhagic disease).[20]

The β-hCG levels after operative treatment should be reduced by 70% after 2 days and by another 70% after 7 days. About 30% of women with a previous ectopic pregnancy have difficulties in conceiving. The conception rate is about 77%, no matter what kind of therapy they receive. The incidence of recurrence is between 5% and 20% and rises up to 32% following two ectopic pregnancies.[5,18,31]

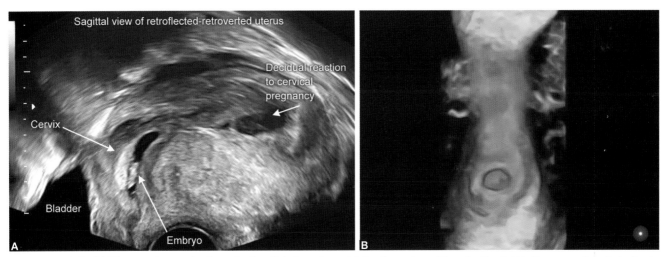

Figs 12A and B: (A) Ultrasound scan clearly marks the dilated cervix containing the embryo. The retention fluid in the corporal cavity is due to a decidual reaction to the cervical pregnancy; (B) 3D reconstruction gives vitality signs in the cervical region

Today, it appears useful to perform routine early ultrasound scans of all women with positive pregnancy tests to check the location of the gestation so that earlier and more conservative treatment options are possible in cases of ectopic pregnancies. Nevertheless, the presence of an intrauterine pregnancy does not exclude the possibility of a heterotopic pregnancy as pregnancies at multiple locations may occur.

ACKNOWLEDGMENTS

The authors thank Dawn Rüther for editing the manuscript.

REFERENCES

1. Bouyer J, Coste J, Fernandez H, et al. Sites of ectopic pregnancy: a 10 year population-based study of 1800 cases. Hum Reprod. 2002;17:3224-30.
2. Murray H, Baakdah H, Bardell T, et al. Diagnosis and treatment of ectopic pregnancy. CMAJ. 2005;173:905-12.
3. Luciano D, Roy G, Luciano A. Ectopic pregnancy. In: Pasic R, Levine R (Eds). A Practical Manual of Laparoscopy: A Clinical Cookbook. Andover: Informa Healthcare; 2007. pp. 155-68.
4. Barbosa C, Mencaglia L. Laparoscopic Management of Ectopic Pregnancy. In: Mencaglia L, Minelle L, Wattiez A (Eds). Manual of Gynecological Laparoscopic Surgery. 11th edition. Schramberg, Germany: Endo Press; 2010. pp. 115-23.
5. Hucke J, Füllers U. Extrauterine Schwangerschaft. Der Gynäkologe. 2005;38(6):535-52.
6. Dericks-Tan JS, Scholz C, Taubert HD. Spontaneous recovery of ectopic pregnancy: a preliminary report. Eur J Obstet Gynecol Reprod Biol. 1987;25(3):181-5.
7. Lipscomb GH, Stovall TG, Ling FW. Nonsurgical treatment of ectopic pregnancy. N Engl J Med. 2000;343(18):1325-9.
8. Marchbanks PA, Annegers JF, Coulam CB, et al. Risk factors for ectopic pregnancy. A population-based study. JAMA. 1988;259(12):1823-7.
9. Nezhat C, Nezhat F, Luciano A, et al. Ectopic Pregnancy. In: Nezhat C, Nezhat F, Luciano A (Eds). Operative Gynecologic Laparoscopy: Principles and Techniques. New York: McGraw-Hill; 1995. pp. 107-20.
10. Kadar N, Romero R. Serial human chorionic gonadotropin measurements in ectopic pregnancy. Am J Obstet Gynecol. 1988;158(5):1239-40.
11. Fritz MA, Guo SM. Doubling time of human chorionic gonadotropin (hCG) in early normal pregnancy: relationship to hCG concentration and gestational age. Fertil Steril. 1987;47(4):584-9.
12. Brennan DF. Ectopic pregnancy--Part I: Clinical and laboratory diagnosis. Acad Emerg Med. 1995;2(12):1081-9.
13. Kurjak A, Zalud I, Schulman H. Ectopic pregnancy: transvaginal color Doppler of trophoblastic flow in questionable adnexa. J Ultrasound Med. 1991;10(12):685-9.
14. Kupesic S. Ectopic pregnancy. In: Kurjak A, Chervenak FA (Eds). Donald School Textbook of Ultrasound in Obstetrics and Gynecology, 2nd ed. New Delhi: Jaypee Brothers Medical Publishers; 2008. pp. 230-43.
15. Honemeyer U. Primary care in obstetrics and gynecology—A place for advanced ultrasound. Donald School Journal of Ultrasound in Obstetrics and Gynecology. 2009;3(3):61-74.
16. Mehta TS, Levine D, Beckwith B. Treatment of ectopic pregnancy: is a human chorionic gonadotropin level of 2,000 mIU/mL a reasonable threshold? Radiology. 1997;205:(2)569-73.
17. Ardaens Y, Guérin B, Perrot N, et al. [Contribution of ultrasonography in the diagnosis of ectopic pregnancy]. J Gynecol Obstet Biol Reprod (Paris). 2003;32:S28-38.
18. Lozeau AM, Potter B. Diagnosis and management of ectopic pregnancy. Am Fam Physician. 2005;72(9):1707-14.
19. Mol BW, Lijmer JG, Ankum WM, et al. The accuracy of single serum progesterone measurement in the diagnosis

of ectopic pregnancy: a meta-analysis. Hum Reprod. 1998;13(11):3220-7.

20. Alkatout I, Honemeyer U, Strauss A, et al. Clinical diagnosis and treatment of ectopic pregnancy. Obstet Gynecol Surv. 2013;68(8):571-81.

21. Koike H, Chuganji Y, Watanabe H, et al. Conservative treatment of ovarian pregnancy by local prostaglandin F2 alpha injection. Am J Obstet Gynecol. 1990;163(2):696.

22. Lang PF, Weiss PA, Mayer HO, et al. Conservative treatment of ectopic pregnancy with local injection of hyperosmolar glucose solution or prostaglandin-F2 alpha: a prospective randomised study. Lancet. 1990;336(8707):78-81.

23. Shamma FN, Schwartz LB. Primary ovarian pregnancy successfully treated with methotrexate. Am J Obstet Gynecol. 1992;167(5):1307-8.

24. Chelmow D, Gates E, Penzias AS. Laparoscopic diagnosis and methotrexate treatment of an ovarian pregnancy: a case report. Fertil Steril. 1994;62(4):879-81.

25. Mashiach S, Carp HJ, Serr DM. Nonoperative management of ectopic pregnancy. A preliminary report. J Reprod Med. 1982;27(3):127-32.

26. Alkatout I, Stuhlmann-Laeisz C, Mettler L, et al. Organ-preserving management of ovarian pregnancies by laparoscopic approach. Fertil Steril. 2011;95(8):2467-70

27. Hoover KW, Tao G, Kent CK. Trends in the diagnosis and treatment of ectopic pregnancy in the United States. Obstet Gynecol.115(3):495-502.

28. Tulandi T. Tubal ectopic pregnancy: salpingostomy and salpingectomy. In: Tulandi T (Ed). Atlas of Laparoscopic Technique for Gynecologists. London: WB Saunders Company Ltd; 1994. pp. 33-42.

29. Advincula AP, Senapati S. Interstitial pregnancy. Fertil Steril. 2004;82(6):1660-1.

30. Ash A, Smith A, Maxwell D. Cesarean scar pregnancy. BJOG. 2007;114(3):253-63.

31. Tay JI, Moore J, Walker JJ. Ectopic pregnancy. BMJ. 2000;320(7239):916-9.

CHAPTER 10

Laparoscopic Hysterectomy

Linda Shiber, Thomas Lang, Resad Pasic

■ INTRODUCTION

Laparoscopic hysterectomy is considered the standard-of-care approach to hysterectomy in most women with benign gynecologic pathology who are not candidates for vaginal hysterectomy.[1] The advantages of a laparoscopic approach are numerous, including a faster recovery time, decreased hospital costs and increased patient satisfaction.

■ INDICATIONS

Laparoscopic hysterectomy is indicated in women with both complicated and straightforward pathology. Women with pelvic pain, large fibroid uteri, multiple prior surgeries or need for concomitant prolapse procedures, such as sacrocolpopexy, may be better served by the laparoscopic approach as it allows close inspection of the abdomen and pelvis for etiologies of pain, such as endometriosis, methodical management of adhesions and, with use of 30° laparoscopes and strategic port placement, can facilitate complex dissections for challenging pathology.

The laparoscopic approach to hysterectomy is generally contraindicated in women who have any condition preventing insufflation of the abdomen or who are medically unstable for surgery. In addition, women who have suspected ovarian/tubal malignancy should be first considered for an open abdominal approach. Traditionally, women with uteri larger than 18 week gestational age have not been considered to be candidates for laparoscopic surgery. However, as techniques have been refined and surgical expertise improves, even larger uteri may be safely removed laparoscopically, provided there is adequate space in the abdomen and pelvis for port placement and dissection.

■ INFORMED CONSENT

As with any surgical procedure, obtaining informed consent is paramount to good patient care. We counsel our patients that along with the general surgical risks of bleeding/transfusion, infection, visceral injury, the laparoscopic approach may also be associated with specific unique risks: i.e., longer operative time, risk of conversion to laparotomy, slightly increased risk of urinary tract injury and potentially increased chance of vaginal cuff dehiscence.[2-8] As important as it is to discuss these risks, it is also important to discuss the modifying effects of surgeon experience on quoted complication rates. In essence, at a center, such as ours, where laparoscopic surgeons have extensive experience managing complex pathology, these risks are typically quoted as far lower.

■ PREOPERATIVE MANAGEMENT

During initial office consultation, work-up depends primarily on presenting symptoms. Assessment begins with a thorough pelvic exam. A pap smear is obtained if indicated. In general, any woman with abnormal bleeding undergoes endometrial biopsy and transvaginal ultrasound or saline infusion sonogram. Ultrasound is not only potentially diagnostic of fibroids, polyps, etc. but is also instrumental in assessing the size and shape of the uterus and planning the surgical approach. In woman with very large uteri or suspected complex pelvic pathology/endometriosis, MRI may be a superior imaging study to obtain during preoperative preparation. After initial diagnostic tests have been performed, we emphasize conservative management plans to our patients prior to moving toward definitive surgical management. Many benign gynecologic problems can now be treated effectively using medical management with hormonal contraceptives, intrauterine devices, hysteroscopic surgery and/or endometrial ablation. These options must, at the very minimum, be addressed with eligible patients.

As with any major elective surgery, patients are encouraged to optimize their pre-existing medical problems prior to going to the operating room. Women with any significant cardiopulmonary disease are specifically referred for anesthesia consultation preoperatively. Women on anticoagulation are advised to consult with their hematologist (as well as their surgeon) regarding cessation of anticoagulation preoperatively, whether perioperative bridging with heparin or lovenox is indicated and to determine when anticoagulation can be resumed postoperatively.

Glycemic control is emphasized in women with diabetes and smoking cessation is encouraged preoperatively to improve wound healing.

Current evidence from both gynecology and general surgery has indicated that preoperative bowel preparation has no benefit in women undergoing hysterectomy.[9,10] In our practice, women are not advised to complete any type of bowel preparation.

Perioperative antibiotics are administered in the operating room prior to initial incision in accordance with surgical care improvement project (SCIP) and guidelines for a Class II/clean-contaminated procedure.[10] For women with no penicillin allergy, 1–2 g cefazolin is given depending on patient weight. In women with a significant penicillin allergy, we typically administer gentamicin and clindamycin.

POSITIONING AND PREPARATION

On arrival to the operating room, the patient is moved to the operating table and is positioned on of a large bean bag. After induction of anesthesia and securing of the endotracheal tube, the legs are placed in yellofins stirrups with care taken to avoid hyperflexion or hyperextension of the hips and knees. The patient is moved down on the table so the buttocks are just over the edge of the bed, ensuring that the sacrum is supported and padded. Arms are tucked at the sides, with the thumbs up and hands padded with foam, using the draw sheet between the patient and the bean bag. Once appropriate positioning is accomplished, the edges of the bean bag are pushed around the patient's arms, shoulders and head and the bag is attached to suction, forming a protective "shell" around the patient. The straps securing the bag to the OR table are tightened and the

anesthesiologist places the patient in steep Trendelenburg position to ensure no sliding occurs.

Other techniques can be utilized to prevent the patient from sliding while in Trendelenburg position. These include using a gel pad beneath the patient or taping the upper chest/shoulders to the bed using a foam pad and velcro strap.

After the patient is anesthetized, she is examined, noting uterine position, mobility and size of cervix. The abdomen is then prepped with chlorhexadine + alcohol and the vagina/perineum is cleansed using betadine scrub and paint solutions.

The patient is draped. A Foley catheter is inserted under sterile conditions. The RUMI uterine manipulator is then placed, securing the cup at the cervix using two sutures of 0-vicryl, one anteriorly and one posteriorly.

A nasogastric or orogastric tube is then placed by the anesthesiologist in preparation for initial trocar placement.

TROCAR PLACEMENT

In patients with prior abdominal surgeries or large uteri, we typically place our initial trocar at Palmer's point in an effort to avoid potential adhesions and obtain a panoramic view of the pelvis. In other cases, the initial trocar can be placed infraumbilically. We typically use a Veress needle to insufflate to a pressure of 25 mm Hg prior to inserting the optiview trocar.

Our general trocar layout is as follows:
- Initial trocar placement: Palmer's point
- 10 mm infraumbilical—camera
- Low lateral ports versus lateral paramedian ports × 2
- +/– suprapubic port

All trocars are placed under direct visualization. The lateral trocars are placed somewhat higher or paramedian to avoid the inferior epigastric vessels which are visualized laparoscopically, coursing medial to the round ligament, within the lateral umbilical folds on the anterior abdominal wall.

PROCEDURE

After trocar placement, a careful laparoscopic survey is made of the abdomen and pelvis, specifically looking for adhesive disease, endometriosis and any other relevant pathology (Fig. 1). The liver edge and appendix, if present, are inspected. The patient is then placed in steep Trendelenburg and the pelvis is carefully examined, noting pelvic sidewalls, adnexa, ovarian fossa, posterior cul-de-sac and bladder peritoneum.

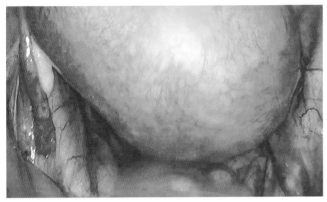

Fig. 1: Uterine survey

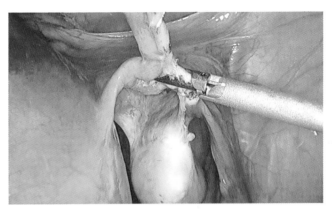

Fig. 2: Salpingectomy

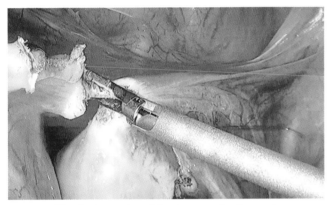

Fig. 3: Coaptation of the utero-ovarian ligament

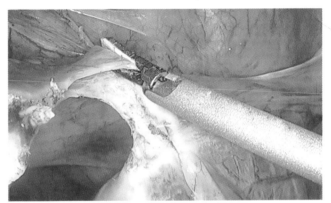

Fig. 4: Broad ligament dissection

Dissection is generally begun on the left side, after identification of the ureter at the pelvic brim. Ureteral identification is usually accomplished transperitoneally. The ureter can be seen medial to the infundibulopelvic ligament with gentle retraction of the sigmoid colon medially. This step is emphasized primarily if salpingo-oophorectomy is planned.

If ovarian preservation is intended, the fallopian tube is still routinely removed. This practice was adopted by our institution in accordance with new information regarding potential origin of some high-grade serous ovarian carcinomas at the fimbriated end of the fallopian tube.[11] The fallopian tube is grasped with a blunt grasper from the contralateral lower quadrant port and is placed on gentle traction to delineate its attachments to the ovary (Fig. 2). The Harmonic scalpel is then used to desiccate and transect these (generally) filmy attachments to the level of the uterus. Care is taken to avoid dissection proximal to the cornua of the uterus, as it is likely to create unnecessary bleeding. The utero-ovarian ligament is then identified, sealed and transected, followed by the round ligament (Fig. 3). If anatomically possible, the round ligament is divided at least 2–3 cm from the uterus to decrease the likelihood

of bleeding at this site; this concept of staying lateral is especially important with large, bulky, fibroid uteri.

Once the round ligament is divided, the anterior and posterior leaves of the broad ligament are identified, and using the narrow, active blade of the Harmonic scalpel, are separated (Fig. 4). The anterior leaf is dissected down to the peritoneal reflection of the bladder on the lower uterine segment and this dissection continues in the correct plane, allowing the bladder to be gently pushed caudad, away from the site of the planned colpotomy. The posterior leaf of the broad ligament is then divided perpendicular and toward to the uterine vessels. Care is taken here to stay close to the lateral aspect of the uterus and not drift lower/more lateral, as this can result in ureteral injury.

At this point, the uterine artery and vein can be easily seen. The areolar tissue surrounding the vascular bundle is gently dissected to decrease the volume of tissue incorporated into the vascular pedicle. Once the vessels are adequately skeletonized, they may be sealed and transected (Fig. 5). In cases with large, fibroid uteri and large diameter vessels, the ROBI bipolar device is used first to aid in sealing these large caliber vessels, following by transection using the Harmonic. In cases with smaller-caliber blood supply,

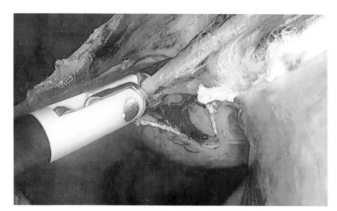

Fig. 5: Coagulation of the uterine vessels

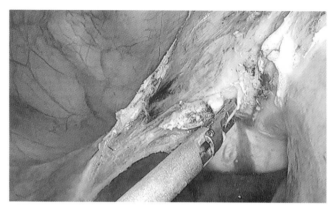

Fig. 6: Lateralizing the uterine vessels

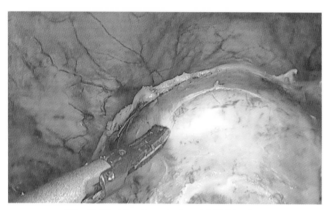

Fig. 7: Bladder dissected and RUMI in view

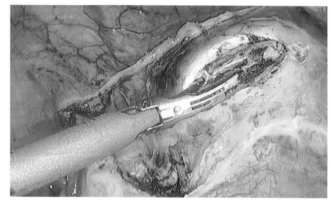

Fig. 8: Anterior colpotomy

the Harmonic scalpel, on "minimum" may be used alone to seal and transect these vessels. It is important when using the Harmonic on a vascular pedicle, to relieve tension on the tissue and allow the ultrasonic energy to slowly seal and divide the tissue (Fig. 6). Once the uterine vessels have been secured and divided, small bites are taken immediately over and medial to the vascular pedicle to lateralize it in preparation for colpotomy. In addition, the peritoneum posterior to the cervix may be incised to delineate the "path" for the posterior colpotomy, allowing this tissue to more easily fall away during that step.

The same dissection is then performed on the right side. When both uterine vessels have been sealed, the uterine fundus and body is noted to blanch significantly, indicating blood supply has been fully interrupted. Preparation is now made for colpotomy.

Depending on the anatomy encountered, colpotomy may be initiated at whichever point is most readily accessible. In the majority of situations, we find it most logical to begin anteriorly. The assistant responsible for manipulating the uterus is asked to push the manipulator cephalad and slightly anteriorly. If the bladder has been

appropriately dissected, the RUMI cup is easily seen beneath the pubocervical fascia (Fig. 7). The active blade of the Harmonic scalpel is used to incise this tissue, staying within the margin of the cup and creating an approximately 2 cm long incision (Fig. 8). Care is taken to avoid lingering in one area too long with an activated instrument in order to prevent tissue damage that may interfere with cuff healing. Once the metal is contacted along this entire opening, the uterus is manipulated to expose the left side and the incision is extended downward, staying medial to the uterine vascular pedicle. The cup outline is then followed posteriorly (also along the previously made peritoneal incision). When creating this posterior colpotomy, the active blade of the instrument may be inserted into the vagina, then moved superiorly to "hug up" to the cervix and the blades can be closed to create better control (Fig. 9). It is important to constantly be aware of the contralateral pelvic sidewall, as it is fairly easy, with the uterine manipulation, to inadvertently contact this area with the Harmonic.

The Harmonic is then inserted into the right lower lateral or paramedian port to complete colpotomy (Fig. 10). Once the uterus and cervix are separated, the assistant removes

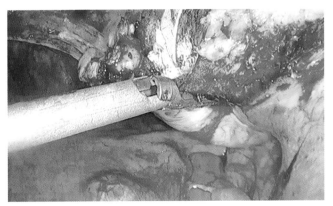

Fig. 9: Posterior colpotomy

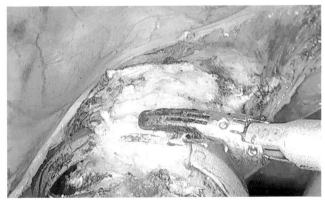

Fig. 10: Completion of colpotomy

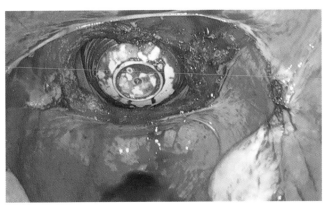

Fig. 11: Use of blue bulb

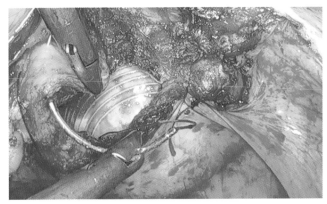

Fig. 12: Colpotomy suturing

the manipulator and grasps the cervix transvaginally with a single tooth tenaculum. If it is a large, bulky specimen, transvaginal morcellation may be performed using right angle and narrow Deaver retractors as well as a weighted speculum to protect the bladder, vagina and rectum. Otherwise, the specimen is removed intact. A blue Asepto bulb is then placed into the vagina with a ring forceps on the end to maintain pneumoperitoneum (Fig. 11).

Cuff closure may be accomplished using several techniques.

For most of our cases, the vagina is closed using 3–4 figure-of-eight sutures. The suture material we typically use is a 2–0 monocryl suture instead of vicryl, as this monofilament material slides more easily through tissue and is easier to use when placing figure-of-eight sutures. Depending on surgeon preference, suturing may be performed using a 10 mm suprapubic port (the surgeon, on the patient's left side, introduces the needle with the left hand through the suprapubic port; the needle holder is introduced through the left low lateral port/paramedian port), ipsilaterally, extending the low left port to 10 mm and placing the needle holder in the left upper quadrant port, or contralaterally, either introducing the needle through the 10 mm infraumbilical port or extending the left low lateral

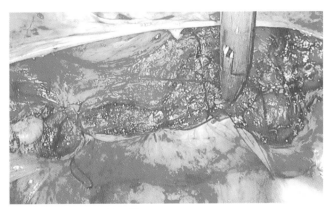

Fig. 13: Closed colpotomy

port and inserting the needle holder in the right low lateral port.

Regardless of the ports utilized, the corners of the vaginal cuff are usually approximated first, incorporating some posterior peritoneum and part of the uterosacral ligament on that side but avoiding the uterine vascular pedicle (Fig. 12). Each suture is placed through the pubocervical fascia (with the bladder retracted caudad) and the vaginal epithelium on both the anterior and posterior cuff, at least a centimeter from the cut edge (Fig. 13).

In some cases, simple interrupted sutures of 0-vicryl may be placed. In other cases, a barbed suture such as v-loc may be used to close the cuff in a running fashion.

The pelvis is then irrigated. All vascular pedicles and areas of dissection are inspected to ensure hemostasis. Cystoscopy is performed routinely after laparoscopic hysterectomy. To decrease the costs of opening an entire cystoscopy set, the Foley catheter is clamped and the bladder is back-filled with ~150 cc of saline. The catheter is removed and then a 5 mm 30° laparoscope is inserted. Both ureteral jets are visualized and the entire bladder is examined, focusing mainly at the dome to ensure no suture material has been placed in the bladder wall. Once cystoscopy is found to be satisfactory, the Foley catheter is replaced. The fascia at the 10 mm port site(s) is closed using either a Carter-Thomason device or interrupted sutures of 0-vicryl on a UR6 needle. Skin is closed with 4-0 monocryl in a subcuticular fashion.

POSTOPERATIVE MANAGEMENT

Following uncomplicated total laparoscopic hysterectomy, we typically admit our patients for 23-hour observation. The Foley catheter is removed within 4–6 hours after surgery to encourage ambulation. Diet is advanced as tolerated. Patients are encouraged to walk, at first with assistance, to use an incentive spirometer at least 10 times per hour and to take oral pain medications (ibuprofen, percocet) as necessary. Thromboembolism-deterrent stockings/ Sequential compression devices (TEDs/SCDs) remain in place while the patient is in bed. Serum labs, complete blood count, basic metabolic panel (CBC, BMP), are drawn early on postoperative day one. Patients are typically discharged postoperative day 1 (POD#1) provided pain is controlled, they are tolerating diet and labs/vitals are within normal limits.

In most patients, pharmacologic thromboembolism prophylaxis is not initiated postoperatively as hospital stay is very brief and ambulation occurs rapidly after surgery. In women with morbid obesity, prolonged hospital stay, incidental malignancy, or other significant risk factors for thromboembolism, prophylaxis, typically with enoxaparin, for 2 weeks postoperatively, may be considered.

Upon discharge to home, pelvic rest is mandated for at least 6 weeks.

FOLLOW-UP

Patients are seen in the outpatient clinic for follow-up at 2 weeks and 6 weeks postoperatively. Speculum exam is performed, typically at the 6 week follow-up visit, to ensure the vaginal cuff is healing appropriately. Return to work and other daily activities may occur by the 2 week mark. Patients may resume sexual activity, provided exam reveals normal healing, after the 6 week follow-up visit.

> **Key Points**
> - The advantages of laparoscopic hysterectomy are numerous and include a faster recovery time, decreased hospital costs and increased patient satisfaction.
> - Preoperative assessment should include routine gynecologic screening, thorough physical exam, endometrial biopsy if abnormal bleeding is a complaint, ultrasound versus MRI imaging and optimization of pre-existing medical comorbidities.
> - Initial trocar placement at Palmer's point is used in patients with prior surgeries and large uteri.
> - Accessory trocar placement is mapped according to pelvic pathology as well as surgeon preference with regard to laparoscopic suturing.
> - Cystoscopy is routinely performed after laparoscopic hysterectomy to ensure bladder integrity and ureteral patency.

REFERENCES

1. Nieboer TE, Johnson N, Lethaby A, et al. Surgical approach to hysterectomy for benign gynaecological disease. Cochrane Database Syst Rev. 2009 Jul 8;(3):CD003677. doi: 10.1002/14651858.CD003677.pub4.

2. Clark-Pearson DL and Gellar EJ. Complications of hysterectomy. Obstet Gynecol. 2013;121(3):654-73.

3. Hur HC, Donnellan N, Mansuria S, et al. Vaginal cuff dehiscence after different modes of hysterectomy. Obstet Gynecol. 2011;118(4):794–801.

4. Kho RM, Akl MN, Cornella JL, et al. Incidence and characteristics of patients with vaginal cuff dehiscence after robotic procedures. Obstet Gynecol. 2009;114:231-5.

5. Uccella S, Ghezzi F, Mariani A, et al. Vaginal cuff closure after minimally invasive hysterectomy: our experience and systematic review of the literature. Am J Obstet Gynecol. 2011;205(2):119 e1–12.

6. Shen CC, Hsu TY, Huang FJ, et al. Comparison of one- and two-layer vaginal cuff closure and open vaginal cuff during laparoscopic-assisted vaginal hysterectomy. J Am Assoc Gynecol Laparosc. 2002;9(4): 474–80.

7. Siedhoff MT, Yunker AC, Steege JF. Decreased incidence of vaginal cuff dehiscence after laparoscopic closure with bidirectional barbed suture. J Minim Invasive Gynecol. 2011;18(2):218–23.

8. Uccella S, Ceccaroni M, Cromi A, et al. Vaginal cuff dehiscence in a series of 12,398 hysterectomies: Effect of different types of colpotomy and vaginal closure. Obstet Gynecol. 2012;120(3):516-23.

9. Siedhoff MT, Clark LH, Hobbs KA, et al. Mechanical bowel preparation before laparoscopic hysterectomy: a randomized controlled trial. Obstet Gynecol 2014;123(3): 562-7.

10. ACOG Committee on Practice Bulletins--Gynecology. ACOG Practice Bulletin No. 104. Antibiotic prophylaxis for gynecologic procedures. Obstet Gynecol. 2009;113(5):1180-9.

11. Society of Gynecologic Oncology (2011). SGO Clinical Practice Statement: Salpingectomy for Ovarian Cancer Prevention. [online] Available from www.sgo.org/clinical-practice/guidelines/sgo-clinical-practice-statement-salpingectomy-for-ovarian-cancer-prevention. [Accessed January 2015].

CHAPTER 11

Laparoscopic Myomectomy

Thomas Lang, Linda Shiber, Resad Pasic

◼ INTRODUCTION

Management of symptomatic uterine leiomyomata, the most common solid tumor in women, is a large part of every gynecology practice. Studies have shown that up to 70% of Caucasian women and 80% of African American women will have uterine leiomyomas by the age of 50 years.[1] Many women experience symptomatic fibroids prior to completing childbearing and desire fertility sparing surgery, i.e., myomectomy. Some women who are beyond their reproductive years may also prefer myomectomy to hysterectomy for a variety of psychosocial and cultural reasons. As a gynecologist, being able to offer these women fertility-sparing surgical options with faster recovery times and improved outcomes is of paramount importance. Laparoscopic myomectomy is a viable surgical option for these women and preserves reproductive capacity as well as providing symptomatic relief.

The most common symptoms experienced by patients with fibroids are abnormal uterine bleeding, pelvic pressure or mass effect symptoms such as urinary frequency and constipation, pelvic pain and infertility. However, having fibroids do not guarantee symptoms; the occurrences of the above symptoms is typically dependent on fibroid size, number and location within the uterus and pelvis.

Regarding women of reproductive age, it is important to note that leiomyomas are present in approximately 5-10% of women with infertility and are the sole factor identified in 1–2.4% of women with infertility.[2-4] However, leiomyomas should not be considered the default cause of infertility without completing a basic evaluation to assess the woman and her partner.[5] This is of primary importance when discussing surgical options with women who have fibroids and infertility but do not have other symptoms usually resultant from fibroids.

◼ PREOPERATIVE CONSIDERATIONS

The indications for myomectomy include abnormal uterine bleeding, pelvic pain and pressure, enlarging leiomyoma and possibility of neoplasia, infertility, and ureteral obstruction resultant from a large broad ligament fibroid. Of course, in all these scenarios, hysterectomy is the most definitive therapy, though it may not be acceptable to certain patients, namely those desiring future pregnancy. To determine if myomectomy is a feasible therapeutic option, it is important to complete a detailed work up including an assessment of patient goals and symptom profile, performing a careful physical exam, obtaining imaging, tissue sampling and extensive patient counseling.

Preoperative imaging is integral to determining what surgical approach will benefit a particular patient. Transvaginal ultrasound or saline infusion sonography is a cost-effective method that provides important information about the size, type and location of uterine

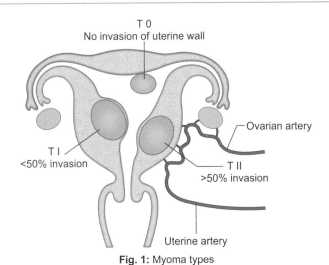

T 0
No invasion of uterine wall

T I
<50% invasion

T II
>50% invasion

Ovarian artery

Uterine artery

Fig. 1: Myoma types

leiomyoma. Saline infusion sonography, in particular, is helpful in identifying intracavitary myomas that can contribute to menorrhagia and infertility; this imaging modality allows the clinician to determine if such lesions are hysteroscopically resectable. For women with larger fibroid uteri or more serious sequelae from their fibroids, such as ureteral obstruction, MRI is a very useful modality. MRI allows planes between normal myometrium and leiomyomata to be clearly identified and provides much more comprehensive information about fibroid location in relation to other abdominopelvic structures. Its higher cost, however, must be taken into consideration during a preoperative work up and must be balanced by logical rationale necessitating such imaging (Fig. 1).

Anemia resulting from abnormal uterine bleeding should be assessed prior to going to surgery. Women can be placed on oral contraceptive pills or gonadotropin-releasing hormone (GnRH) agonists such as Depot-Lupron. While a GnRH agonist can decrease the size of the myoma, improve anemia and decrease the need for transfusion, it can make the surgical planes difficult to identify intraoperatively. A simple and effective means of increasing hemoglobin preoperatively is oral iron therapy. Alternatively, in women with severe anemia, preoperative blood transfusion versus intravenous iron infusions can optimize anemia. It is important to remember that pRBC transfusion should be done at least 24 hours before planned surgery date as stored pRBC's do not contain 2,3 diphosphoglycerate (DPG) and require approximately 24 hours to become optimally effective.

Preoperative counseling is extremely important. The patient must understand the risks of laparoscopy (including damage to bowel, bladder and blood vessels), as well as the risk of conversion to laparotomy and hysterectomy. She must also understand that a myomectomy may not improve her symptoms and, with regard, to infertility, she may not become pregnant after surgery. The risk of uterine rupture and a discussion of route of delivery (i.e. requiring cesarean section) with future pregnancies needs to be addressed and documented in the medical record. Risk of recurrence of fibroid tumors, especially in younger women, should also be discussed. A large retrospective series of 512 patients reported a leiomyoma recurrence rate of 11.7% after 1 year and up to 84.4% after 8 years, but a reoperation rate for recurrence of 6.7% at 5 years and 16% at 8 years.[6]

The use of power morcellation has become an issue of concern. As per the AAGL statement, they agree that "morcellation is generally contraindicated in the presence of documented or highly suspected malignancy. Meticulous adherence to preoperative screening guidelines, including endometrial biopsy and cervical cytology, to exclude coexisting uterine or cervical malignancy or premalignancy is imperative".[7] "Power morcellation is an important tool in treating symptomatic uterine fibroids which allows up to 150,000 women each year to undergo minimally invasive surgery when they would otherwise require laparotomy for an abdominal hysterectomy. While research, education and improved tissue extraction techniques can probably further enhance the safety profile of power morcellation, the elimination of power morcellation and conversion of these women to open surgery would likely increase morbidity and mortality from open surgery and cause harm to more patients".[8]

It is also important to remember that surgical expertise/ technique can play a big role in surgical outcome. A surgeon who is just beginning to do laparoscopic myomectomies should be selective of their surgical cases and begin small.

Room Setup
• Trocars (2 × 5 mm, 1 × 12 mm)
• Sutures/Needles (Discussed later)
• Needle drivers × 2
• 5 and 10 mm myoma screw
• Manipulator with chromotubation capabilities.

■ INTRAOPERATIVE CONSIDERATIONS

The patient should be placed in the dorsal lithotomy position with the arms tucked at her sides and adequately padded with foam. Proper patient positioning is discussed

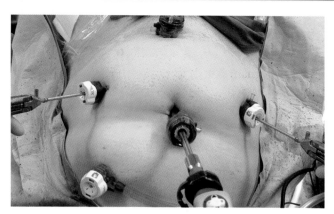

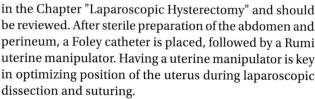

Fig. 2: Port configuration

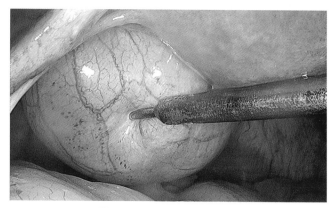

Fig. 3: Injection of vasopressin

in the Chapter "Laparoscopic Hysterectomy" and should be reviewed. After sterile preparation of the abdomen and perineum, a Foley catheter is placed, followed by a Rumi uterine manipulator. Having a uterine manipulator is key in optimizing position of the uterus during laparoscopic dissection and suturing.

Preoperative antibiotics are not indicated for all laparoscopic myomectomies. If there is strong likelihood that the endometrial cavity will be opened during the case, making it clean-contaminated, we typically do administer prophylactic antibiotics either prior to incision or intraoperatively if this occurs.

Primary port entry though Palmer's point should be considered if the myoma/pathology is large or if the patient has had prior abdominal surgery. Peritoneal access is also discussed in Chapter: Laparoscopic Hysterectomy or Chapter: Peritoneal Access in Laparoscopy (Fig. 2).

Various port configurations can be used for laparoscopic myomectomy, depending primarily on the comfort and expertise of the surgeon. In patients who are not massively obese, contralateral suturing through a right and left lower quadrant (LLQ) port is feasible and has the advantage of improved triangulation for intracorporeal knot tying. Depending on the location of the fibroid to be resected and its accessibility, suturing can also occur using a lower quadrant port and a midline suprapubic port, ipsilateral ports, or a lower quadrant and suprapubic port. A suprapubic port can serve a dual purpose; in addition to suturing, it is also helpful for aiding with uterine manipulation using a myoma screw or tenaculum.

When suturing contralaterally, the surgeon typically stands on the patient's left side. Needles are introduced through the LLQ port and, assuming a horizontal incision on the uterus, each suture is placed forehand, from the top layer of the defect to the bottom. If the ipsilateral technique or the suprapubic port is preferred, the surgeon, standing on the patient's left side, places each suture in a forehand manner, from bottom to top.

The initial step in performing a laparoscopic myomectomy is preparing and preventing excessive blood loss. We typically begin with infiltration of dilute vasopressin in the serosa and myometrium surrounding the fibroid of interest. A dilution of 20 units vasopressin in 100 cc saline versus 20 units vasopressin in 200 cc saline, depending on the volume that will be needed for the injection, is typically used. A 20 gauge spinal needle or a laparoscopic needle with a syringe attached is passed through the trocar closest in proximity to the fibroid. As the uterus is stabilized, a laparoscopic needle driver is used to guide the needle into the tissue. The goal with the injection of the vasopressin is to infiltrate the pseudocapsule of the leiomyoma. This helps facilitate both vasoconstriction of the capillary bed for hemostasis as well as aiding in hydrodissection (Fig. 3).

If vasopressin is not available, bilateral uterine artery clipping using vascular clips can be performed to decrease surgical blood loss. These clips can remain in place or be removed at the end of the procedure. If fertility is desired, removal of the clips on completion of the case is recommended.

Once the myometrium and pseudocapsule have been infiltrated with dilute vasopressin, the myometrial incision is made. The length and axis of the incision will depend on the location and size of the leiomyoma as well as the surgeon's preference for port placement. The incision can be made with monopolar, bipolar or ultrasonic energy. The incision is extended deeply until the pseudo capsule is entered (Fig. 4). The myoma is then visualized and enucleation is begun by grasping the myoma with a laparoscopic tenaculum (or myoma screw) for traction. A combination of blunt and surgical energy is used to separate the myoma from the surrounding myometrium and thus complete the enucleation. If the surgeon maintains dissection in the pseudocapsule, then blood loss will be minimized. This, however, can be rather difficult in cases involving irregularly shaped leiomyomas, adenomyomas

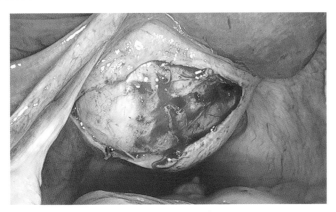

Fig. 4: Initial dissection

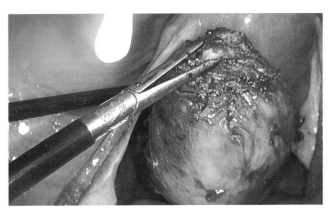

Fig. 5: Enucleation

and in women treated preoperatively with Lupron (Figs 5 and 6).

After excision of the myoma, the first step in repairing the uterus is to assess the integrity of the endometrial cavity. This is easily done if a Rumi uterine manipulator has already been placed. Sterile saline stained with indigo carmine dye can be infused through the manipulator and the bed of the defect inspected laparoscopically for leakage of blue fluid. If a defect is noted, it is repaired with either single interrupted sutures of 3-0 Monocryl or a continuous running suture of 3-0 Monocryl. Given the delicacy of this tissue, the needle of choice for this is typically an SH or CT2.

❑ The angle of the endometrial defect is identified and the suture is placed just lateral to it to ensure a strong tissue purchase. We prefer intracorporeal knot tying here to decrease the likelihood of tearing the delicate endometrial tissue.

❑ Suturing is then continued, incorporating both edges of the endometrium and, if possible, avoiding full thickness passes. Instead, effort is taken to skim the endometrium, decreasing the amount of exposed suture in the cavity and the chance of subsequent intrauterine adhesive disease. At the same time, inversion of the endometrium should also be avoided to decrease the theoretical likelihood of subsequent adenomyosis.

❑ Each suture should be placed approximately 0.5 cm apart and 0.5 cm from the edge of the defect.

❑ When the opposite angle is reached, the suture can be tied intracorporeally. Some surgeons prefer to place a second layer of suture in the opposite direction for additional reinforcement. Once the endometrium has been closed satisfactorily, infusion of indigo tinted saline is again performed through the Rumi manipulator to confirm adequate closure.

If the endometrium is intact, or, conversely, when the endometrium has been closed, attention is turned to

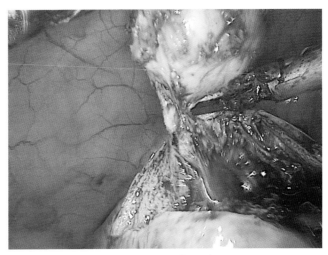

Fig. 6: Myoma dissection

closure of the myometrial defect. Maintaining symmetry of both sides of the myometrium as well as ensuring closure of the dead space is the key to a hemostatic repair and to easy placement of subsequent layers. There is no magic number of layers that must be placed to ensure ideal future pregnancy outcomes. Uterine rupture has been described in pregnancy even after myomectomy with three layer closure.[9] It is up to the surgeon to determine what approach is ideal for a particular patient.

When closing the myometrium, two common suture materials are used:

❑ 2-0 Vicryl with a CT-1 needle

❑ *Barbed suture (It is Important to go up one size in suture caliber as the barbs are cut into the suture making there effective diameter less)*

❑ V-Loc 90, (90 37 mm ½ Circle Taper Point on GS21 needle, 15cm)

❑ Quill 0, (36 mm ½ Circle Taper point PDO, 14 cm × 14 cm)

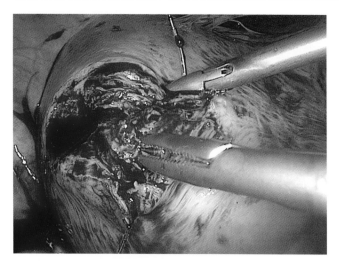

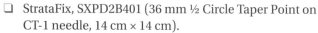

Fig. 7: Myometrial closure

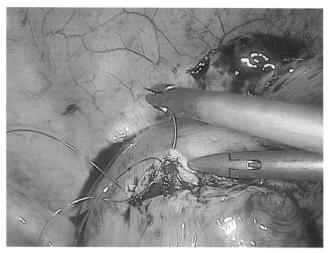

Fig. 8: Baseball stitch

❑ StrataFix, SXPD2B401 (36 mm ½ Circle Taper Point on CT-1 needle, 14 cm × 14 cm).

Prior to the introduction of barbed sutures, 2-0 Vicryl with a CT-1 needle was used by many to re-approximate the myometrium in two layers. Suturing occurs in a typical angle-to-angle continuous running fashion, being careful not to incorporate endometrium into the closure (Fig. 7).

❑ The initial angle stitch is tied intracorporeally. Alternatively, a LAPRA-TY can be placed at the end of the suture, tightening it down once the angle is purchased. If VLoc is being used, the angle stitch is placed and the needle is passed through the loop and pulled through, eliminating the need for knot tying.

❑ Suturing is then continued in a continuous running fashion, spacing each pass approximately 1 cm apart and tucking raw muscle edges in as progress is made. Once again, symmetry is essential, as it will ease the placement of each successive layer. In the case of barbed suture, tensioning the suture after each throw is necessary. This should be done by pushing the myometrial tissue down rather than simply tugging on the suture (which can result in frustrating breakage).

❑ Once the opposite angle is reached, the suture can be either tied intracorporeally (in the case of Monocryl) or, if using barbed suture, several sutures can be placed in the opposite direction to prevent unraveling of the repair. The barbed suture is then tensioned and cut flush with the tissue surface.

❑ When the bidirectional Quill or StrataFix suture materials are used for myometrial closure, suturing is begun in the middle of the defect. Each half of the suture is then run in opposite directions. Again, no knot is necessary.

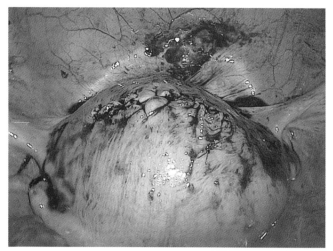

Fig. 9: Hemostatic closure

After the myometrium is reapproximated and hemostatic, the serosa is closed. Debate exists as to the optimal technique for serosal closure: continuous running suture versus the 'in-to-out' baseball technique. At our institution, the baseball technique is preferable as this minimizes suture exposure and may decrease adhesion formation. Regardless of the technique chosen, each stitch must be placed 0.5–1.0 cm apart and approximately 0.5 cm deep. The LAPRA-TY or intracorporeal knot can be placed at the last stitch. The suture material used for the serosal layer is typically a monofilament such as 3-0 Monocryl on a CT-1 or SH needle (Fig. 8).

Once the serosa is closed, careful inspection for hemostasis is performed (Fig. 9). Any areas with persistent bleeding are typically managed using a bipolar electrosurgical device (if superficial and focal) or by placing additional figure-of-eight sutures. The pelvis is irrigated and when no further bleeding is noted, an adhesion barrier, such as Interceed, may be placed over the suture line to decrease adhesion formation.

Pedunculated Fibroids/Small Defects

If the defect is small, such as after resection of a small, pedunculated fibroid, single interrupted sutures with 2-0 Monocryl or Vicryl on a CT-1 needle can be placed for hemostasis. It is adequate hemostasis and lack of exposed raw edges that will decrease adhesion formation.

Once the defect is completely repaired, the myoma itself must be removed from the peritoneal cavity. This can be done in one of three ways. The myoma can be removed via a mechanical morcellator from the LLQ port. Another option is to extend a laparoscopic port site to allow removal of the myoma or morcellation at the skin. Finally, a posterior colpotomy can be made and the tumor can be removed through this. It is paramount to thoroughly inspect the peritoneal cavity to ensure that no residual fragments of myoma remain within the cavity. Morcellating within a retrieval bag can help limit this.

■ POSTOPERATIVE CONSIDERATIONS

Depending on the extent of the surgery and the patient's medical comorbidities, she may be discharged home from the postanesthesia care unit (PACU), or the recovery unit, or kept for observation overnight. Our practice is to admit these patients for 23 hours observation and to ensure immediate postoperative milestones are met. A complete blood count (CBC) is checked in the morning of postoperative day one. Combination of pain control with nonsteroidal anti-inflammatory drugs (NSAIDs) and oral narcotics along with ice packs to the abdomen seems to improve patient pain scores and satisfaction. We have found that ice packs placed on incision sites, in particular, have decreased narcotic use in the immediate postoperative period. A Foley catheter is typically removed 4–6 hours after surgery.

In general, patients are seen in the office at 2 weeks and 6 weeks postoperatively. Attempts at pregnancy should be deferred for 2–3 months after the initial recovery period.

> **Key Points**
> - The advantages of laparoscopic myomectomy are numerous and include a faster recovery time, decreased hospital costs and increased patient satisfaction.
> - A thorough preoperative evaluation is paramount, including endometrial biopsy and imaging, to aid in surgical planning.
> - Primary port entry through Palmer's point should be considered if the myoma/pathology is large or if the patient has had prior abdominal surgery.
> - When dissecting the myoma, care should be taken to keep the endometrium intact if possible.
> - Depending on the extent of the surgery and the patient's medical comorbidities, she may be discharged home from the PACU, or kept for observation overnight.

■ REFERENCES

1. Day Baird D, Dunson DB, Hill MC, et al. High cumulative incidence of uterine leiomyoma in black and white women: ultrasound evidence. Am J Obstet Gynecol. 2003;188:100-7.
2. Buttram VC Jr, Reiter RC. Uterine leiomyomata: etiology, symptomatology, and management. Fertil Steril. 1981;36: 433-45.
3. Manyonda I, Sinthamoney E, Belli AM. Controversies and challenges in the modern management of uterine fibroids. BJOG. 2004;111:95-102.
4. Olufowobi O, Sharif K, Papaionnou S, et al. Are the anticipated benefits of myomectomy achieved in women of reproductive age? A 5-year review of the results at a UK tertiary hospital. J Obstet Gynaecol. 2004;24:434-40.
5. American College of Obstetricians and Gynecologists. ACOG Practice Bulletin. 96. Alternatives to Hysterectomy in the Management of Leiomyomas, 2008;112(2 Pt 1):387-400.
6. Yoo EH, Lee PI, Huh CY, et al. Predictors of leiomyoma recurrence after laparoscopic myomectomy. J Minim Invasive Gynecol. 2007;14:690-7.
7. AAGL-Advancing Minimally Invasive Gynecology Worldwide. Member update #5: AAGL Response to FDA Guidance on Use of Power Morcellation during tissue extraction for uterine fibroids. 43rd AAGL Global Congress in Vancouver; 2014.
8. AAGL-Advancing Minimally Invasive Gynecology Worldwide. AAGL Statement to the FDA on Power Morcellation, July 2014.
9. Parker WH, Einarsson J, Istre O, et al. Risk factors for uterine rupture after laparoscopic myomectomy. J Minim Invasive Gynecol. 2010;17(5):551-4.

CHAPTER 12

Adenomyosis—Management and Laparoscopic Surgery

Grigoris Grimbizis, Themistoklis Mikos

▮ INTRODUCTION

Adenomyosis is an enigmatic condition in etiology, perplexing in diagnosis, unspecified in clinical significance and challenging in treatment. It has been described in the mid-19th century and since then numerous studies consistently report liaison of adenomyosis with a variety of benign gynecological symptoms.

Adenomyosis is defined as the presence of endometrial tissue (glands and stroma) within the uterine smooth muscle layers of the myometrium; heterotopic endometrial tissue foci are surrounded from myometrial areas characterized by a variable degree of smooth muscle cell hyperplasia. The adenomyotic glands penetrate within the muscular uterine wall at least 2.5 mm beyond the endometrial-myometrial interface. The disease is characterized as diffuse or localized (focal) depending on the extent of myometrial invasion. Moreover, adenomyotic lesions manifest with a histological spectrum ranging from mostly solid to mostly cystic generating an inconsistent pathologic profile.[1]

Currently, there are four distinct theories for the *pathogenesis* of adenomyosis that have been proposed. The *endometrial invagination theory* is the more accepted one, and it is based on the hypothesis of myometrial invasion from endometrium basalis. A disruption of the endometrial—myometrial barrier is supposed to be the underlying factor that enables invagination of endometrial glands within the myometrium. Uterine "trauma" (surgery, cesarean section, pregnancy, etc.) and endometrial interventions (curettage, ablation, etc.) associated with altered immunoreaction and/or increased invasiveness of endometrium basalis, all seem to be crucial predisposing factors.[2] *De novo development of ectopic endometrium* from Müllerian remnants within the myometrium or metaplasia of pluripotent immature cells of Müllerian origin that are misplaced into the myometrium represents the second hypothesis. This theory explains better the types of adenomyosis at extrauterine sites (e.g. rectovaginal septum disease), and it is supported by the differences in the biological characteristics observed between ectopic and eutopic endometrium.[3,4] *Invagination* of junctional zone and myometrium by endometrial cells *through the lymphatic system* is the third explanation. This hypothesis stands along with the potential pathogenesis of endometriosis, as proposed and documented by Sampson.[5] According to the fourth theory, adenomyosis is caused from bone marrow stem cells that could evolve to endometrial cells and are displaced through the vasculature. It is presumed that bone marrow-derived stem cells could repopulate within the myometrium causing adenomyosis with local proliferation of the glands and the stroma.[6]

The *prevalence* of adenomyosis in the general and in selected populations is still not exactly known. As histology was the only "diagnostic" tool before the era of ultrasound and magnetic resonance imaging (MRI), the prevalence of adenomyosis was estimated between 20 and 30% on hysterectomy series but, depending on the presenting symptoms, it varies widely between 5 and 70%. The disease is mostly diagnosed between 30 and 45 years of age.[7-9] Recently, in a prospective study of women attending a gynecologic clinic, the frequency of adenomyosis diagnosed with the aide of structured 2D ultrasound was 20.9%.[10]

Clinical presentation is respectively capricious. Women with extensive adenomyosis may have no clinical burden, whereas patients with localized disease may present with a variety of gynecological problems. Although an unknown proportion of patients with adenomyosis could be asymptomatic, the disease is mainly related to abnormal uterine bleeding, pelvic pain (usually dysmenorrhea), pressure symptoms on bladder and/or bowel, and impaired reproductive performance.[11]

Women with mild to severe disease are complicated with abnormal uterine bleeding in 23–82% of the cases.[11] It seems that there is a positive, although not absolute, relation between severity of menorrhagia and the extent of adenomyosis.[8,12,13] Dysmenorrhea, affecting up to 50% of women with adenomyosis, is also related with the extent of myometrial penetration.[11,12] There is evidence to support a causal association between adenomyosis and impaired fertility potential.[14] Patients with adenomyosis who underwent in vitro fertilization experienced lower pregnancy and increased miscarriage rates.[15,16] It seems, also, that late pregnancy outcome is impaired in patients with adenomyosis with increased preterm delivery and preterm rupture of membranes.[17] Due to the increasing trend of getting pregnant at a later age, adenomyosis could increasingly complicate the fertility potential of women in this age group.[18] Therefore, screening for adenomyosis before initiation of any assisted reproductive procedure might be useful.[16]

RECENT GUIDELINES AND MANAGEMENT

Although, currently, there is no generally accepted consensus, a *classification of adenomyosis* is a prerequisite for its management. The classification should express the disease extent, severity and histological diversity, should be correlated with symptomatology, should be fitted to the needs of the treatment and should be comprehensive, clear and as simple as possible. However, this task is not easy due to the histological diversity of adenomyosis, the variety of the locations and the differences in the extent of the disease as well as the plurality of its symptoms.

A first attempt of classification was the disease categorization in three distinct groups based on MRI findings: (1) *junctional zone hyperplasia*, characterized by junctional zone thickness up to 12 mm; (2) *adenomyosis (obviously diffuse),* characterized by junctional zone thickness less than or equal to 12 mm and/or various degree of outer myometrium's; (3) *adenomyoma*, characterized by myometrial mass with indistinct margins.[19] Another approach was the subclassification of the surgically treated adenomyosis according to the disease topography on MRI into *the intrinsic, extrinsic, intramural and indeterminate* forms, trying to link the disease categorization with its potential pathogenesis.[20]

Nevertheless, in order to evaluate the results of any treatment (medical, conservative surgery or even definitive surgery) a more clinical categorization of the disease is necessary. Hence, taking into account the extent of the myometrial invasion and the histological characteristics as well as the needs of the treatment, the following *clinical/ histological classification* of adenomyosis has been proposed:[21]

Class I. Diffuse adenomyosis, including the following subclasses, *(Ia)* smooth muscle hyperplasia with ectopic endometrium (increased junctional zone) and, (Ib) micro-dilated ectopic endometrial glands throughout hyperplastic myometrium

Class II. Focal adenomyosis, further subdivided in *(IIa) adenomyoma, (IIb) cystic adenomyosis* including, also, *(IIba) juvenile cystic adenomyosis*

Class III. Polypoid adenomyomas, further subdivided in *(IIIa) typical polypoid* and *(IIIb) atypical polypoid adenomyomas*

Class IV. Other forms, including *(IVa) adenomyomas of endocervical type* and *(IVb) retroperitoneal adenomyomas.*

Precise *diagnosis* is essential for treatment. Clinical suspicion based on patient's history and clinical examination is the first step. Although, myometrial biopsy provides definite identification of the disease, it is interventional and it is not indicated in young and/or subfertile patients for the design of their treatment. Thus, nowadays, diagnosis should be based on noninvasive imaging using ultrasound and MRI.[22]

Ultrasound assists gynecologists to set diagnosis globally. The application of the vaginal probes that beam to the uterus closely is a major advantage of ultrasound. Moreover, recent advances in ultrasound technology (Doppler technology, three-dimensional imaging, high resolution, off-line analysis, etc.) further increased its diagnostic capabilities. Asymmetrical thickening of myometrium in the absence of uterine fibroids, parallel shadowing, linear striations, myometrial cysts, hyperechoic islands, ill-defined nodular heterogeneous myometrial mass and irregular endometrial–myometrial junction seems to be ultrasound findings in adenomyosis.[10,23-25] The accuracy of the ultrasound in the diagnosis of adenomyosis is high with a mean sensitivity of 0.72 (95% CI: 0.65-0.79), specificity of 0.81 (95% CI: 0.77-0.85), and area under the curve (AUC) of 0.85;[22] however, its diagnostic performance is biased by the experience of the examiner.

Magnetic resonance imaging has, also, high diagnostic accuracy with a pooled sensitivity of 77% (95% CI 67–85%), specificity of 89% (95% CI 84–92%) and AUC of 0.92.[22,26] When comparing ultrasound and MRI, an advantage of MRI is that the diagnosis is based on "hard" standard imaging findings non-depended on the examiners experience and that fibroids do not affect their reading.[22] Another advantage of MRI is the excellent correlation between imaging findings and histology, which is very important for implementing a surgical treatment strategy.[27,28] The spectrum of described MRI findings includes diffuse or focal thickening (>12 mm) of the junctional zone, ill-defined myometrial nodules within myometrium, punctuate foci of high intensity within the myometrium or within the low intensity lesions, and linear striation radiating out of the endometrium.[29]

Adenomyosis is a benign disease. Hence, *treatment strategy* is aiming only to the control of clinical symptomatology of patients (Flow chart 1). Adenomyotic tissue invades the uterine muscle layer with unclear borders of the lesion and, thus, complete excision of the affected area remains inaccurate.[30] Therefore, it is well accepted that only hysterectomy is a definite treatment for patients with adenomyosis. However, it is invasive and associated with reproductive amputation. Thus, conservative treatment options in patients wishing fertility should be selected. Excision of adenomyotic tissue is always accompanied with excision of myometrium being partly destructive for the uterine wall: one has to balance between the advantages of removing an affected area and the disadvantages of a possibly defected uterine wall. As a result, conservative surgery has not become the standard treatment for adenomyosis.

It is generally accepted that *medical treatment* options that could lead to an effective control of clinical symptoms and to a potential regression of the disease should be applied in symptomatic patients as a first-line treatment. In patients not wishing pregnancy and presenting with pelvic pain and/or abnormal uterine bleeding, the levonorgestrel intrauterine system (LNG-IUS) represents a potential efficacious treatment option. It seems that it is associated with 70–90% bleeding control and pelvic pain relief. Furthermore, a regression of the disease process was observed during the first 2–3 years, with a relapse thereafter. In infertile patients wishing pregnancy who are treated with in vitro fertilization, the administration of gonadotropin-releasing hormone analogs in the long or extra-long protocol seems to represent an option reversing the adverse effect of adenomyosis on IVF outcome.[16]

The concept of *conservative, uterine-sparing surgery* for adenomyosis is kept as the last option when medical manipulations fail to provide a successful control of symptoms and the disease could be excised surgically. Nowadays, this option seems to represent an effective alternative indeed, as fertility preservation and quality of life improvement, can be achieved in this group of patients.[30]

FERTILITY SPARING LAPAROSCOPIC SURGERY IN ADENOMYOSIS

Classification of Uterine-sparing Surgery

For the most of the cases of adenomyosis, the disease involves a minor or major degree of myometrial infiltration; in these cases, removal of healthy myometrium happens inevitably during excision of the lesion. The proposed classification of the currently available surgical techniques regarding the excision of adenomyosis is based on the extent of removal of the adjacent healthy myometrium and the preservation of the integrity (and subsequently the functionality) of the uterine wall. The currently available uterine preserving surgical options for adenomyosis could be classified as following:

❑ *Complete excision of adenomyosis or adenomyomectomy:* Adenomyomectomy is presumed to be the most advantageous technique for the treatment of adenomyosis because during these operations the adenomyotic lesions are radically excised. The subtraction of the disease is expected to lead to subsequent dissolution of the symptoms and treatment.

 ❖ *Adenomyomectomy:* This technique is applied in cases of localized adenomyosis (adenomyoma) but also in a number of selected cases of more diffuse adenomyosis with reconstruction of the uterine wall. It is characterized by the (1) *complete* removal of *all clinically recognizable non-microscopic* lesions, and (2) maintenance of uterine wall's integrity in spite of the removal of large amount of myometrium.[31-33]

 ❖ *Cystectomy:* This technique is applied in cases of cystic focal adenomyosis. It includes the entire removal of the adenomyotic cyst.[34,35] Although cystic adenomyomas are rare entities, the possibility of complete excision and restoration of normal uterine anatomy is of great importance specifically for symptomatic women including those with poor reproductive history.

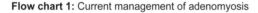

Flow chart 1: Current management of adenomyosis

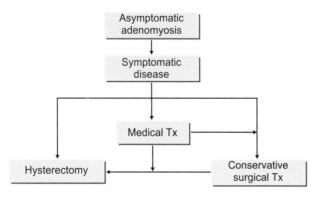

❏ *Cytoreductive surgery/partial adenomyomectomy:* This technique is applied in cases of diffuse adenomyosis, including the *partial* removal of the *clinically recognizable non-microscopic* lesions. The reason is that complete removal of the lesion would lead to the concomitant excision of critical amount of healthy myometrium that could lead to "functional" hysterectomy.[36,37] Theoretically, the partial adenomyomectomy appears to be less effective approach compared to the complete adenomyomectomy. The residual adenomyotic tissue could postoperatively cause persistence and recurrence of symptoms.

❏ *Non-excisional techniques:* This is a heterogeneous group that includes endoscopic interventions where removal of adenomyotic tissue is *not* included.[37-39]

Currently Available Methods of Uterine-sparing Surgical Treatment

Adenomyosis is a disease with a nonuniform anatomical appearance. Therefore, depending on the anatomical manifestation of the lesion, the surgeon should carefully select the appropriate uterine-sparing option. Apparently, preoperative diagnostic imaging is of paramount importance for this decision. As mentioned above, the combination of ultrasound and MRI have a high sensitivity for the correct depiction of adenomyotic lesions. Based on this information, surgery is personalized for the individual patients' needs. Adenomyomectomy, either for diffuse or focal adenomyosis, cytoreductive surgery (partial adenomyomectomy) and a variety of non-excisional techniques, have all been described thoroughly in the literature for the uterine-sparing surgical treatment of adenomyosis.

The described proposals, classified according to the radicality of the excision of the adenomyotic tissue, have been as followed.

Complete Excision of Adenomyosis/Adenomyomectomy

Classical technique: This technique applies mainly in cases where adenomyosis presents with the form of an adenomyoma; this is a lesion resembling a leiomyoma and in the majority of the cases the surgeon suspects adenomyosis intraoperatively, because of the surgically ill-defined margins of the adenomyoma, the absence of the pseudo-capsule of the leiomyoma, but also the difficulty that it encounters because of the nonuniformity of the lesion. An adenomyomectomy (open or laparoscopic)

follows the same steps as myomectomy (open or laparoscopic) (Figs 1A to F): (1) recognition of the lesion's location and borders by inspection and/or palpation, (2) longitudinal incision of the uterine wall along the lesion, (3) sharp and blunt dissection of the adenomyoma with scissors, graspers and/or diathermy similarly to the removal of a fibroid, (4) approximation of the uterine wall in a seromuscular layer[32,40] or in single or multiple layers[31,41] and suturing of the endometrial cavity with absorbable suture when necessary; in cases of laparoscopic adenomyomectomy, the adenomyotic mass is removed with the use of morcellator.[32] In cases where intraoperative recognition of the adenomyotic lesion is laborious, *the use of ultrasound guidance* has been proposed, either in the form of hydroultrasonographic monitoring or in the form of transtrocar ultrasonography.[42,43]

Modification in wall reconstruction (U-shaped suturing): This is a technique described mainly for the conservative surgical management of diffuse adenomyosis. According to this technique, after removal of adenomyomatous tissue, U-shape sutures at the muscle layer approximate the wall's cave-like wound; the seromuscular layer is closed by figure-of-eight suture.[44]

Modification in wall reconstruction (overlapping flaps): This is another technique for the conservative surgical management of diffuse adenomyosis. According to this technique, a transverse incision is made in the adenomyotic tissue and the lesion is excised with monopolar needle; the remaining seromuscular layers are overlapped and sutured to counteract the lost muscle layer of the uterus.[45]

Triple-flap method: This is another technique for the conservative surgical management of diffuse adenomyosis, as well. It has been described mainly as a laparotomic procedure and involves: (1) extraperitonealization of the uterus and rubber tourniquet placement for hemostasis, (2) bisection of the uterus in the midline and in the sagittal plane with a scalpel until the uterine cavity is encountered, (3) opening of the endometrial cavity to permit the insertion of the index finger to guide during excision of adenomyotic tissues, (4) use of Martin forceps to grasp adenomyotic tissues and to excise them from surrounding myometrium leaving a myometrial thickness of 1 cm from serosa above and endometrium below, (5) closure of the endometrium with 3-0 vicryl, (6) approximation of the flaps of the uterine wall closing the myometrium and serosa of the bisected uterus' one side in the anteroposterior plane with interrupted 2-0 vicryl, whereas the contralateral side of the uterine wall is brought over the reconstructed first side in such a way as to cover it.[33]

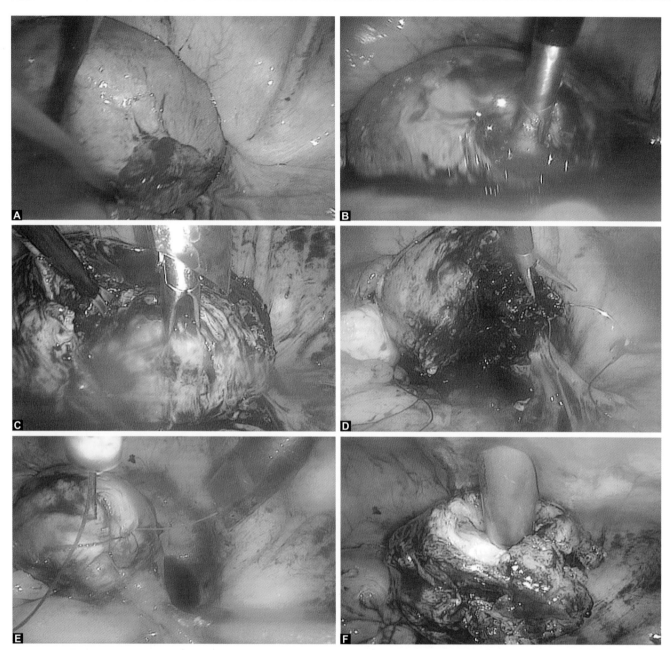

Figs 1A to F: Operative steps of adenomyomectomy: (A) Adenomyotic uterus: an adenomyoma is diagnosed during laparoscopy, (B) The surgeon grasps the adenomyoma and pulls it to start dissect healthy myometrium around it, (C) The adenomyoma is retracted and the surgeon, using scissors, separates the lesion from healthy tissue, (D) The adenomyoma is removed and the surgeon starts suturing the uterus, (E) Suturing is complete; uterine traumatic surfaces are appropriately approximated and hemostasis secured, and (F) The adenomyoma is taken out of the peritoneal cavity with the use of morcellator

Cytoreductive Surgery/Partial Adenomyomectomy

Classical technique (excision of diffused adenomyosis): Cytoreductive surgical approaches imply that a percentage of adenomyotic tissue remains unexcised. This theoretically poses the notion that these techniques are followed by inferior postoperative results compared to the techniques where complete excision of adenomyotic tissue takes place. However, the truth is that these techniques may account for a more realistic approach of the disease. The reason is that, apart from the cases of adenomyomas, adenomyosis commonly has a universal impact on the myometrium. Thus, complete excision of the disease is frequently impossible, unless a hysterectomy takes place.

Cytoreductive techniques for adenomyosis involve the following steps: (1) a vertical or transverse incision is applied in the middle of the anterior or the posterior uterine wall; (2) Ford T-clamps (or an equivalent instrument) are applied to the wound edges so as myometrium of the subserous layer, which is rarely affected by adenomyosis (up to ~10 mm), can be later preserved; (3) the uterine wall is inspected for clinically recognizable non-microscopic adenomyotic lesions (coarse, white trabeculations) which are excised piecemeal, paying attention to preserve as much of the adjacent normal myometrium as possible; (4) if adenomyosis is extended to the contralateral wall of the uterus as well, the incision is extended over the top of the uterus and down toward the urinary bladder of the pouch of Douglas. Approximation of myometrium is performed in a single or multiple layers and of the serosa in one layer with interrupted sutures. Attention is taken as to secure that no uterine defects are left that could increase the risk of hematoma.[46]

Transverse H-incision technique: This is cytoreductive technique described for the management of diffuse adenomyosis and is performed mainly by laparotomy. It has been described for the treatment of anterior uterine wall adenomyosis. Initially, the surgeon places a tourniquet at the uterine cervix and vasoconstricting agents are used in order to minimize blood loss. A vertical incision is performed in the uterine wall and two transverse incisions are made perpendicularly to the initial incision along the upper and lower edges of the uterus (H-incision). A 5 mm thickness of the uterine serosa is cut out from uterine myometrium along the vertical incision. The surgical field is extended and the uterine serosa is widely opened bilaterally at the area under the H-incision. Then, adenomyotic tissue is removed bit by bit, using manual palpation to define the borders of healthy myometrium. Chromopertubation test using indigo-carmine permits assessment of endometrial perforation. As above, approximation of the myometrium is performed in a single or multiple layers and of the serosa in a single layer with interrupted sutures.[46]

Wedge resection of the uterine wall: This is another technique described for the management of diffuse adenomyosis. According to this technique (open or laparoscopic), the part of the seromuscular layer where adenomyosis is located is removed by wedge resection of the uterine wall. The operation is completed with traditional closure of the uterine wounds as described in the classical technique of partial adenomyomectomy.[44]

Asymmetric dissection of uterus: This is another technique described for the management of diffuse adenomyosis.

It is described as a laparotomic technique: the uterus is dissected longitudinally with surgical electric knife in an asymmetrical fashion to divide the inside from outside, preserving both the uterine cavity and bilateral uterine arteries. Because of this asymmetric approach, the myometrium is dissected diagonally, as if hollowing out the uterine cavity. Then, the uterine cavity is transversely incised and subsequently entered; the index finger is introduced into the cavity and adenomyotic lesions are excised using a loop electrode to a thickness of 5 mm of the inner myometrium. The procedure continues with subtraction of adenomyosis to a thickness of 5 mm of the serosal myometrium, Then the endometrial cavity is approximated and the uterine flaps are rejoined in layers (muscle and serosa).[36]

Laparoscopically-assisted Vaginal Excision

This is another technique described for the management of diffuse adenomyosis. According to this technique, the surgeon initially creates pneumoperitoneum and confirms that the uterus is free of any adhesions. A laparoscopic bilateral uterosacral ligament removal is carried out and a posterior colpotomy follows. Through the vaginal incision, the uterus is extracted and under direct manipulation the surgeon subtracts adenomyotic fragments verified by touch using monopolar cautery. Residual myometrium is approximated in two layers. The advantage of excising adenomyotic tissue distinguished by manual contact as well as knotting manually with adequate tension secures the non-inferiority of this method compared to open adenomyomectomy.[47]

Non-excisional Techniques

It is presumed that non-excisional techniques apply better to diffuse adenomyosis. The laparoscopic non-excisional approaches have the advantage of fertility sparing. On the contrary, hysteroscopic or ablative techniques, without being contraceptive *per se*, they annihilate the fertility potential and therefore are not suitable for patients seeking pregnancy. The following groups of non-excisional techniques have been illustrated in the literature for the uterine-sparing management of adenomyosis:

❑ *Combination of excisional and non-excisional techniques:* Kang et al. described a series where laparoscopic resection of diffuse adenomyosis after laparoscopic uterine artery occlusion was performed.[48] This approach is suitable for fertility sparing.

❑ *Laparoscopic non-excisional techniques:* Laparoscopic electrocoagulation of the myometrium[37,38] and laparoscopic uterine artery ligation[39] have been described. These approaches permit further pregnancy as well.

❏ *Hysteroscopic non-excisional techniques:* Operative hysteroscopy,[49] rollerball endometrial ablation,[50] transcervical resection of the endometrium[51,52] and endomyometrial resection[37] have been proposed. All these techniques hamper the fertility potential of the patients.

❏ *Other techniques:* Ablation of focal adenomyosis with high frequency ultrasound,[53] alcohol instillation under ultrasound guidance for the treatment of cystic adenomyosis,[54] radiofrequency ablation of focal adenomyosis,[55] microwave endometrial ablation[56] and balloon thermoablation[57] for diffuse adenomyosis have been also described.

Results after Uterine-sparing Surgical Treatment for Adenomyosis

Current literature suggests that uterine-sparing treatment of adenomyosis appears to be feasible and efficacious. However, the main problem of an attempt to systematically review this type of procedures is that there are only a few studies with good quality data and, therefore, the cumulative results could easily be criticized. In fact, the prospective studies dealing with the conservative surgical treatment of adenomyosis are not many, and there is no uniform design and/or outcome, so the feasibility of pooling the results is suboptimal.

In a systematic review of uterus-sparing surgery results, complete excision of adenomyosis, partial excision of adenomyosis and complete excision of cystic adenomyomas, yield a reduction of *dysmenorrhea* in 80–85% of the treated cases.[21] These results indicate that the excision of the bulk of adenomyosis ensues pain control, even if some amount of residual lesion has been left, as it happens in cases of cytoreductive surgery.[21]

In terms of *abnormal bleeding* control, complete excision of adenomyosis results in approximately 70% menorrhagia reduction, notably better compared to partial excision of adenomyosis resulting in approximately 50% reduction.[21] It seems, therefore, that after partial excision of adenomyosis, the residual adenomyotic tissue adjacent continues to cause bleeding symptoms. This implies that in cases of diffuse adenomyosis with menorrhagia, cytoreductive partial excision of the lesion is less effective comparable to complete excision techniques. After non-excisional techniques, the observed approximately 75% regulation of menorrhagia appears to be better compared to partial excision techniques, and comparable to complete excision techniques.[21] However, the control of bleeding is achieved indirectly through the destruction/excision of endometrium, without treatment of the primary disease, resulting in loss of the fertility of the patient.

Uterus-sparing surgery for adenomyosis involves techniques that modify the anatomy of the uterus and the surgery itself may concomitantly cause deformities (i.e. pelvic adhesions, uterine cavity deformities, intrauterine adhesions, reduced uterine capacity) that may contribute to a declined postoperative pregnancy rate.[36] Nevertheless, it seems that, after uterine-sparing surgery, not only *fertility* is finally preserved, but also subfertility related to adenomyosis could potentially be treated; conception rates appears to be approximately 50% after partial and approximately 65% after complete excision of adenomyosis with approximately 70% crude delivery rates in patients achieving a pregnancy.[21]

Pregnancy-related Issues and Potential Complications

Commenting about the appropriate time between uterine-sparing surgery and conception, most of the studies dealing with pregnancy after surgery for adenomyosis, attempts for conception were permitted at least 3 months after intervention.[36] After adenomyomectomy, it is speculated that subsequent uterine scars may conceal dense residual adenomyotic foci and, as a consequence, the tensile strength of the uterus may be impaired leading to possible rupture during pregnancy.[47,58] However, the real risk is not still known and the one out of eight pregnant women reported risk seems to be simply an overestimation.[59]

It has been shown that ART methods show increased pregnancy rates compared to natural cycles after operative intervention for adenomyosis.[44] Moreover, a single embryo transfer policy minimizes the risk of uterine rupture, because a twin pregnancy generates uterine activity at an earlier gestational age, which may lead to this catastrophic event.[47]

Although most of the reported deliveries have been completed with cesarean section, there are few reports where vaginal deliveries were permitted. Sporadic reports have outlined the risk of pungent atonic postpartum hemorrhage in women with known adenomyosis that can necessitate peripartum hysterectomy.[60] Due to the absence of data and experience, it seems that in terms of patient safety, it would be desirable to perform an elective cesarian section after adenomyomectomy, especially in non-organized centers.

Laparotomy or Laparoscopy

Traditionally, laparotomy has been used for the surgical treatment of adenomyosis, because of the extension of the disease within the myometrium and the difficulty in suturing of the remaining uterine wedges after the abscission. The leading merit of laparotomy remains the ability of the surgeon to palpate and recognize the adenomyotic lesions during the operation. However, when the adenomyotic lesion can be clearly outlined in the MRI, laparoscopy is attainable either for ablation of the adenomyotic foci or for excision of adenomyomas, whereas laparoscopic suturing presents no more arduousness compared to suturing after myomectomy.[32,61]

No evidence can indicate the technique that secures the better clinical and reproductive performance. Each author describes the theoretical benefits of his technique, but in practice the results have no considerable clinical differences. Mainly, most of the modifications aim (1) to maximize the amount of adenomyotic tissue excised during the operation by offering an augmented area where surgical manipulations can be performed, (2) to equip the uterine wall integrity, so future pregnancy can be sustained without uterine rupture.

■ CONCLUSION

Adenomyosis is a disease of the myometrium with unclear clinical presentation and still unknown etiology that hampers women's reproductive years. Uterine-sparing techniques offer the possibility of controlling the symptoms while maintaining the uterus along with improving the fertility potential of the patient. The optimal technique has still not been established, although numerous interventions have been described.

Laparoscopy holds a major part in the actualization of the majority of these techniques. Knowledge about the epidemiology and the natural history of the disease, improving the surgical skills, and defining the limits of the operating capabilities of the surgeon, are the important steps for improving gynecological health in this intriguing clinical field.

■ REFERENCES

1. Farquhar C, Brosens I. Medical and surgical management of adenomyosis. Best Pract Res Clin Obstet Gynaecol. 2006;20:603-16.
2. Wang JH, Wu RJ, Xu KH, et al. Single large cystic adenomyoma of the uterus after cornual pregnancy and curettage. Fertil Steril. 2007;88(4):965-7.
3. Matsumoto Y, Iwasaka T, Yamasaki F, et al. Apoptosis and Ki-67 expression in adenomyotic lesions and in the corresponding eutopic endometrium. Obstet Gynecol. 1999;94(1):71-7.
4. Propst AM, Quade BJ, Gargiulo AR, et al. Adenomyosis demonstrates increased expression of the basic fibroblast growth factor receptor/ligand system compared with autologous endometrium. Menopause. 2001;8(5):368-71.
5. Sampson JA. Metastatic or embolic endometriosis, due to the menstrual dissemination of endometrial tissue into the venous circulation. Am J Pathol. 1927;3:109.
6. Garcia L, Isaacson K. Adenomyosis: review of the literature. J Minim Invasive Gynecol. 2011;18(4):428-37.
7. Fedele L, Bianchi S, Frontino G. Hormonal treatments for adenomyosis. Best Pract Res Clin Obstet Gynaecol. 2008;22(2):333-9.
8. Levgur M, Abadi MA, Tucker A. Adenomyosis: symptoms, histology, and pregnancy terminations. Obstet Gynecol. 2000;95(5):688-91.
9. Sammour A, Pirwany I, Usubutun A, et al. Correlations between extent and spread of adenomyosis and clinical symptoms. Gynecol Obstet Invest. 2002;54(4):213-6.
10. Naftalin J, Hoo W, Pateman K, et al. How common is adenomyosis? A prospective study of prevalence using transvaginal ultrasound in a gynaecology clinic. Hum Reprod. 2012;27(12):3432-9.
11. Peric H, Fraser IS. The symptomatology of adenomyosis. Best Pract Res Clin Obstet Gynaecol. 2006;20(4):547-55.
12. Bird CC, McElin TW, Manalo-Estrella P. The elusive adenomyosis of the uterus-revisited. Am J Obstet Gynecol. 1972;112(5):583-93.
13. Naftalin J, Hoo W, Pateman K, et al. Is adenomyosis associated with menorrhagia? Hum Reprod. 2014;29(3):473-9.
14. Tomassetti C, Meuleman C, Timmerman D, et al. Adenomyosis and subfertility: evidence of association and causation. Semin Reprod Med. 2013;31(2):101-8.
15. Maubon A, Faury A, Kapella M, et al. Uterine junctional zone at magnetic resonance imaging: a predictor of in vitro fertilization implantation failure. J Obstet Gynaecol Res. 2010;36(3):611-8.
16. Vercellini P, Consonni D, Dridi D, et al. Uterine adenomyosis and in vitro fertilization outcome: a systematic review and meta-analysis. Hum Reprod. 2014;29(5):964-77.
17. Juang CM, Chou P, Yen MS, et al. Adenomyosis and risk of preterm delivery. BJOG. 2007;114(2):165-9.
18. Leyendecker G, Kunz G, Kissler S, et al. Adenomyosis and reproduction. Best Pract Res Clin Obstet Gynaecol. 2006;20:523-46.
19. Gordts S, Brosens JJ, Fusi L, et al. Uterine adenomyosis: a need for uniform terminology and consensus classification. Reprod Biomed Online. 2008;17(2):244-8.
20. Kishi Y, Suginami H, Kuramori R, et al. Four subtypes of adenomyosis assessed by magnetic resonance imaging and their specification. Am J Obstet Gynecol. 2012;207(2):114.e1-7.

21. Grimbizis GF, Mikos T, Tarlatzis B. Uterus-sparing operative treatment for adenomyosis. Fertil Steril. 2014;101(2):472-87.

22. Champaneria R, Abedin P, Daniels J, et al. Ultrasound scan and magnetic resonance imaging for the diagnosis of adenomyosis: systematic review comparing test accuracy. Acta Obstet Gynecol Scand. 2010;89:1374-84.

23. Reinhold C, Tafazoli F, Mehio A, et al. Uterine adenomyosis: endovaginal US and MR imaging features with histopathologic correlation. Radiographics. 1999;19:147-60.

24. Dueholm M. Transvaginal ultrasound for diagnosis of adenomyosis: a review. Best Pract Res Clin Obstet Gynaecol. 2006;20(4):569-82.

25. Exacoustos C, Brienza L, Di Giovanni A, et al. Adenomyosis: three-dimensional sonographic findings of the junctional zone and correlation with histology. Ultrasound Obstet Gynecol. 2011;37(4):471-9.

26. Stamatopoulos CP, Mikos T, Grimbizis GF, et al. Value of magnetic resonance imaging in diagnosis of adenomyosis and myomas of the uterus. J Minim Invasive Gynecol. 2012;19:620-6.

27. Dueholm M, Lundorf E, Hansen ES, et al. Magnetic resonance imaging and transvaginal ultrasonography for the diagnosis of adenomyosis. Fertil Steril. 2001;76:588-94.

28. Bazot M, Cortez A, Darai E, et al. Ultrasonography compared with magnetic resonance imaging for the diagnosis of adenomyosis: correlation with histopathology. Hum Reprod. 2001;16:2427-33.

29. Tamai K, Koyama T, Umeoka S, et al. Spectrum of MR features in adenomyosis. Best Pract Res Clin Obstet Gynaecol. 2006;20(4):583-602.

30. Koo YJ, Im KS, Kwon YS. Conservative surgical treatment combined with GnRH agonist in symptomatic uterine adenomyosis. Pak J Med Sci. 2011;27:365-70.

31. Wang PH, Fuh JL, Chao HT, et al. Is the surgical approach beneficial to subfertile women with symptomatic extensive adenomyosis? J Obstet Gynaecol Res. 2009;35(3):495-502.

32. Grimbizis GF, Mikos T, Zepiridis L, et al. Laparoscopic excision of uterine adenomyomas. Fertil Steril. 2008;89(4):953-61.

33. Osada H, Silber S, Kakinuma T, et al. Surgical procedure to conserve the uterus for future pregnancy in patients suffering from massive adenomyosis. Reprod Biomed Online. 2011;22(1):94-9.

34. Protopapas A, Millingos S, Markaki S, et al. Cystic uterine tumors. Gynecol Obstet Invest. 2008;65:275-80.

35. Takeuchi H, Kitade M, Kikuchi I, et al. Diagnosis, laparoscopic management, and histopathologic findings of juvenile cystic adenomyoma: a review of nine cases. Fertil Steril. 2010;94:862-8.

36. Nishida M, Takano K, Arai Y, et al. Conservative surgical management for diffuse uterine adenomyosis. Fertil Steril. 2010;94:715-9.

37. Wood C. Surgical and medical treatment of adenomyosis. Hum Reprod Update. 1998;4:323-36.

38. Phillips DR, Nathanson HG, Milim SJ, et al. Laparoscopic bipolar coagulation for the conservative treatment of adenomyomata. J Am Assoc Gynecol Laparosc. 1996;4:19-24.

39. Wang CJ, Yen CF, Lee CL, et al. Laparoscopic uterine artery ligation for reatment of symptomatic adenomyosis. J Am Assoc Gynecol Laparosc. 2002;9:293-6.

40. Dubuisson JB, Fauconnier A, Deffarges JV, et al. Pregnancy outcome and deliveries following laparoscopic myomectomy. Hum Reprod. 2000;15:869-73.

41. Hyams LL. Adenomyosis; its conservative surgical treatment (hysteroplasty) in young women. N Y State J Med. 1952;52:2778-84.

42. Nabeshima H, Murakami T, Terada Y, et al. Total laparoscopic surgery of cystic adenomyoma under hydroultrasonographic monitoring. J Am Assoc Gynecol Laparosc. 2003;10:195-9.

43. Nabeshima H, Murakami T, Nishimoto M, et al. Successful total laparoscopic cystic adenomyomectomy after unsuccessful open surgery using transtrocar ultrasonographic guiding. J Minim Invasive Gynecol. 2008;15:227-30.

44. Sun AJ, Luo M, Wang W, et al. Characteristics and efficacy of modified adenomyomectomy in the treatment of uterine adenomyoma. Chin Med J (Engl). 2011;124:1322-6.

45. Takeuchi H, Kitade M, Kikuchi I, et al. Laparoscopic adenomyomectomy and hysteroplasty: a novel method. J Minim Invasive Gynecol. 2006;13:150-4.

46. Fujishita A, Masuzaki H, Khan KN, et al. Modified reduction surgery for adenomyosis. A preliminary report of the transverse H incision technique. Gynecol Obstet Invest. 2004;57:132-8.

47. Wada S, Kudo M, Minakami H. Spontaneous uterine rupture of a twin pregnancy after a laparoscopic adenomyomectomy: a case report. J Minim Invasive Gynecol. 2006;13:166-8.

48. Kang L, Gong J, Cheng Z, et al. Clinical application and midterm results of laparoscopic partial resection of symptomatic adenomyosis combined with uterine artery occlusion. J Minim Invasive Gynecol. 2009;16:169-73.

49. Fernandez C, Ricci P, Fernandez E. Adenomyosis visualized during hysteroscopy. J Minim Invasive Gynecol. 2007;14:555-6.

50. Preutthipan S, Herabutya Y. Hysteroscopic rollerball endometrial ablation as an alternative treatment for adenomyosis with menorrhagia and/or dysmenorrhea. J Obstet Gynaecol Res. 2010;36:1031-6.

51. Kumar A, Kumar A. Myometrial cyst. J Minim Invasive Gynecol. 2007;14:395-6.

52. Maia H Jr, Maltez A, Coelho G, et al. Insertion of mirena after endometrial resection in patients with adenomyosis. J Am Assoc Gynecol Laparosc. 2003;10:512-6.

53. Yang Z, Cao YD, Hu LN, et al. Feasibility of laparoscopic high-intensity focused ultrasound treatment for patients

with uterine localized adenomyosis. Fertil Steril. 2009;91:2338-43.

54. Furman B, Appelman Z, Hagay Z, et al. Alcohol sclerotherapy for successful treatment of focal adenomyosis: a case report. Ultrasound Obstet Gynecol. 2007;29:460-2.

55. Ryo E, Takeshita S, Shiba M, et al. Radiofrequency ablation for cystic adenomyosis: a case report. J Reprod Med. 2006;51:427-30.

56. Kanaoka Y, Hirai K, Ishiko O. Successful microwave endometrial ablation in a uterus enlarged by adenomyosis. Osaka City Med J. 2004;50:47-51.

57. Chan CL, Annapoorna V, Roy AC, et al. Balloon endometrial thermoablation - an alternative management

of adenomyosis with menorrhagia and dysmenorrhoea. Med J Malaysia. 2001;56:370-3.

58. Levgur M. Therapeutic options for adenomyosis: a review. Arch Gynecol Obstet. 2007;276:1-15.

59. Wang CJ, Yuen LT, Chang SD, et al. Use of laparoscopic cytoreductive surgery to treat infertile women with localized adenomyosis. Fertil Steril. 2006;86:462.e5-8.

60. Coghlin DG. Pregnancy with uterine adenomyoma. Can Med Assoc J. 1947;56:315-6.

61. Morita M, Asakawa Y, Nakakuma M, et al. Laparoscopic excision of myometrial adenomyomas in patients with adenomyosis uteri and main symptoms of severe dysmenorrhea and hypermenorrhea. J Am Assoc Gynecol Laparosc. 2004;11:86-9.

CHAPTER 13

Laparoscopic Management of Endometriosis

Stephan Gordts

■ INTRODUCTION

The estimated incidence of endometriosis in the general population is 2–22% with a reported incidence between 20–50% in patients with infertility.[1]

Based on epidemiological data, it is generally accepted that endometriotic implants are related to an impaired reproductive outcome, although the causal relationship between endometriosis and infertility has not clearly been proven so far. As long as there is no proven causal relationship, treatment of these lesions will remain debatable. The gold standard for diagnosis is laparoscopy and the staging is based on the criteria of the revised American Fertility Society (r-AFS).[2] By exclusion of male factor infertility and looking at the pregnancy rates in patients using donor insemination, a significant reduction of fertility in laparoscopic-proven cases of minimal and mild endometriosis versus normal controls has been shown by Toma et al.[3] (0.14 versus 0.06, respectively). Jansen[4] has reported the same findings with an average fecundability of 0.12 in normal women versus 0.036 in women with minimal endometriosis. Endometriosis is a pleiotropic reproductive condition and the lesions visualized at laparoscopy are only one aspect of this disease process. At present, there is no evidence that surgery for endometriosis can cure infertility. In advanced stages, infertility is at least partially due to the disturbed tubo-ovarian relationship, but in minimal and mild stages, the cause is unknown.

■ PATHOGENESIS

Thomas Cullen described for the first time under the name of "adenomyoma" the full morphological and clinical picture of what today is identified as endometriosis and adenomyosis.[5,6] The term "endometriosis" was first mentioned by Sampson[7] in 1927, postulating that the presence of ectopic endometrium outside the uterus was due to the tubal regurgitation and dissemination of endometrial cells. These regurgitated endometrial cells may implant on the ovarian surface, causing local bleeding and adhesions.[8] Hughesdon[3] investigated a series of ovaries with the endometrioma in situ and demonstrated the invaginated cortex with fibrosis and adhesion formation. Although the hypothesis of menstrual regurgitation and subsequent angiogenesis and implantation is being the most widely accepted, other theories are tissue metaplasia of invaginated coelomic epithelium or Müllerian remnants.[9,10] In a recent paper, Vercellini et al.[11] concluded that bleeding from corpus luteum appears to be a critical event in the development of endometriomas. Communicating luteal cysts have been observed by Sampson[12] in 9% of his cases. The presence of peritoneal and ovarian endometriosis in premenarchal girls without an obstructive anomaly has supported the concept that endometriosis may result from an etiology other than retrograde menses as proposed by Sampson in 1927. Batt and Mitwally[13] have argued for recognition of embryonic müllerian rests as the pathogenesis in cases of early endometriosis not explained by accepted theories. Ectopic endometrium in human female fetuses at different gestational ages has been described by Signorile et al.[14] and Bouquet de Jolinière et al.[15] referring to the possible theory of involvement of Müllerian or Wolffian cell rests in the pathogenesis of endometriosis. Recently, Brosens and Benagiano[16] formulated the hypothesis that perinatal uterine bleeding occurring in some newborns—a phenomenon that is routinely discounted as insignificant—may be a cause of premenarchal and adolescent endometriosis. More recently, mesenchymal stem cells[17] and endometrial stem cells[18] may be involved in the origin of endometriosis.

DIAGNOSIS

Transvaginal sonography (TVS) is considered as a useful method for early detection of the ovarian endometrioma and seems a reliable screening technique to exclude significant ovarian endometriosis in infertile patients. However, sensitivity and specificity can show important variations between ultrasonographists as it has been shown in the publication of Raine-Fenning[19] with a sensitivity varying between 64–89 and a specificity of 89–100. A systematic review by Moore et al.[20] concluded that ultrasound was an effective tool to confirm and exclude the diagnosis of an endometrioma with moderate accuracy. In the study of Holland et al.[21] the sensitivity and specificity of preoperative ultrasound for the detection of ovarian endometrioma is respectively 84.0 (95% CI 73.7–91.4) and 95.6 (95% CI 92.8–97.6). The positive likelihood ratio (LR+) was very useful (>10) for the TVS diagnosis of ovarian endometriomas, moderate or severe ovarian adhesions, pouch of Douglas adhesions and deeply infiltrating endometriosis of bladder, rectum, sigmoid and sacrouterine ligaments. The indirect imaging techniques [ultrasound and magnetic resonance imaging (MRI)] are certainly offering a benefit in the diagnosis and extension of DIE (Deep Infiltrating Endometriosis). Laparoscopy remains the golden standard in the diagnosis of peritoneal endometriotic lesions. This endoscopic exploration however, in absence of clinical symptoms, is frequently postponed in patients searching fertility care, due to its invasiveness. Furthermore, patients are easily referred to an IVF program without endoscopic investigation.

Delay of Diagnosis

The Endometriosis Association survey (www.endometriosisassn.org) reported an average time of 9.3 years between the onset of the first symptoms and the final diagnosis of endometriosis with an average time of 4.6 years before the first medical consult. Also Arruda et al.[22] found that the median time between onset of symptoms and diagnosis was 4.0 (2.0–6.0) years for women whose main complaint was infertility, but 7.4 (3.6–13.0) years for those with pelvic pain. There are several reasons to explain this delay. There is first the attitude to reveal the symptoms and to be convinced that it is not abnormal that menstruations are painful. Secondly, also at a first consult by the general practitioners, the symptoms are frequently minimized and

finally there is the invasiveness of the standard laparoscopy necessary for a final diagnosis. Although we cannot predict the progressivity of the disease there is a serious risk of progression of the disease with an impairment of the fertility potential in young women. The incidence of endometriosis in adolescents can be compared with the incidence in adults and is reported to be, by age 20 years or less, 35% stage III or IV, although severity greatly differed among studies.[23]

PERITONEAL AND OVARIAN ENDOMETRIOSIS

Peritoneal Endometriosis

Peritoneal lesions can be present in different forms: as active glandular or vesicular red lesions, as black advanced and older lesions and as white healed lesions. These different lesions can be subtle and very superficial, while others can be more typical lesions with deeper invasion in the subperitoneal layers. Red lesions can be polyps, vesicles or flame-like lesions (Fig. 1). They mostly show a strong neoangiogenesis. Most frequently, they are seen in young patients while the black and white lesions are more frequently present in older women.[24,25] In his study[24] comparing the reoperation rate of endometriosis in adolescents, the rate was significantly lower following resection of these lesions compared to superficial ablation (14.2%> <42.8%). The subtle superficial lesions can appear and disappear like mushrooms and it has been suggested that this is a normal event in menstruating women.[26] As such, the clinical significance of these lesions is yet not fully

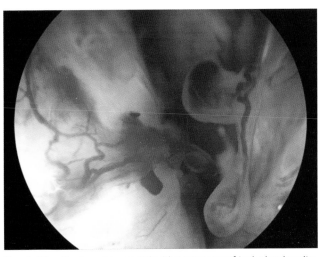

Fig. 1: Visualization at transvaginal laparoscopy of typical peritoneal lesion and presence on the ovarian surface of adhesions. On both sides a distinct neoangiogenesis is present

understood. Due to the high intra-abdominal pressure at standard laparoscopy, some of these lesions can be missed. A more accurate detection is obtained by inspection of these lesions under water like at transvaginal laparoscopy.[27] Some of the lesions remain undiagnosed; biopsies of normal looking peritoneum in patients with endometriosis showed histologic presence of endometriosis.[28] Also Nisolle et al.[29] and Belasch et al.[30] found a histologic confirmation of the presence of endometriosis in normal looking sacrouterine ligaments in patients with and without endometriosis.

Minimal and Mild Endometriosis

The necessity of surgical treatment in case of minimal and mild endometriosis has been highly controversial. The randomized Endocan study[31] demonstrated a modest beneficial effect on fertility of laparoscopic surgery. However, the beneficial findings of surgery in this group were not confirmed by the Italian study.[32] A review combining the results of both trials into a meta-analysis showed that surgical treatment is more favorable than expectant management (odds ratio for pregnancy 1.7; 95% confidence interval 1.1–2.5).[33] Current practice when minimal or mild endometriosis is diagnosed at laparoscopy is to surgically treat it where excision is preferred above ablation.[24]

Ovarian Endometrioma

Although an ovarian endometrioma is described as an ovarian cyst, its structure is different from other benign ovarian cysts. Sampson[7] was the first to suggest that ovarian endometriotic cysts originate from the outside of the ovary. He suggested that the endometrioma had an extra-ovarian origin and was caused by adhesions and bleeding of surrounding peritoneal implants. Regurgitated endometrial cells may implant on the ovarian surface, causing local bleeding and adhesions. Hughesdon[8] investigated a series of ovaries with the endometrioma in situ and demonstrated the invaginated cortex with fibrosis and adhesion formation. In contrast with other benign ovarian cysts, the ovarian endometrioma is formed as a pseudocyst. In situ ovarian cystoscopy and selected biopsies by Brosens et al.[34] confirmed these findings. As such, the basis and wall of this cyst is formed by inverted ovarian cortex, harboring primordial and primary follicles. With the aging of the endometrioma, the invaginated cortex gradually thickens by smooth muscle metaplasia and fibrosis, and its appearance at cystoscopy changes from pearl-white to yellow-white and finally black and fibrotic.[35] As disease and diameter progresses, the negative impact of fibrosis and smooth

muscle metaplasia upon the ovarian reserve are becoming more important.[36] Pathological progression occurs in the interstitial endometrioma bed and is manifested by smooth muscle metaplasia and hyperplasia, devascularization and follicle loss. In a recent study, Kuroda et al.[37] evaluated biopsies from healthy adherent ovarian tissue in women with endometrioma and in those with nonendometriotic cysts. The study demonstrated that the density of follicles in ovarian tissue from the endometrioma bed is approximately one- to two-thirds of adjacent to a nonendometriotic cyst in women younger than 35 years. The study suggests that ovarian endometriomata have a detrimental impact of follicle reserve in younger women and that cystectomy in young patients with an endometrioma may be particularly detrimental on the follicle reserve. Kityama et al.[38] described in their paper the presence of structural tissue alterations, such as formation of fibrosis and concomitant loss of cortex-specific stroma, in endometriotic cysts smaller than 4 cm and with apparently normal ovarian cortex responsible for the reduced ovarian reserve. Schubert et al.[39] concluded that endometriosis appeared to be a different disease from the other kind of cysts. It did not seem to be restricted only to the cyst, but rather invaded the surrounding cortex, and was responsible for the fibrotic reaction. In their study, fibrosis on the histology of the endometriotic cysts was frequently observed (n=9/13). Impaired ovarian reserve has also been reported in the study of Pacchiarotti et al.[40] with a significantly different lower Anti-Müllerian Hormone (AMH) concentration in patients with stage III–IV endometriosis versus fertile patients ($0.97 \pm 0.59 > < 1.72 \pm 0.63$; p = 0.001).

Ovarian Endometrioma and Surgery

Surgery in the more advanced stages of endometriosis aims for the restoration of normal tubo-ovarian anatomy and the elimination of endometrial implants in order to restore fertility. Several publications claim the beneficial effect of conservative surgery for moderate and severe forms of endometriosis.[41-43] This beneficial effect of surgery has to be balanced against the growing concern of damaging the ovarian reserve. The risk of premature ovarian failure after surgery for ovarian endometrioma has extensively been discussed in the recent literature. Coccia[44] showed that women previously submitted to bilateral cystectomy for ovarian endometrioma were younger at menopause than those with monolateral endometrioma (42.1 ± 5.1 years versus 47.1 ± 3.5 years, p = 0.003). The relationship between the preoperative ovarian endometriomas, total diameter and menopausal age was significant in case of surgery for bilateral endometriomas ($R^2 = 0.754$, p = 0.002). In the study of Takae et al.[45] out of 75 patients with premature ovarian failure, 66 patients (88.0%) underwent cystectomy for ovarian endometriosis. As there is no real plane of cleavage in endometriotic cysts, cystectomy of the pseudocyst wall will remove primordial follicles. In addition, extensive coagulation of the ovarian bed and more specifically at the hilus will destroy more follicles and damage the blood supply with an irreversible damage. This will result in a premature ovarian failure with unresponsiveness to ovarian stimulation and premature onset of menopause. The Cochrane review[46] comparing excisional surgery versus ablation recommends cystectomy because of a lower recurrence rate and a higher change for a spontaneous conception. It should be reminded that this study of Hart is based upon three randomized controlled trial (RCT) in only two centers and on 245 patients. Although, it is the only randomized available study Donnez et al.[47] questioned if the conclusion that excision was better than ablation was not too hasty concluded. Recent data on ablative surgery using plasma jet show lesser damage of the ovarian reserve than cystectomy.[48] In an attempt to lower the risk of ovarian damage a combination of an excisional and ablative surgery has been described[49] and in case of larger endometrioma (>5 cm) a two-step procedure has been advocated.[50,51] A recent study concludes that the operation-related damage to the ovarian reserve was positively related to whether the endometriomas were bilateral, as well as cyst size.[52] It is obvious that with the available surgical procedures damage will be done to the ovarian reserve. Some authors are therefore referring patients directly to an IVF program instead of surgical correction. Garcia Velasquez[53] recommends proceeding directly to IVF to reduce time to pregnancy, to avoid potential surgical complications and to limit patient costs. His indication for surgery is limited to large ovarian cysts, concomitant pain symptoms or when malignancy cannot reliably be ruled out. The increased use of assisted reproduction technology has led to higher fertility rates in patients with endometriosis. Presence of ovarian endometrioma in spontaneously conceived pregnancies is a rare event, but a 4-fold increase has been reported in recent years, making it today the most common adnexal mass detected during pregnancy.[54] The number of pregnant women with endometriosis and associated complications may rise, particularly when they are no longer operated on before pregnancy occurs. Up till now there are no follow-up studies available of patients referred to IVF programs without surgical correction of endometriotic cysts.

Postoperative adhesion formation is another concern of ovarian surgery. Several papers are discussing the potential of adhesion prevention mainly focusing on barrier agents or gel.[55,56] Also temporary postoperative ovarian suspension is reported to minimize adhesion formation.[57,58]

Place of Transvaginal Laparoscopy

Atraumatic ovarian surgery to avoid loss of ovarian reserve is based on early-stage diagnosis when cystectomy can be avoided. Although laparoscopy is traditionally recommended, transvaginal endoscopy has been shown to be safe and most effective in ablating ovarian endometriomas that are not larger than 3 cm. in diameter.[59,60] It is questionable on which basis the European Society of Human Reproduction and Embryology (ESHRE) guidelines[61] recommend that removal of endometriomas before IVF should be considered if more than 3 cm. There is no consensus on a cut-off value above which surgical treatment is warranted. The intracystic exploration at transvaginal laparoscopy shows clearly the aggressiveness of the lesions by the presence of neoangiogenesis and active endometrial-like tissue (Fig. 2). As the transvaginal laparoscopy is performed using a watery distension medium it enables accurate visualization of the vascularization of superficial implants and adhesions covering the site of small endometriotic lesions. The tubo-ovarian organs can be inspected in their natural position with easy exploration of the fossa ovarica without need of extra manipulation. Ovarian surface adhesions and the place of invagination can clearly be identified. By the use of a bipolar needle, the pseudocystic invagination is opened. At the basis of these small invaginations, endometrial-like tissue is identified. After rinsing and identification of the endometrial-like tissue lining the wall, full ablation is easily performed using a 5-Fr. bipolar coagulation probe. As endometriosis is a progressive disease, we suggested in a recent paper an early diagnosis and a surgical treatment as early as possible in adolescents.[62] As ablative surgery of small endometrioma intends to be more accurate and complete, reasonably we could expect, although not proven, that this will result in a lower recurrence rate, being easier to perform and minimal invasive.

■ CONCLUSION

The complexity of endometriosis as a disease does not allow an easy answer on the kind of treatment to perform. It can affect women during their all life span from adolescents until the menopause and treatment will differ according to age, complaints and symptoms. An individualized approach is mandatory. In adolescents and women in their reproductive life span, decision-making should always be based upon the principle of minimal invasiveness balancing treatment against the possible risk of surgery by damaging the ovarian reserve causing resistance to ovarian stimulation or premature ovarian failure. The

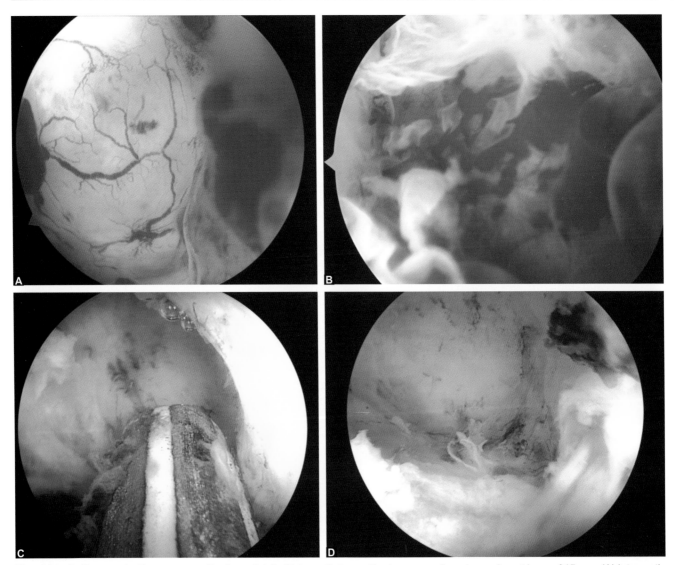

Figs 2A to D: Transvaginal laparoscopy allowing a detailed intracystic inspection in a case of ovarian endometrioma of 15 mm. (A) Intracystic visualization of distinct neoangiogenesis and at the site wall the presence of endometrial-like tissue; (B) Identification of active endometrial like tissue insight the ovarian cyst; (C) Ablation of wall endometriotic cyst using a 5 Fr bipolar probe; (D) View after ablation using the bipolar probe; remark the absence of carbonization and the white color of the insight of the cyst comparable with the aspect of a normal ovarian cortex

possible advantages of diagnosis and treatment of ovarian endometrioma in an early stage are, apart from a possible relief of pain, prevention of more damage to the ovary caused by the disease itself and avoiding damage of an invasive operative procedure. The ovarian endometrioma is not a simple benign ovarian cyst. In contrast to other cysts, it has an extraovarian localization and it affects the surrounding ovarian cortex resulting in smooth muscle metaplasia and fibrosis causing depletion of ovarian follicles. Further research is necessary to elucidate if an early treatment will result in lower recurrence rates and less severe forms of the disease. Endometriosis is a progressive disease; as until now there are no markers identifying the possible risk of progressivity of the disease in individual women; accurate hormonal or surgical treatment should be done when diagnosed. Used as a first-line diagnostic procedure,[63] the transvaginal laparoscopic approach provides through its direct access to the ovary and the fossa ovarica, the possibility of an early diagnosis and a minimal invasive treatment. The accuracy provided using a watery distension medium and the possibility of exploring the ovaries in their natural position without the necessity of extra manipulation, the structure of the endometrioma can be recognized as an inverted pseudocyst with normal cortex at the base of the cyst. At these early stages and as there is no cleavage plane ablative surgery should be performed.

■ REFERENCES

1. Moen MH. Endometriosis in women at interval sterilization. Acta Obstet Gynecol Scand. 1987;66(5):451-4.

2. Anonymous. Revised American Society for Reproductive Medicine classification of endometriosis 1996. Fertil Steril. 1997;67:817-21.

3. Toma SK, Stovall DW, Hammond MG. The effect of laparoscopic ablation or danocrine on pregnancy rates in patients with stage I or II endometriosis undergoing donor insemination. Obstet Gynecol. 1992;80:253-6.

4. Jansen RP. Minimal endometriosis and reduced fecundability: prospective evidence from an artificial insemination by donor program. Fertil Steril. 1986;46:141-3.

5. Cullen TS. The distribution of adenomyomata containing uterine mucosa. Arch Surg. 1920;1:215-83.

6. Benagiano G, Brosens I. Who identified endometriosis? Fertil Steril. 2011;95:13-6.

7. Sampson JA. Peritoneal endometriosis due to the menstrual dissemination of endometrial tissue into the peritoneal cavity. Am J Obstet Gynecol. 1927;14:422-69.

8. Hughesdon PE. The structure of endometrial cysts of the ovary. J Obstet Gynaecol Br Emp. 1957;44:481-7.

9. Nisolle M, Donnez J. Peritoneal endometriosis, ovarian endometriosis, and adenomyotic nodules of the rectovaginal septum are three different entities. Fertil Steril. 1997;68:585-96.

10. Cornillie FJ, Oosterlynck D, Lauweryns JM, et al. Deeply infiltrating pelvic endometriosis: histology and clinical significance. Fertil Steril. 1990;53:978-83.

11. Vercellini P, Somigliana E, Vigano P, et al. 'Blood On The Tracks' from corpora lutea to endometriomas. BJOG. 2009;116:366-71.

12. Sampson JA. Perforating hemorrhagic (chocolate) cysts of the ovary. Arch Surg. 1921;3:245-323.

13. Batt RE, Mitwally MF. Endometriosis from thelarche to midteens: pathogenesis and prognosis, prevention and pedagogy. J Pediatr Adolesc Gynecol. 2003;16(6):337-47.

14. Signorile PG, Baldi F, Bussani R, et al. Embryologic origin of endometriosis: analysis of 101 human female fetuses. J Cell Physiol. 2012;227(4):1653-6.

15. Bouquet de Jolinière J, Ayoubi JM , Lesec G, et al. Identification of displaced endometrial glands and embryonic duct remnants in female fetal reproductive tract: possible pathogenetic role in endometriotic and pelvic neoplastic processes. Front Physiol. 2012;3:444

16. Brosens I, Benagiano G. Is neonatal uterine bleeding involved in the pathogenesis of endometriosis as a source of stem cells? Fertil Steril. 2013;100:622-3.

17. Lin J, Xiang D, Zhang JL, et al. Plasticity of human menstrual blood stem cells derived from the endometrium. J Zhejiang Univ Sci B. 2011;12:372-80.

18. Gargett CE, Ye L. Endometrial reconstruction from stem cells. Fertil Steril. 2012;98:11-20.

19. Raine-Fenning N, Jayaprakasan K, Deb S. Three-dimensional ultrasonographic characteristics of endometriomata. Ultrasound Obstet Gynecol. 2008;31: 718-24.

20. Moore J, Copley S, Morris J, et al. A systematic review of the accuracy of ultrasound in the diagnosis of endometriosis. Ultrasound Obstet Gynecol. 2002;20:630-4.

21. Holland TK, Cutner A, Ertan Saridogan E, et al. Ultrasound mapping of pelvic endometriosis: does the location and number of lesions affect the diagnostic accuracy? A multicentre diagnostic accuracy study. BMC Women's Health. 2013;13:43.

22. Arruda MS, Petta CA, Abrao MS, et al. Time elapsed from onset of symptoms of endometriosis in a cohort study of Brazilian women. Hum Reprod. 2003;18:756-9.

23. Brosens I, Gordts S, Benagiano G. Endometriosis in adolescents is a hidden, progressive and severe disease that deserves attention, not just compassion. Hum Reprod. 2013;28:2026-31.

24. Kalu E, McAuley W, Richardson R. Teenagers, adolescents, endometriosis and recurrence: a retrospective analysis of recurrence following primary operative laparoscopy. Gynecol Surg. 2008;5:209-12.

25. Vasquez G, Cornillie F, Brosens IA. Peritoneal endometriosis: scanning electron microscopy and histology of minimal pelvic endometriotic lesions. Fertil Steril. 1984;42(5):696-703.

26. Evers JL. The second-look laparoscopy for evaluation of the result of medical treatment of endometriosis should not be performed during ovarian suppression. Fertil Steril. 1987;47:502-4.

27. Campo R, Gordts S, Rombauts L, et al. Diagnostic accuracy of transvaginal hydrolaparoscopy in infertility. Fertil Steril. 1999;71:1157-60.

28. Murphy AA, Green WR, Bobbie D, et al. Unsuspected endometriosis documented by scanning electron microscopy in visually normal peritoneum. Fertil Steril. 1986;46(3):522-4.

29. Nisolle M, Paindaveine B, Bourdon A, et al. Histologic study of peritoneal endometriosis in infertile women. Fertil Steril. 1990;53(6):984-8.

30. Balasch J, Creus M, Fábregues F, et al. Visible and non-visible endometriosis at laparoscopy in fertile and infertile women and in patients with chronic pelvic pain: a prospective study Hum Reprod. 1996;11(2):387-91.

31. Marcoux S, Maheux R, Berube S. Laparoscopic surgery in infertile women with minimal or mild endometriosis. The Canadian Collaborative Group on endometriosis. N Engl J Med. 1997;337:217-22.

32. Parazzini F. Ablation of lesions or no treatment in minimal-mild endometriosis in infertile women: a randomized trial. Gruppo Italiano per lo Studio dell'Endometriosi. Hum Reprod. 1999;14:1332-4.

33. Olive DL, Pritts EA. The treatment of endometriosis: a review of the evidence. Ann N Y Acad Sci. 2002;955:360-72.

34. Brosens IA, Puttemans PJ, Deprest J. The endoscopic localization of endometrial implants in the ovarian chocolate cyst. Fertil Steril. 1994;61:1034-38.

35. Darwish AM, Amin AF, El-Feky MA. Ovarioscopy, a technique to determine the nature of cystic ovarian tumors. J Am Assoc Gynecol Laparosc. 2000;7:539-44.

36. Fukunaga M. Smooth muscle metaplasia in ovarian endometriosis. Histopathology. 2000;36:348-52.

37. Kuroda M, Kuroda K, Arakawa A, et al. Histological assessment of impact of ovarian endometrioma and laparoscopic cystectomy on ovarian reserve. J Obstet Gynaecol Res. 2012;38:1187-93.

38. Kitajima M, Defrère S, Dolmans MM, et al. Endometriomas as a possible cause of reduced ovarian reserve in women with endometriosis. Fertil Steril. 2011;96(3):685-91.

39. Schubert B, Canis M, Darcha C, et al. Human ovarian tissue from cortex surrounding benign cysts: a model to study ovarian tissue cryopreservation. Hum Reprod. 2005;20:1786-92.

40. Pacchiarotti A, Frati P, Milazzo GN, et al. Evaluation of serum anti-Mullerian hormone levels to assess the ovarian reserve in women with severe endometriosis. Eur J Obstet Gynecol Reprod Biol. 2014;172:62-4.

41. Adamson GD, Hurd S, Pasta D. Laparoscopic endometriosis treatment: is it better? Fertil Steril. 1993;59:35-44.

42. Donnez J, Nisolle M, Gillet N, et al. Large ovarian endometriomas. Hum Reprod. 1996;11:641-6.

43. Murphy A, Schlaff W, Hassiakos D, et al. Laparoscopic cautery in the treatment of endometriosis-related infertility. Fertil Steril. 1991;55:246-51.

44. Coccia MA, Rizzello F, Mariani G, et al. Ovarian surgery for bilateral endometriomas influences age at menopause. Hum Reprod. 2011;26(11):3000-7.

45. Takae S, Kawamura K, Sato Y, et al. Analysis of late onset ovarian insufficiency after ovarian surgery: retrospective study with 75 patients of post-surgical ovarian insufficiency. PLoS One. 2014;5:1-6.

46. Hart R, Hickey M, Maouris P, et al. Excisional surgery versus ablative surgery for ovarian endometriomata: a Cochrane Review. Hum Reprod. 2005;20:3000-7.

47. Donnez J, Squifflet J, Donnez O. Minimally invasive gynecologic procedures. Curr Opin Obstet Gynecol. 2011;23:289-95.

48. Roman H1, Auber M, Mokdad C, et al. Ovarian endometrioma ablation using plasma energy versus cystectomy: a step toward better preservation of the ovarian parenchyma in women wishing to conceive. Fertil Steril. 2011;96:1396-400.

49. Donnez J, Lousse JC, Jadoul P, et al. Laparoscopic management of endometriomas using a combined technique of excisional (cystectomy) and ablative surgery. Fertil Steril. 2010;94(1):28-32.

50. Tsolakidis D, Pados G, Vavilis D, et al. The impact on ovarian reserve after laparoscopic ovarian cystectomy versus three-stage management in patients with endometriomas: a prospective randomized study. Fertil Steril. 2010;94(1):71-7.

51. Donnez J, Squifflet J, Donnez O. Minimally invasive gynecologic procedures. Curr Opin Obstet Gynecol. 2011;23(4):289-95.

52. Chen Y, Pei H, Chang Y, et al. The impact of endometrioma and laparoscopic cystectomy on ovarian reserve and the exploration of related factors assessed by serum anti-Mullerian hormone: a prospective cohort study. J Ovarian Res. 2014;7:108.

53. Garcia-Velasco JA, Somigliana E. Management of endometriomas in women requiring IVF: to touch or not to touch. Hum Reprod. 2009;24(3):496-501.

54. Ueda Y, Enomoto T, Miyatake T, et al. A retrospective analysis of ovarian endometriosis during pregnancy. Fertil Steril. 2010;94:78-84.

55. Ahmad G, Duffy JM, Farquhar C, et al. Barrier agents for adhesion prevention after gynecological surgery. Cochrane Database Syst Rev. 2008;(2):CD000475.

56. Metwally M, Cheong Y, Li TC. A review of techniques for adhesion prevention after gynaecological surgery. Curr Opin Obstet Gynecol. 2008;20(4):345-52.

57. Seracchioli R, Di Donato N, Bertoldo V, et al. The role of ovarian suspension in endometriosis surgery: a randomized controlled trial. J Minim Invasive Gynecol. 2014;21(6):1029-35.

58. Pellicano M, Giampaolino P, Tommaselli GA, et al. Efficacy of ovarian suspension to round ligament with a resorbable suture to prevent postoperative adhesions in women with ovarian endometrioma: follow-up by transvaginal hydrolaparoscopy. Gynecol Surg. 2014;11:261-6.

59. Gordts S, Campo R, Puttemans P, et al. Transvaginal access: a safe technique for tubo-ovarian exploration in infertility? Review of the literature. Gynecol Surg. 2008;5:187-91.

60. Gordts S, Campo R, Brosens I. Experience with transvaginal hydrolaparoscopy for reconstructive tubo-ovarian surgery. Reprod Biomed Online. 2002;4(3):72-5.

61. Dunselman G, Vermeulen N, Becker C, et al. ESHRE guideline: management of women with endometriosis. Hum Reprod. 2014;29(3):400-12.

62. Gordts S, Puttemans P, Gordts S, et al. Ovarian endometrioma in the adolescent: a plea for early-stage diagnosis and full surgical treatment. Gynecol Surg. 2014. (in press.)

63. Tanos V, Bigatti G, Paschopoulos M, et al. Transvaginal endoscopy: new technique evaluating female infertility. Three Mediterranean countries' experiences. Gynecol Surg. 2005;2:241-3.

CHAPTER 14

Laparoscopic Colposuspension

Guenter K Noé

■ INTRODUCTION

The lateral repair and colposuspension are accepted methods for the repair of paravaginal defects and the treatment of female incontinence. Several open or vaginal approaches have been described, but there is still no standardized, reproducible laparoscopic technique. Thus only a few clinics perform the laparoscopic approach although it offers several advantages compared to open or vaginal surgery.

The major form of a cystocele is originated from a midline defect of the cystovaginal fascia. A reduction of the vaginal rugae is a clinical sign for this type of cystocele.

In 1909, White described another type of cystocele with sustained rugae.[1] This defect we find more lateral and characterized by elapsed sulci. White called this type of a cystocele "lateral" or "paravaginal" defect. The anatomic correlate is a rupture or a dilatation of the adjacent fascia. Although White suggested a vaginal approach containing a suture as an effective therapy for a durable repair, this method could not accomplish until Richardson revived this method.[2] Richardson described four predilection areas: the arcus tendineus (lateral defect), the midline (classical cystocele), the pubovesical fascia (transversal defect) and the ureterocele (distal defect).

Various open and vaginal approaches have been reported.[3-6] The laparoscopic approach came into focus during the last decade. Success rates of about 90 percent have been reported in some articles but there is a lack of controlled trials.[5,7] According to our experience the repair of the lateral defect and the stabilization of the paraurethral tissue can be performed laparoscopicaly with a high success rate and a high satisfaction rate of the patients.

■ INDICATION

We use the colposuspension as a first choice for the surgical therapy of stress urinary incontinence (SUI). The second indication is a clinical relevant cystocele because of a lateral defect. Relevant means symptoms like vaginal pressure, sexual difficulty or associated symptoms of the urinary bladder (urinary incontinence or overactive bladder). Often we combine the technique with other surgical procedures according to the stage and type of the prolapse. A perineal ultrasound is performed regularly to differentiate the forms of the vaginal prolapse. It helps to use reproducible reference points in order to compare the preoperative and postoperative situation. In literature, the assessment of the extension of the paravaginal defect is via ultrasound by the relation of the vesical floor and the lower edge of the symphysis pubis as a reference point is required.[8,9] Most important are at least the physical examination and the anamnesis of the patient. To avoid overcorrection, it is important not to cure the anatomy but the complaints of the patient.

If only a treatment of SUI or the "lateral defect" alone is required, we perform the procedure completely retroperitoneal. If the colposuspension is combined with other procedures, it is performed as a last step.

■ PREOPERATIVE TREATMENT

We never use a special diet or bowel preparation. A subcutaneous injection of an antithrombotic agent is given routinely but no prophylactic antibiotics are used.

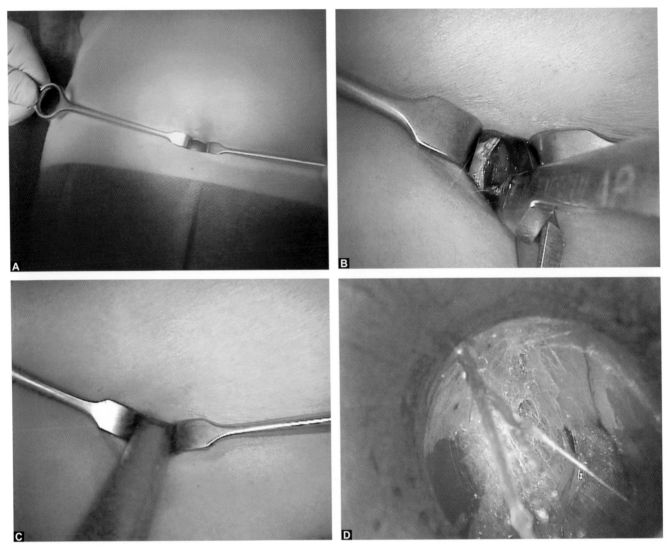

Figs 1A to D: (A) Umbilical incision; (B) Extension of the fascia; (C) Access port 10 mm; (D) Blunt preparation

Preparation in the Theater

The patient is placed in a dorsal lithotomy position with both arms tucked to her side. A 16-F catheter with a 5 mL balloon tip is inserted into the bladder and attached to a continuous drainage. The catheter remains until the next morning to avoid an overflow bladder.

Procedure

Step One

As mentioned the beginning of the procedure is different according to the accompanying surgery. If the colposuspension is performed, alone it is carried out completely retroperitoneal. Therefore, an incision is made in the lower two-thirds of the umbilicus. With a clamp or

small hooks, we retract the wound and open the two fascial layers. When we reach the retroperitoneal fatty tissue, a 10 mm port is bluntly pushed in the direction of the symphysis (Figs 1A to D).

Routinely two additional 5 mm ports are inserted. The placement is 2 to 3 cm superior the symphysis in the midline and 2 to 4 cm medial and inferior the anterior superior ischiatic spine on the left side. In a difficult field, a third port can be placed on the right side either. The CO_2 insufflation follows to an intra-abdominal pressure of 10–12 mm Hg.

When another procedure is performed first, the left access port is pushed back behind the peritoneum and a grasper is inserted. Now it is possible to perform a blunt preparation retroperitoneal in the direction of the umbilicus. In most cases, it is possible to reach the camera port, push back the peritoneum with the optic and insufflate

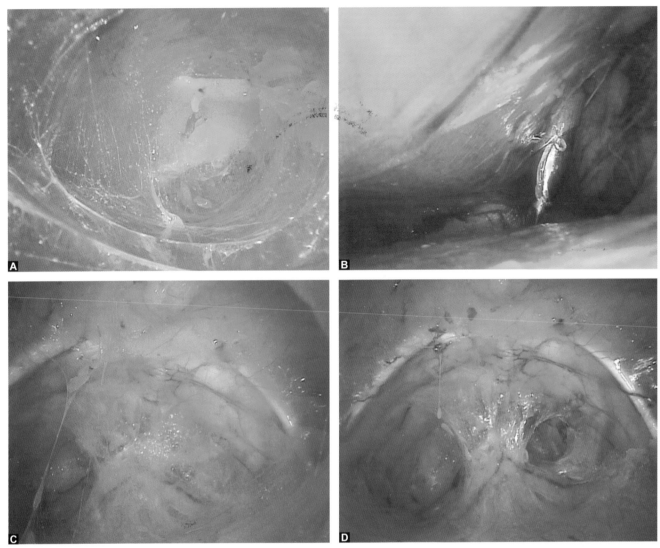

Figs 2A to D: (A) Extension of space of rezius; (B) Introducing midline access port; (C) Identification of the symphysis; (D) Preparation of ligament and pubovesical fascia

the retroperitoneum. Now the midline access port is retracted and with an additional grasper, the preparation of the space of Retzius is performed (Figs 2A and B).

Step Two

With a bipolar grasper, the iliopectineal (Cooper) ligament and the paravaginal fascia are cleared. The visualization of the ligament is to perform thoroughly to avoid orientation problems while the later stitching (Figs 2C and D). The complete clearing of the fascia is performed later when the left hand is inserted into the vagina.

Step Three

According to the planed procedure (incontinence or cystocele), a 2-0 nonabsorbable woven suture of 45–60 cm length is inserted through the 10 mm port. The first stich is performed caudal at the Cooper's ligament. The thread is prepared with nods at the end so that it is not necessary to perform nod tying. The suspension is performed with a running suture. The stitches in the paravaginal fascia as well as the traction of the tissue are controlled by the left hand in the vagina. To treat incontinence we perform three stitches triangular, laterally of the urethra (Figs 3A and B).

According to the degree of the defect we perform additional stitches (3–6) and combine it with a gathering of the fascia if there is a lot of widened material (Figs 4A and B).

It is useful to clear the fascia with a bipolar clamp when the hand is in the vagina. Therefore, the surgeon gets a good control of the thickness of the tissue. The preparation should always been performed from lateral to the middle.

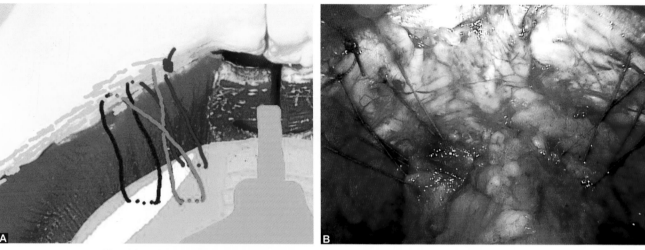

Figs 3A and B: (A) Suspention triangular in the paraurethral fascia; (B) Laparoscopic view of 3A

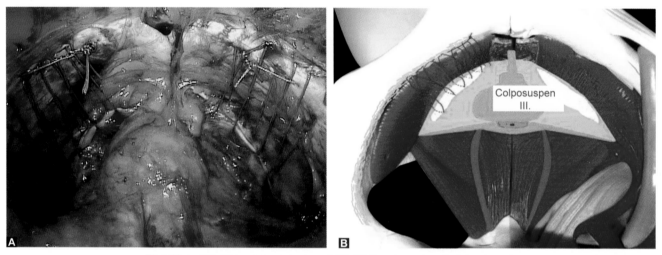

Figs 4A and B: (A) Laparoscopic view of 4B; (B) Running suture for lateral repair

Step Four

Needles can be removed through the abdominal wall. A closure of the peritoneum is not necessary. After careful hemostasis the ports are removed and the CO_2 gas is sucked off.

■ POSTOPERATIVE TREATMENT

The catheter is removed in the morning of the first postoperative day. We routinely perform an ultrasound of the bladder after urinating the next day.

We have an experience by more than 400 procedures. The mean operation time is 30–40 minutes. We had two hematomas, which had to be removed. One bladder defect had to be sutured. In a small study with 55 patients, we found a cure rate of 98% after a mean time of 29 months.[6]

The running suture provides a good traction control and the opportunity to perform a correction. The technique is executable with three ports and less foreign material. As we have a good experience, the colposuspension is our first choice for the treatment of SUI and the lateral defect.

■ REFERENCES

1. White GR. Cystocele—a radical cure by suturing lateral sulci of the vagina to the white line of pelvic fascia. 1909. Int Urogynecol J Pelvic Floor Dysfunct. 1997;8(5):288-92.

2. Richardson AC, Edmonds PB, Williams NL. Treatment of stress urinary incontinence due to paravaginal fascial defect. Obstet Gynecol. 1981;57(3):357-62.

3. Young SB, Daman JJ, Bony LG. Vaginal paravaginal repair: one-year outcomes. Am J Obstet Gynecol. 2001;185(6):1360-6. discussion 1366-7.

4. Demirci F, Ozdemir I, Somunkiran A, et al. Abdominal paravaginal defect repair in the treatment of paravaginal defect and urodynamic stress incontinence. J Obstet Gynaecol. 2007;27(6):601-4.

5. Miklos JR, Kohli N. Laparoscopic paravaginal repair plus burch colposuspension: review and descriptive technique. Urology. 2000;56(6 Suppl 1):64-9.

6. Banerjee C, Noe KG. Endoscopic cystocele surgery: lateral repair with combined suture/mesh technique. J Endourol. 2010;24(10):1565-9. discussion 1569.

7. Behnia-Willison F, Seman EI, Cook JR, et al. Laparoscopic paravaginal repair of anterior compartment prolapse. J Minim Invasive Gynecol. 2007;14(4):475-80.

8. Martan A, Masata J, Halaska M, et al. Ultrasound imaging of paravaginal defects in women with stress incontinence before and after paravaginal defect repair. Ultrasound Obstet Gynecol. 2002;19(5):496-500.

9. Ostrzenski A, Osborne NG, Ostrzenska K. Method for diagnosing paravaginal defects using contrast ultrasonographic technique. J Ultrasound Med. 1997;16(10):673-7.

Section 4

SPECIAL SITUATIONS FOR MINIMALLY INVASIVE APPROACH

- Laparoscopic Subtotal Hysterectomy
- Laparoscopy in Pregnancy
- Non-Descent Vaginal Hysterectomy

"Intelligence is the ability to adapt to change."

Stephen Hawking

CHAPTER 15

Laparoscopic Subtotal Hysterectomy

Ibrahim Alkatout, Liselotte Mettler

■ GENERAL INTRODUCTION

Hysterectomy is the most commonly performed gynecological surgical procedure. Nevertheless, the rates of hysterectomy appear to be decreasing, with a peak in 2002, possibly due to the advent of less invasive therapies for management of conditions previously treated with hysterectomy.

Once the decision has been made to proceed with hysterectomy, the surgeon and patient must decide whether the procedure will be performed abdominally, vaginally, or with laparoscopic or robotic assistance. The route chosen depends upon the woman's clinical circumstances and the surgeon's technical expertise. Furthermore, the surgeons personal preference also plays a major role. Within today's multiple treatment possibilities for myomas/fibroids as surgical, medical or interventional imaging advances, there is still some room left for total hysterectomy (TH) and subtotal hysterectomy (SH) (Fig. 1). Laparoscopic hysterectomy was first performed in 1989. The impetus for trying a new approach to a common gynecologic procedure was to reduce the morbidity and mortality of abdominal hysterectomy to the level observed with vaginal hysterectomy. Particularly the laparoscopic approach for both techniques on the benign side as well as for radical hysterectomies in malignancies of the genital tract becomes more accepted and important. As it is less the invasive procedure, indicated patients with myomas and/or bleeding disorders can consider a subtotal approach [laparoscopic subtotal hysterectomy (LSH)]. However, only laparoscopic total hysterectomies (LTH) can protect 100% from new fibroid formations, avoid later cervix carcinoma or sarcoma formation, uncontrolled bleedings or any other problems arising from the uterus.

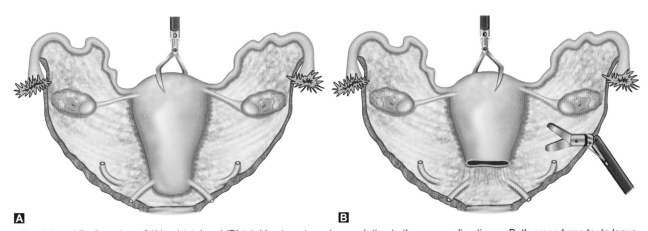

Figs 1A and B: Overview of (A) subtotal and (B) total hysterectomy in correlation to the surrounding tissue. Both procedures try to leave out the sacrouterine ligaments

ETIOLOGY

The etiology of fibroid formation remains unclear in spite of numerous theories. Nevertheless, a genetic disposition must be given, as Africans have in a much higher frequency of multiple myomas than Caucasians. Although certain upregulations and downregulations in the genes of patients with and without myomas have been described, no clear prevention for fibroids is available. It is known that patients who have close relatives with fibroids are more likely to develop fibroids themselves (family aggregation). In some patients, fibroids are clustered with other disorders. Hereditary leiomyomatosis and renal cell carcinoma syndrome is a rare syndrome involving fibroids. Individuals with the gene that leads to both fibroids and skin leiomyomas are at increased risk for a rare case of kidney cell cancer (papillary renal cell carcinoma).

Understanding which genes are involved in fibroids do not automatically tell us why fibroids develop or how to control them. From our understanding of fibroid behavior, we would guess that genes involved in estrogen or progesterone production, metabolism, or action would be involved. There are also small variations called polymorphisms in genes that may play a role in influencing the risk of fibroids. Both polymorphisms and mutations are changes in the sequence of genes, but the difference is in the degree of change.

THE GENETICS OF FIBROIDS, GENOTYPE AND PHENOTYPE

The discovery of the structure of DNA (deoxyribonucleic acid) by Watson and Crick revolutionized biology and medicine. They discovered that DNA carries the code for life in a ladder-like structure and the genes from a single person has been found to take up the space of 400,000 times the distance from the earth to the moon or 1,000 times the distance from the earth to the sun = 150 billion kilometers.[1-3]

We believe that fibroids are a common phenotype that represents many different underlying genotypes. In other words, in our view, fibroids can arise through multiple different pathways. This information would be most helpful in advances of treatment, so that the woman who carried a high-risk of recurrent fibroids and had completed their family might even choose to have a hysterectomy because their chance of having an additional surgery was so high. We currently have some clinical information (based on physicians' clinical experience with many patients) to predict prognosis for recurrence after abdominal myomectomy, but our clinical information for alternative forms of treatment options is limited.

Finally, understanding the underlying genotype would open up important possibilities for the future. It may, for example, point two ways in which women can modify their risk of disease and lead to prevention of disease. If, for example, a major protein involved in body fat metabolism was found to be abnormally sensitive in women with fibroids, weight loss or preventing weight gain might be an effective strategy for decreasing the risk of fibroids. Now, new therapies can be developed that are targeted to specific abnormalities.

Studies of women with fibroids suggest several reasons to suspect that genes play a role in fibroid formation. The first is that both women in a pair of identical twins are twice as likely to have had a hysterectomy as both women in a pair of fraternal (nonidentical) twins. This suggests that the genes that identical twins share make them more likely to form fibroids, since both identical and nonidentical twins have equal exposure to environmental factors. This difference between identical and fraternal twins has been observed in a general population of women undergoing hysterectomy and a population of women with fibroids leading to hysterectomy.[4,5]

There is also evidence that women who have close relatives, such as a mother or sister, with fibroids are much more likely to have fibroids themselves.[6,7] This propensity is called familial aggregation.

Understanding which genes are involved in fibroids do not automatically tell us why fibroids develop or how to control them. From our understanding of fibroid behavior, we would guess that genes involved in estrogen or progesterone production, metabolism, or action would be involved.[8-11]

MICROSCOPIC FACTS AND FIBROID VIABILITY

Fibroids are composed primarily of smooth muscle cells. The uterus, stomach and bladder are all organs made of smooth muscle. Smooth muscle cells are arranged so that the organ can stretch, instead of being arranged in rigid units like the cells in skeletal. In women with fibroids, tissue from the endometrium typically looks normal under the microscope. Sometimes, however, there is an unusual type of uterine lining over submucosal fibroids that do not have the normal glandular structures. The presence of this abnormality, called aglandular functionalis, in women having bleeding disorders, is sometimes a clinical clue for their doctors to look more closely for a submucosal fibroid.[12] A second pattern of endometrium, termed chronic endometritis, can also suggest that there may be a submucosal fibroid, although this pattern can also be associated with other problems such as retained products of conception and various infections of the uterus. Once we move beyond hysterectomy as a one-size-fits-all solution to fibroids, distinctions in size, position and appearance will likely be important for treating fibroids.

COSTS OF FIBROIDS

In fact, accurately capturing all the costs attributable to uterine fibroids will help us move toward more effective and innovative therapies. When deciding whether to launch a new concept, companies typically look at the amount currently spent for other treatments. The economics of fibroids has chiefly been discussed in terms of the health care costs of hysterectomy. This in itself is a huge amount of money. According to a recent estimate, in the United States, more than $2 billion every year is spent on hospitalization costs due to uterine fibroids alone.[13] Additionally, one study estimates that the healthcare costs due to uterine fibroids are more than $4,600 per woman per year.[14]

When you incorporate all the costs of fibroids, however, the total is even more significant.

❑ The costs of myomectomy, uterine artery embolization (UAE) and other minimally invasive therapies
❑ The costs of birth control pills and other hormonal treatments to control bleeding
❑ The costs of tampons, pads, and the adult diapers, many women require to contain the bleeding
❑ The costs of alternative and complementary therapies
❑ The cost of doing nothing (for many women, this means missing work or working less productively during their period).

Why should a patient have a hysterectomy today when so many alterative treatment structures are given? Firstly, up to a certain size of the enlarged uterus, laparoscopic subtotal hysterectomy completely solves the problem and if women want to eliminate every risk of recurrent fibroids, hysterectomy is their only choice. Of course, hysterectomy also eliminates coexisting problems such as adenomyosis, endometriosis and endometrial polyps or cervical dysplasia.

WILL THE OVARIES BE REMOVED OR LEFT IN PLACE?

The ovaries generally are not removed when a hysterectomy is performed for uterine fibroids. Removing the uterus alone will cure the bleeding and the size-related symptoms caused by the fibroids. Removing the ovaries is, thus, not required in treating fibroids as it is sometimes for other diseases like endometriosis or gynecologic cancers.

Many physicians were taught that at a set age (which varies between 35 and 50) women should be told that removal of the ovaries is recommended as part of the surgery, with the speculation of "while we are there, we may as well". The general teaching had been that ovaries do not have any function after menopause and the risk of ovarian cancer increases with increasing age, so removing the ovaries near the time of menopause was a no-lose proposition. This was especially true if hormone replacement therapy could be used to help younger women transition to the time when they would naturally go through menopause.

However, recent research suggests that although after menopause the ovaries do not make much estradiol, they make a tremendous amount of androgens.[15] It is thought that these androgens may be important in maintaining mood and sex drive.[16-18] In addition, the risks of hormone replacement have become clearer, and many women choose to use hormones following menopause.[19,20] However, it is not widely known that the risks for postmenopausal complications after hormone replacement are lower for women without a uterus, who are able to take estrogen alone.[20] Recently, the association of premature loss of ovarian function and the increasing risk of heart disease has also been explored.[21]

Considering all these factors, there are good reasons to retain the ovaries, if possible.

RESECTION OF FALLOPIAN TUBES IN CASES OF HYSTERECTOMY

Once the reproductive function is completed, the tubes of a female should be removed within the reproductive age. Beyond the reproductive age, tubes should always be removed with the uterus while ovaries, as previously discussed, are routinely removed only above the age of 65 years.

According to new research presented today at the Annual Clinical Meeting of the American College of Obstetricians and Gynecologists, bilateral salpingectomy during hysterectomy while preserving the ovaries is considered a safe way of potentially reducing the development of ovarian serous carcinoma. Removing the Fallopian tubes does not cause the onset of menopause, as does the removal of the ovaries.

Furthermore, prophylactic removal of the Fallopian tubes during hysterectomy or sterilization would rule out any subsequent tubal pathology, such as hydrosalpinx, which is observed in up to 30% of women after hysterectomy. Women undergoing hysterectomy with retained Fallopian tubes or sterilization have at least a doubled risk of subsequent salpingectomy. Removal of the Fallopian

Table 1: Broad diagnostic categories of indications for hysterectomy

Uterine leiomyomas
Pelvic organ prolapse
Pelvic pain or infection (e.g. endometriosis, pelvic inflammatory diseases)
Abnormal uterine bleeding
Malignant and premalignant disease

tubes at hysterectomy should, therefore, generally be recommended.[22,23]

There are five broad diagnostic categories of indications for hysterectomy (Table 1).

TOTAL VERSUS SUBTOTAL (SUPRACERVICAL) HYSTERECTOMY

Some women desire to retain the cervix believing that it may affect sexual satisfaction after hysterectomy. It has been postulated that removal of the cervix causes excessive neurologic and anatomic disruption, thereby leading to increased operative and postoperative morbidity, vaginal shortening, subsequent vault prolapse, abnormal cuff granulations and the potential for Fallopian tube prolapse. These issues were addressed in a systematic review of three randomized trials that evaluated TH versus SH for benign gynecological conditions, which reported the following findings:

❑ There was no difference in the rates of incontinence, constipation or measures of sexual function (sexual satisfaction and dyspareunia).
❑ Length of surgery and amount of blood lost during surgery were significantly reduced during SH compared with TH, but there was no difference in the likelihood of transfusion.
❑ Febrile morbidity was less likely and ongoing cyclical vaginal bleeding one year after surgery was more likely after SH.
❑ There was no difference in the rates of other complications, recovery from surgery, or readmission rates.

In the short-term, randomized trials have shown that cervical preservation or removal does not affect the rate of subsequent pelvic organ prolapse.

There is an opinion that the cervix absolutely does not need to be removed to cure the symptoms caused by uterine fibroids. The advantage of the cervix left in place is that cardinal and uterosacral ligaments remain in place.

Advantages to supracervical hysterectomy include shorter operative time than total abdominal hysterectomy, decreased length of hospital stay if performed laparoscopically. Some studies have reported a shorter recovery period following SH, but this finding is not supported by data from randomized trials. In a prospective cohort study, supracervical hysterectomy was associated with greater improvement in short-term quality of life scores compared with TH, but no differences were found in postoperative pain or return to daily activities. There may also be fewer injuries to the urinary tract because the procedure does not dissect as close to the cervix or as deep into the pelvis as TH. However, clinical trials have not been sufficiently powered to demonstrate this clinical observation.

Other differences include posthysterectomy body image and health status. In a randomized, nonblinded study of women undergoing TH versus SH, the patients completed questionnaires regarding postoperative quality of life, body image and sexual activity. Women in the SH versus the TH group reported significantly improved body image and health-related quality of life. Both groups reported improvements in sexual satisfaction.

The only absolute contraindication to SH is the presence of a malignant or premalignant condition of the uterine corpus or cervix. Extensive endometriosis is a relative contraindication as these women may have persistence of dyspareunia if the cervix is retained.

The risks and benefits of retaining the cervix should be included as part of the preoperative informed consent. We suggest that women should be informed that retaining the cervix does not appear to confer any medical or sexual benefits. Although the vagina receives some part of its lubrication from the cervical glands (in addition to transudate through the vaginal walls), there is no evidence that TH versus SH adversely affects vaginal lubrication or leads to dyspareunia. Disadvantages of conserving the cervix include cyclic vaginal bleeding in some patients (7 to 11%), the need for routine screening for cervical cancer, and the potential need for subsequent trachelectomy (e.g. because of bleeding, prolapse, or precancer/cancer). Thus, on balance, there is no compelling reason to retain the cervix if it can be easily removed with the corpus.

Elective supracervical hysterectomy should be preceded by cervical cytology confirming absence of cervical intraepithelial neoplasia. Women who have had a supracervical hysterectomy should be screened for cervical cancer according to standard guidelines for their age and risk status. In women with abnormal uterine bleeding, endometrial cancer should be excluded prior to performing a supracervical hysterectomy.

For an overview, see Table 2.

Table 2: Vaginal versus abdominal versus laparoscopic hysterectomy

Vaginal hysterectomy compared to abdominal hysterectomy

Shorter hospitalization (mean difference 1 day, 95% CI 0.7–1.2)

Speedier return to normal activities (mean difference 9.5 days, 95% CI 6.4–12.6)

Fewer infections or fevers [odds ratio (OR) 0.42, 95% CI 0.21–0.83]

Laparoscopic hysterectomy compared to abdominal hysterectomy

Less blood loss (mean difference 45.3 minutes, 95% CI 17.9–72.7)

Shorter hospital stay (mean difference 2 days, 95% CI 1.9–2.2)

Speedier return to normal activities (mean difference 13.6 days, 95% CI 11.8–15.4)

Fewer wound infections or fevers (OR 0.32, 95% CI 0.12–0.85)

Longer operating time (mean difference 10.6 minutes, 95% CI 7.4–13.8)

More urinary tract injuries (OR 2.61, 95% CI 1.22–5.60)

Laparoscopic hysterectomy compared to vaginal hysterectomy

Similar outcomes except longer operating time (mean difference 41.5 minutes, 95% CI 33.7–49.4)

Total laparoscopic hysterectomy compared to laparoscopically assisted vaginal hysterectomy

Similar outcomes except longer operating time (mean difference 25.3 minutes, 95% CI 10–40.6)

Supracervical hysterectomy—laparoscopic supracervical hysterectomy (LSH) was first described by the present author in 1990.[24] At approximately the same time, another type of subtotal hysterectomy, the classic intrafascial Semm hysterectomy (CISH) was described by Kurt Semm.[25] These two procedures are performed differently and will be described separately.

LSH is performed in an identical fashion to TLH, but after occluding the ascending uterine vascular pedicles, the cervix is amputated in a coring fashion, beginning at the level of the internal os, down into the endocervical canal.

The CISH procedure requires a combined vaginal and laparoscopic technique, using the serrated-edge macromorcellator (SEMM) device to core out the uterine canal from below while applying endoloops around the lower segment of the uterus to control bleeding from the uterine vessels.[8] Upper pedicles are traditionally suture ligated using laparoscopic suturing techniques. Alternatively, cutter/stapling devices or bipolar vessel sealing/cutting devices may be used to occlude the upper vascular supplies.

Operative Technique

General Aspects

Until we have long-term outcome studies, every patient will need to make an informed decision along with her doctor to be executed based on individual needs and availability. A woman who routinely undergoes preventive medical care is a better candidate for a LSH than a woman who is unlikely to go for a Pap smear annually following LSH. Likewise, if pressure against the cervix is a critical part of a woman's sexual response—very few women are aware of this—an LSH may be a better choice. We counsel woman that there is a chance of formation of cervical fibroids following a subtotal/supracervical hysterectomy although this is really a small risk. Sometimes, the cervix needs to be removed surgically later in separate procedure. Being aware, however, of a less invasive procedure in the beginning, this is accepted easily. For patients who want to really minimize their chances of later surgeries, a laparoscopic total hysterectomy (LTH) may be preferable. Furthermore, suspicion of adenomyosis uteri is an important factor for the decision toward LTH, as we know that the risk of persisting bleeding and dysmenorrhea is higher after LSH with the detection of adenomyosis. In all hysterectomies, there must be an antibiotic coverage, e.g. with a cephalosporin in second generation. The antibiotic should be applied about 30 minutes before the start of the operation.

Preoperative Preparation

The exclusion of any cervical pathology or infection is important. Endometriotic lesions around the cervix require cervical resection along with the uterus as a part of LTH. The patient has to be ready for regular gynecologic screening twice a year.

Instruments and Equipment

The instrument set consists of trocars, a uterine manipulator (for LTH only), needle holders, a cutting electrique loop, sutures and a morcellator. In addition to the basic set of laparoscopic instruments, there is a requirement of a coagulation or thermofusion device with integrated knife, graspers, scissors, biopsy forceps and window forceps and a suction irrigation unit. If a robotic set up is available, the instruments have to be adjusted.

Prerequisites

Stable health condition, indication for myomectomy-hysterectomy, full consent of the patient after detailed explanation of the operative procedure. A large uterus or a uterus with multiple myomas is no contraindication for a laparoscopic procedure. Solely, the placement of the trocars might be set higher in the abdominal wall and there might be a need of more than the usually used two ancillary trocars. The use of a uterine manipulator is not necessary but can be very helpful.

Steps of Surgery

Port Placement

According to the size of the uterus with the fibroids, the trocar placement points are selected.

Once the cutaneous region has been determined from the outside with the aid of diaphanoscopy, the safe distance to the plica umbilicalis lateralis can be verified by palpation. The correct point of insertion is usually about two thumbs medial of the anterior superior iliac spine. Being distant to the plica, the trocar is placed at a 90° angle and pushed forward until the tip of the trocar can be seen with the laparoscope (Figs 2A to D).

Precondition for safe trocar insertion is the elevation of the abdominal wall by means of a sufficient pneumoperitoneum (excluding blind entry without pneumoperitoneum). Therefore, an extensive insufflation pressure up to 20 mm Hg can be tolerated.

Optic Trocar

Insertion of the optic trocar is performed in two steps. During the first step, a 5 mm optic trocar and laparoscope are inserted to confirm the correct pneumoperitoneum and the absence of local adhesions. In the second step, dilation to 10 mm occurs, either under sight or blindly, which guarantees an optimal overview during all operations.

First Step: Entry is performed by a Z technique in the following manner: After proceeding with the trocar forward horizontally for about 1.5 cm, the tip of the trocar is moved to the right at a 90° angle for about 1.5 cm. After lifting the abdominal wall in the same manner as when inserting the Veress needle, the trocar is screwed with the dominant hand straight into the abdominal wall at a 90° angle, toward the hollow of the os sacrum.

The sign for correct placement of the trocar is the hissing sound created when gas escapes through the open valve of the trocar. The obturator is then removed and the trocar is held in place. Before dilating to 10 mm, a 5 mm laparoscope is introduced and rotated through 360° to check visually for any bleeding, intraabdominal abnormality and adherent bowel loops. If there is concern that the bowel might be adherent in the umbilical region, the primary trocar site

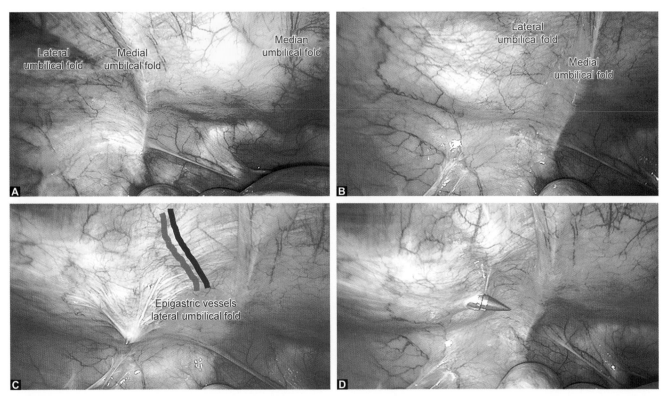

Figs 2A to D: Secondary trocar placement, left lower abdominal entry. (A) The three different plicae are visualized; (B) The palpating finger is showing the area lateral to the lateral umbilical fold; (C) Entry of the sharp ancillary trocar laterally to the lateral umbilical fold; (D) Once the peritoneum is penetrated, the trocar is heading to the fundus of the uterus to avoid injuring of the major vessels and bowel

needs to be visualized from a secondary port site, e.g. in the lower abdominal wall with a 5 mm laparoscope.

Second Step: A blunt palpation probe is placed in the 5 mm trocar and the shaft is pulled over the palpation probe and taken out. A 10 mm trocar is then screwed into the abdominal cavity.[26]

Ancillary Trocars

All ancillary trocars must be inserted with an intraabdominal pressure of 15–20 mm Hg under direct vision. The inferior epigastric vessels are visualized laparoscopically whereas the superficial vessels can be visualized by diaphanoscopy.

Once the tip of the trocar has pierced through the peritoneum, it should be angled in the direction of the uterine fundus under visual control until the port is placed correctly and the sharp tip can be removed.

Before any ancillary trocars are inserted, the patient is moved into the Trendelenburg position. Premature Trendelenburg position can also increase the risk of retroperitoneal vascular injury as the iliac vessels lay right in the axis of a preconceived 45° insertion angle, especially in thin patients with minimal retroperitoneal fat. The number of ancillary trocars is variable but they all must be inserted under direct view. If two working trocars are needed, they should be placed in the lower quadrant above the pubic hairline lateral to the deep epigastric vessels from the interior view. From the exterior view, the trocars are placed two fingers medial of the spina iliaca anterior superior. For safe insertion, the two major superficial vessels in this region have to be avoided. These are the superficial epigastric artery and the superficial circumflex iliac artery. These two superficial vessels can be visualized by diaphanoscopy. If a third ancillary trocar is needed, the suprapubic midline is the most common site. Diaphanoscopy cannot be relied upon to locate the deep vessels, especially in obese patients (Figs 2A to D and 3A to D).

Finger tapping from the outside can identify the right area of trocar placement, and a small skin incision should be made before the trocar sleeve is inserted. The trocars must be inserted by the shortest route at a 90° angle to the skin surface so that the risk of injuring structures on the way to the abdominal wall is minimized. For the use of trocars in the midline, the Foley catheter must be identified to avoid accidental bladder perforation.[24-26]

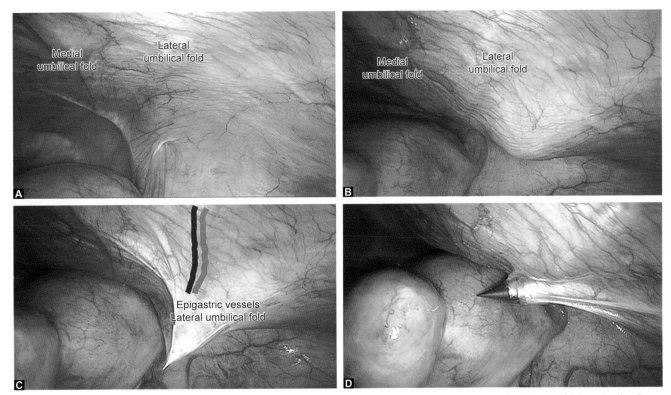

Figs 3A to D: Secondary trocar placement, right lower abdominal entry; (A) The three different plicae are visualized; (B) The palpating finger is showing the area lateral to the lateral umbilical fold; (C) Entry of the sharp ancillary trocar laterally to the lateral umbilical fold; (D) Once the peritoneum is penetrated the trocar is heading to the fundus of the uterus to avoid injuring of the major vessels and bowel

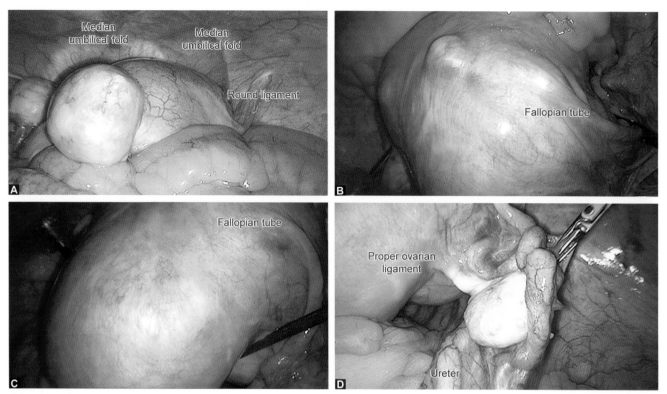

Figs 4A to D: First inspection of the uterus and the surrounding organs. The lower pelvis as well as the ligaments and vessels and the ureter can be differentiated in relation to the uterus

1. Laparoscopic Subtotal Hysterectomy

Steps of surgery

1.1. Inspection of the pelvis, tracing of the ureters and planning of the surgery (Figs 4A to D)

1.2. Pushing the uterus into the opposite direction of separating the adnexas or the ligaments from the pelvic side wall with the assistance of the intrauterine manipulator or by traction (Figs 4A to D and 5)

1.3. Division of the infundibulopelvic ligament and round ligament from the pelvic side wall or in cases the adnexas remain, division of the adnexas from the uterus (Figs 6 to 10)

1.4. Dissection of broad ligament: The broad ligament is opened and each leaf separately coagulated (Figs 11A to D and 12A to D). This is not possible if a sealing and cutting instrument is used as both leafs of the broad ligament are sealed together.

1.5. Separation of the bladder from the uterus by opening the vesicouterine ligament and pushing the bladder downward for about 1–2 cm (Figs 13A to D)

1.6. Presentation of the ramus ascendens of the uterine artery and division of uterine pedicles (Figs 14A to D)

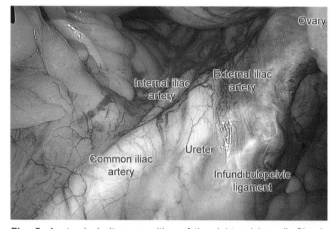

Fig. 5: Anatomical site recognition of the right pelvic wall. Clearly visible are the bifurcation of the common iliac artery and the crossing of the ureter. Lateral to ureter, the infundibulopelvic ligament is situated including the ovarian vessels. This ligament can be fixed to the bowel (especially on the left side) and cause problems in preparation of the adnexa

1.7. The same stepwise dissection of the left adnexas (Figs 15A to D and 16A to D), opening of the bladder peritoneum and broad ligament (Figs 17A to D) and dissection of uterine vessels (Figs 18 to 20) are performed on the left side, thorough inspection all around the cervix.

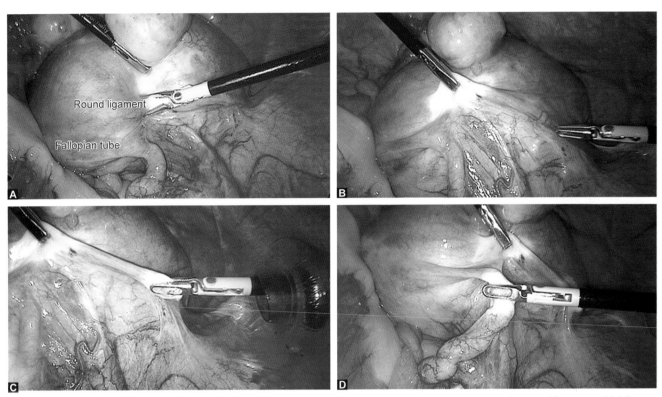

Figs 6A to D: Stepwise bipolar coagulation of right tube and right round ligament. Figures A and B show the round ligament, which is coagulated so that a sharp instrument can pull on the tissue without causing bleedings that worsen the sight

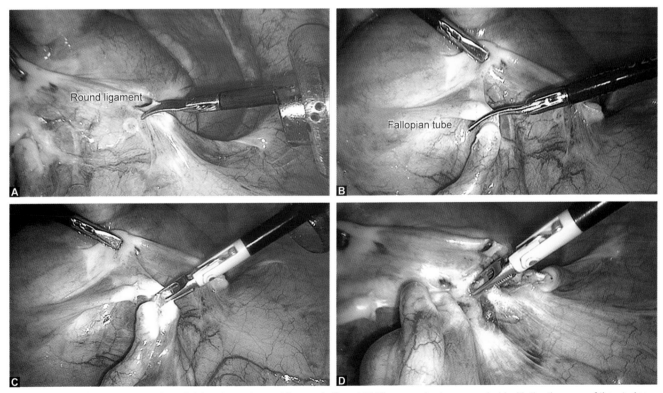

Figs 7A to D: Stepwise dissection of right tube and round ligament. (A and B) The curved scissors are held with the tip away of the uterine wall; (C and D) After dissecting the Fallopian tube, the underneath running vessels must be coagulated before further cutting

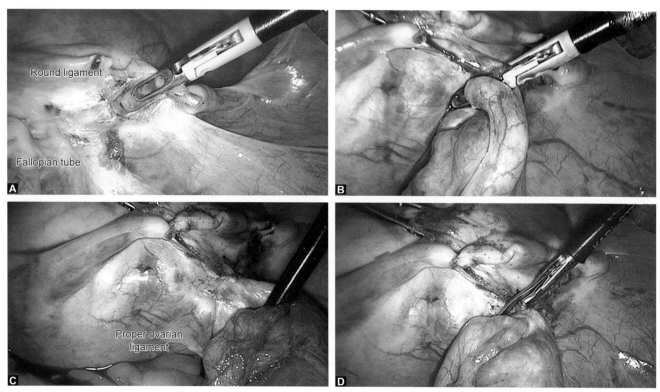

Figs 8A to D: Continuous stepwise dissection and beginning of opening the broad ligament. (A and C) With traction on the tissue, the line of preparation can easily be demarcated; (B and D) Coagulation is involving the whole tissue but the cutting line is strictly omitting the uterine wall

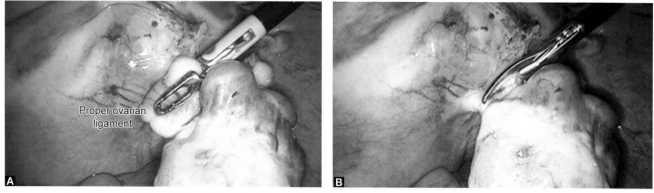

Figs 9A and B: Coagulation of the ovarian ligament and dissecting without involving the uterine or the ovarian wall

1.8. Separation of cervix from the uterus with the help of the electric cutting loop (Figs 21 to 24)

1.9. Coagulation of the cervical canal and remaining cervical stump for adhesion prevention (Figs 25A to D)

1.10. Closure of the peritoneum over the cervical stump with help of a purse string or figure of eight suture (Figs 26 to 29)

1.11. Morcellation of the uterine body, if adnexas are also resected, they should be put into an Endobag for extraction (Figs 30A to D and 31A to D).

▌ COMPARISON TO LTH

2. **Laparoscopic Total Hysterectomy (LTH)**[27,28]

Total hysterectomy—with total laparoscopic hysterectomy (TLH), the entire procedure is performed laparoscopically and the uterus is extracted vaginally or removed abdominally using morcellation techniques. After the uterus is removed, the vaginal cuff is closed using laparoscopic suturing techniques.

TLH is used to treat a number of benign disorders, as well as endometrial cancer and some ovarian cancers.[26]

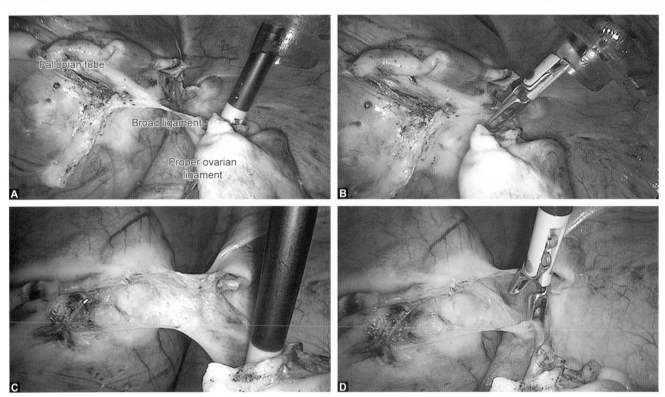

Figs 10A to D: Dissection of the proper ovarian ligament and opening of the broad ligament. (A) After the proper ovarian ligament is dissected, the adnexa falls to the lateral side; (B to D) Thereafter, the broad ligament can pointedly be identified and separated in its two leafs

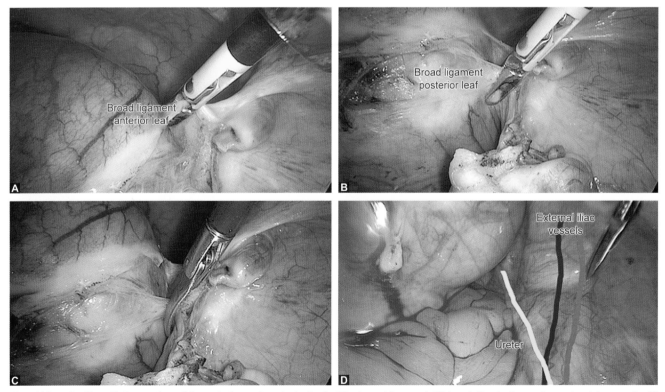

Figs 11A to D: (A to C) Separation of the anterior and posterior leaf of the broad ligament (D) in relation to the ureter and pelvic vessels; (A to C) The broad ligament is coagulated and dissected as close to the uterus as possible without affecting the uterine artery. As both leafs are separated, the ascending branch of the uterine artery can easily be visualized and left out; (D) The tip of the scissors is heading strictly away of the uterine wall using the curved blade

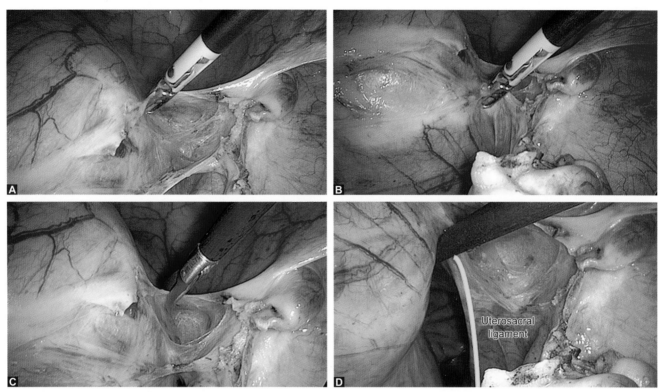

Figs 12A to D: (A to C) Final separation of the leafs of the broad ligament coming closer to the pelvic floor (D) up to the uterosacral ligament (D); (A to C) The uterus is tracted toward the left side and the bladder peritoneum is already expected to be closeby; (D) By blunt manipulation, the curse of the sacrouterine ligament can be visualized and the coagulation line should be leaving this part out

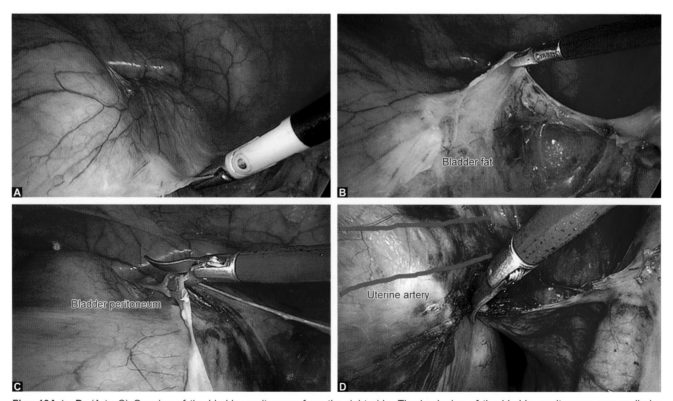

Figs 13A to D: (A to C) Opening of the bladder peritoneum from the right side. The beginning of the bladder peritoneum can easily be demarcated and the cutting line should not be above this zone neither be too far caudal of it. The gas is entering the created space and showing the beginning of the bladder pillar; (D) Freeing the uterine vessel bundle by coagulating and dissecting above and underneath it. The ureter is in a safe distance lateral to this preparation area

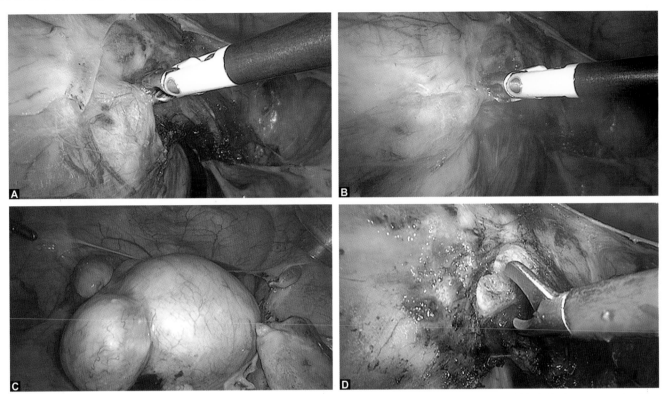

Figs 14A to D: Bipolar coagulation and dissection of the uterine vessels. (A and B) The coagulation area should include the upper parts of the artery to avoid any retrograde bleeding after dissecting the vessel; (C) The uterus changes its color to whitish/grey; (D) Using the hook scissors a deeper cut can be avoided and the uterine artery is dissected in two steps. Herewith, a further coagulation of the tissue part lying just behind the artery is possible and annoying venous bleedings can be avoided

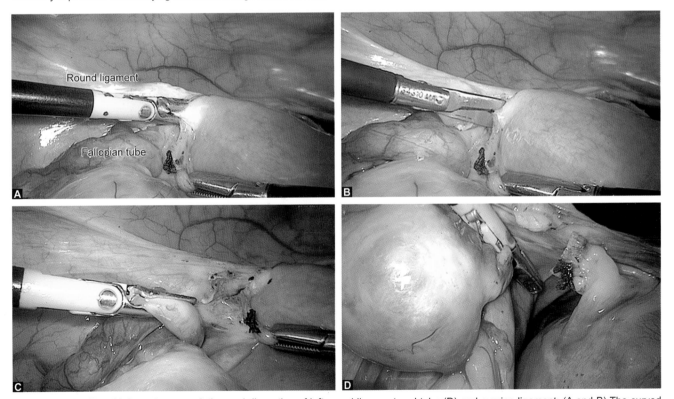

Figs 15A to D: (A to C) Stepwise coagulation and dissection of left round ligament and tube (D) and ovarian ligament; (A and B) The curved scissors are held with the tip away of the uterine wall; (C and D) After dissecting the Fallopian tube, the underneath running vessels must be coagulated before further cutting; (D) By blunt manipulation, the curse of the sacrouterine ligament and the uterus in case of lateral lying myomas can be visualized and the coagulation line should be leaving this part out

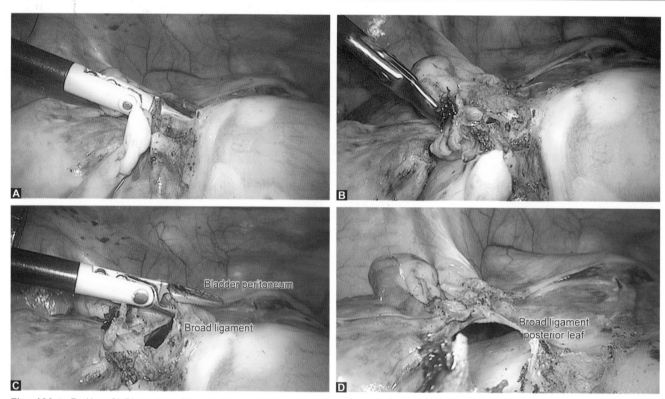

Figs 16A to D: (A to C) Dissection of the bladder peritoneum as well as the anterior and posterior leaf of the broad ligament of the left side; (D) The bladder peritoneum has already been opened from the right side and the posterior leaf of the broad ligament serves as an anatomic landmark toward the uterine vessels

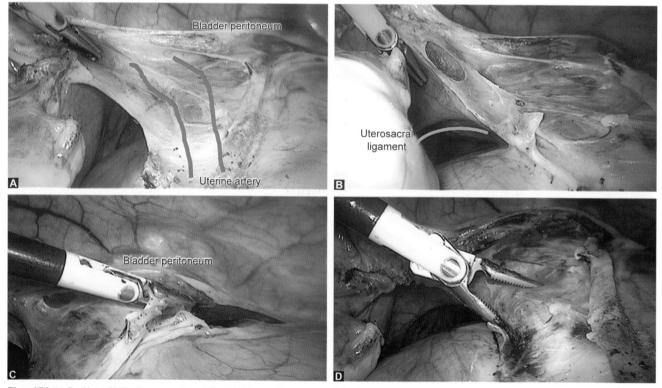

Figs 17A to D: (A to C) Further opening of the bladder peritoneum and the broad ligament (D), and beginning coagulation of the left uterine vessels; (A) The uterine artery is functioning as an anatomic landmark leading downward; (B to D) The intermediate glance to the back of the uterus allows the cutting edge being above the conjunction of the sacrouterine ligaments

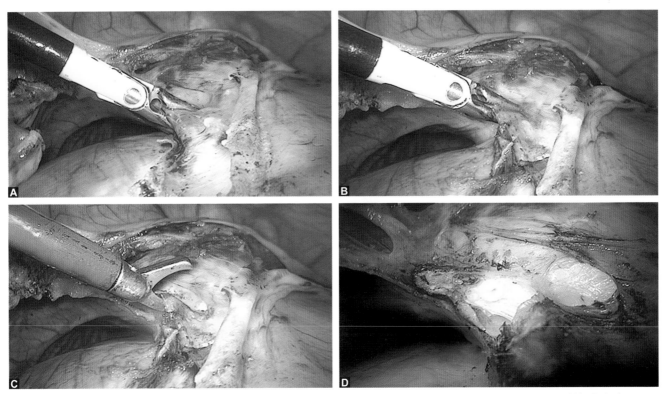

Figs 18A to D: (A) Bipolar coagulation and separation of the uterine vessels on the left side; (B) The coagulation area should include the upper parts of the artery to avoid any retrograde bleeding after dissecting the vessel. The uterus changes its color to whitish/grey; (C and D) Using the hook scissors, a deeper cut can be avoided and the uterine artery is dissected in two steps. Herewith, a further coagulation of the tissue part lying just behind the artery is possible and annoying venous bleedings can be avoided

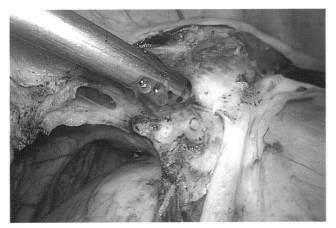

Fig. 19: Visualization of the separated left uterine pedicles. Some drops of normal saline allow the bipolar coagulation to work more effectively because of the electrolyte flow. Especially if the operating field is very dry

However, morcellation is not performed if uterine cancer is suspected. When surgical staging is indicated, evaluation of the abdomen and pelvis, washings, salpingo-oophorectomy, lymph nodes dissection, tissue biopsies and omentectomy can be performed in addition to laparoscopic hysterectomy.

General Aspects

Laparoscopic total hysterectomy today is an easy procedure and can be performed by using suture techniques alone, a combination of suture and coagulation techniques or by applying bipolar coagulation or any of the modern thermofusion, ultrasound and combined instruments for hemostasis.

Preoperative Preparation

The patient is placed in lithotomy position with the buttocks at the end of the table. A uterine manipulator, like the HOHL or the Mangeshikar manipulator is fixed to the cervix after a standard Foley catheter is placed into the bladder. The purpose of the manipulator is to move the uterus in the abdominal cavity for better exposure for its resection.

Instruments and Equipment

The uterine manipulator is used as a third hand of the surgeon in cases of hysterectomy for multiple fibroids. We do not insist on its use in cancer surgery. The vagina has to be closed after the necessary colpotomy at LTH either by

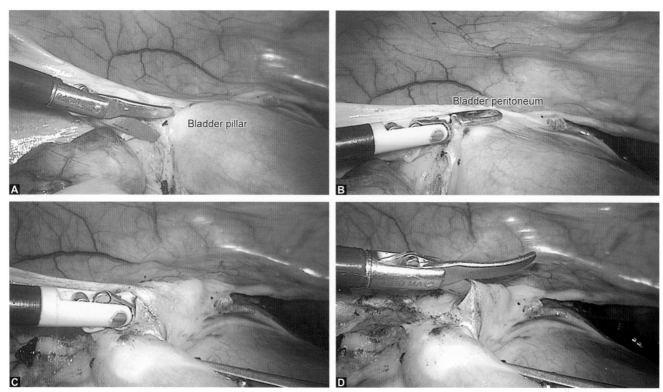

Figs 20A to D: Final dissection of the bladder pillar and the bladder peritoneum from left to right, letting the CO_2 distension medium lead the path. Therewith, the bladder is pushed safely downward out of the operating field and the peritoneal line of the vesicouterine fold is easily being recognized

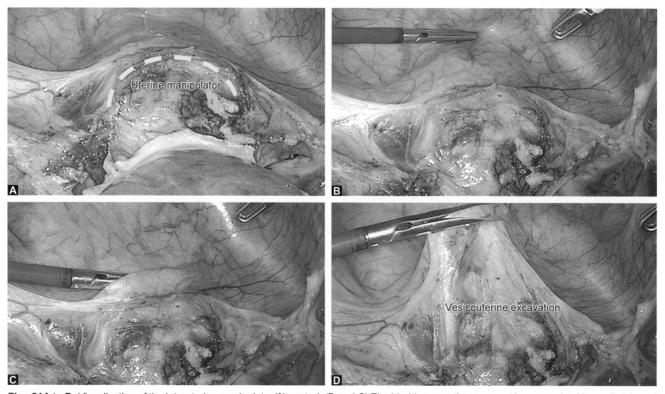

Figs 21A to D: Visualization of the intrauterine manipulator if inserted. (B and C) The bladder sometimes cannot be recognized immediately and left out safely. Therefore, the exact localization of the bladder is possible if a blunt instrument pushes the estimated bladder toward the cervix from the balloon of the Foley catheter. After recognition, the bladder is elevated and the vesicouterine excavation can be opened to push the bladder further down

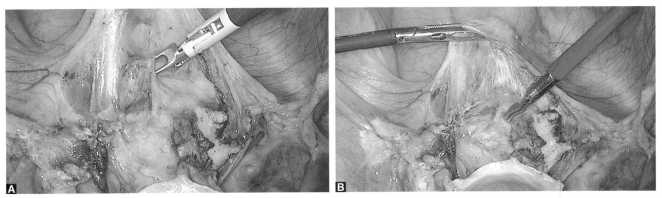

Figs 22A and B: Minimal dissection of the bladder peritoneum of about 1 cm for LSH and 2–3 cm for LTH by opening the vesicouterine excavation. This is easier if a manipulator is inside the vagina and the cervix pushed upward but it is also possible by traction only. Once the vesicouterine space is created, the preparation is easy to be performed with a blunt instrument without any bleeding

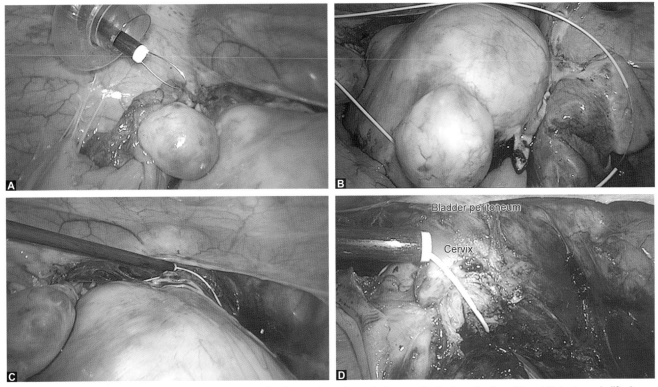

Figs 23A to D: Introduction of a monopolar cutting loop for the cervix and exact placement prior to activation. The whitish uterus is lifted over the loop and the loop is tightened softly. The exact placement is controlled and should be between the stumps of the uterine artery and above the conjunction of the sacrouterine ligaments

a continuous suture, interrupted sutures, barbed sutures, or by sutures for extracorporeal knotting after they have been prepared. The prepared needle holders should be well known to the surgeon. In addition to these, the instruments detailed above are necessary.

Steps for Surgery

2.1 to 2.5 are identical to 1.1 to 1.5 (Figs 2 to 21).

2.6 At separation of the bladder from the uterus, the bladder is pushed and dissected down 2–3 cm to clearly visualize the rim of the cervical cap. In cases of postcesarean section, a careful and gentle blunt and intermediate sharp dissection has to be carried out (Figs 32A to D).

While lateralizing the ureter by pushing up the manipulator, the uterine artery and vein with its collaterals are totally coagulated near the cervix and dissected.

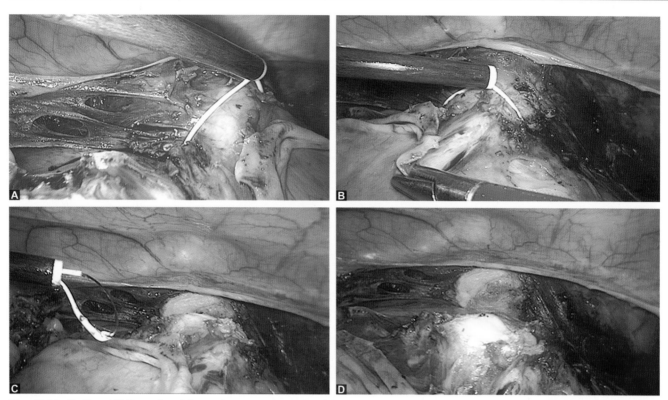

Figs 24A to D: (A and B) Resection of the uterine corpus from cervix after placing the cutting loop with the cutting point on the posterior cervix. The exact placement is controlled and should be between the stumps of the uterine artery and above the conjunction of the sacrouterine ligaments; (C and D) The dissection of cervix and uterus is performed in this case of LSH by monopolar current running in the non-isolated field only. While cutting the uterine corpus is pulled upward to a ire a retrograde conus

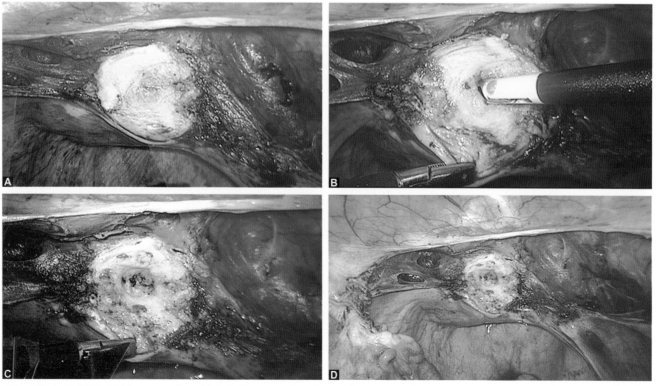

Figs 25A to D: LSH: (A) After separation of the uterine corpus from the cervix, a retrograde conus is achieved; (B) Afterwards, coagulation of inner cervical canal and (C and D) final inspection of the cutting and preparing operating field

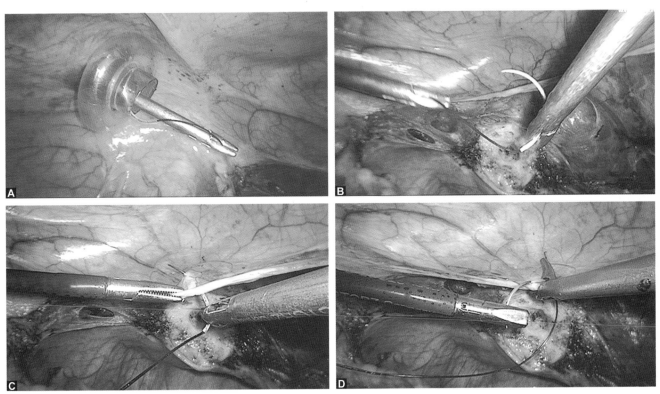

Figs 26A to D: (A) LSH: Introduction of peritoneal suture; (B to D) closure of the peritoneum over the cervical stump with a continuous PDS suture

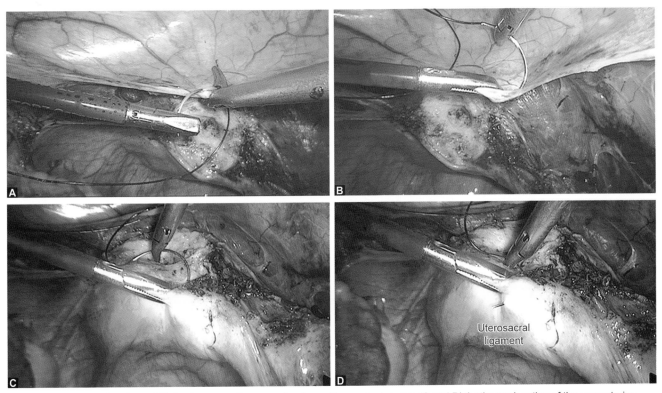

Figs 27A to D: LSH: (A and B) Continuous suture covering the entire cervical stump; (C and D) As the conjunction of the sacrouterine ligaments has been left out, the two ligaments are grabbed and included in the suture to achieve a cervicosuspension

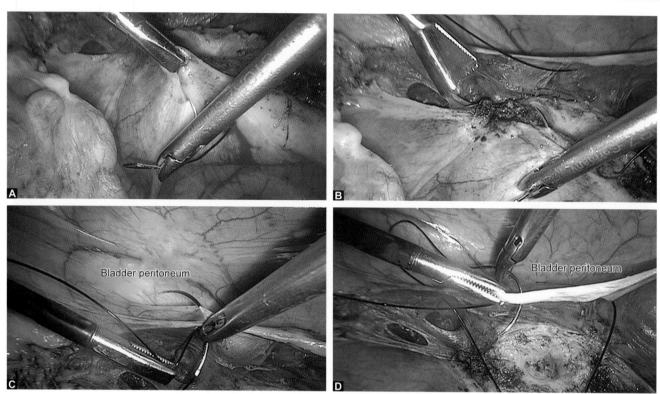

Figs 28A to D: LSH: (A and B) As the conjunction of the sacrouterine ligaments has been left out the two ligaments are grabbed and included in the suture to achieve a cervicosuspension; (C and D) Connecting the bladder peritoneum to the posterior peritoneum in terms of a purse-string suture

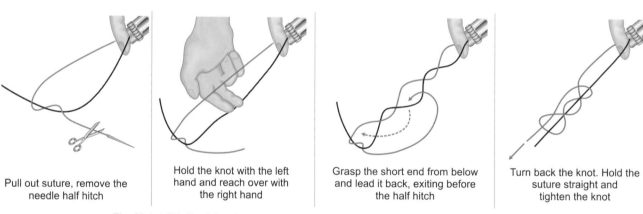

Pull out suture, remove the needle half hitch

Hold the knot with the left hand and reach over with the right hand

Grasp the short end from below and lead it back, exiting before the half hitch

Turn back the knot. Hold the suture straight and tighten the knot

Fig. 29.1: LSH: Finalizing the extracorporeal knot of the PDS suture by the "von Leffern knot"

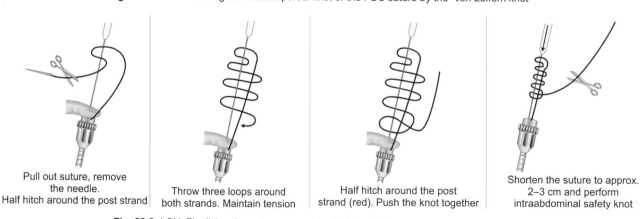

Pull out suture, remove the needle.
Half hitch around the post strand

Throw three loops around both strands. Maintain tension

Half hitch around the post strand (red). Push the knot together

Shorten the suture to approx. 2–3 cm and perform intraabdominal safety knot

Fig. 29.2: LSH: Finalizing the extracorporeal knot of the PDS suture by the "Roeder's knot"

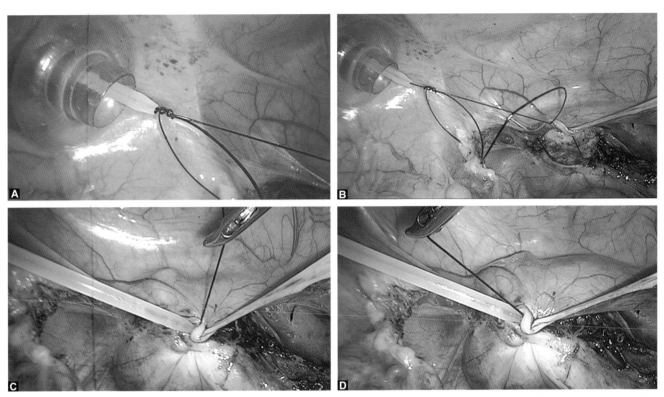

Figs 29.3A to D: With either extracorporeal knot, the peritoneum is closing the cervical channel functionally and leads to a cervicosuspension. Nevertheless, the left out sides allow draining, if necessary

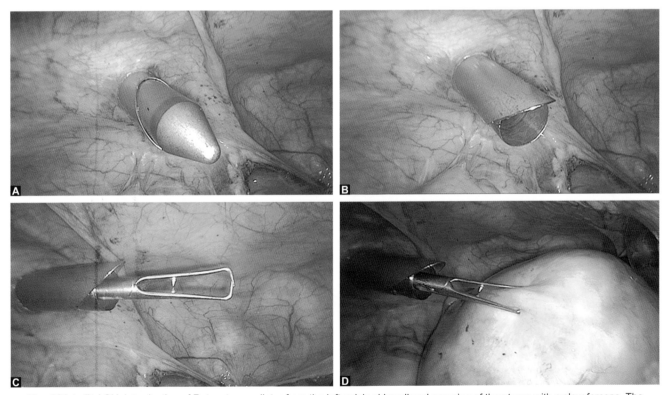

Figs 30A to D: LSH: Introduction of Rotocut morcellator from the left pelvic sidewall and grasping of the uterus with a claw forceps. The Rotocut morcellator exists in 10 mm and 15 mm size

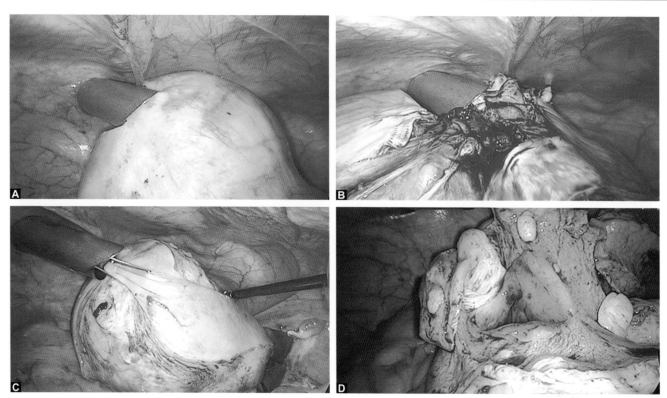

Figs 31A to D: LSH: Morcellation of the myomatous uterus (850 g) under continuous observation of the rotating cutting edge and protection shield of the morcellator. The protection shield is leading upward to the abdominal wall to avoid cutting in the abdominal wall vessels. Nevertheless, the lower part, especially the small bowel has to be exposed to be kept out of the operating area. Cutting into the bowel is one of the major complications in the LSH procedure of a surgeon being too impatient or being too inobservant

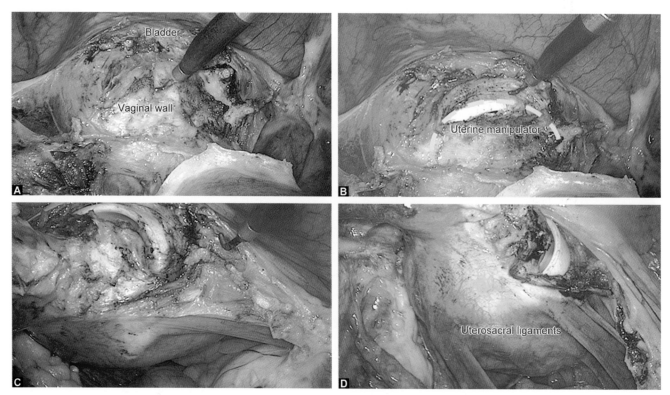

Figs 32A to D: (A) In this case of LTH, the distance between the vagina and bladder is increased due to the preparation of the bladder peritoneum, (B to D) the intrauterine manipulator is firmly pressed into the abdomen and the uterine dissection from the vagina is performed stepwise. The conjunction of the sacrouterine ligaments is kept in place

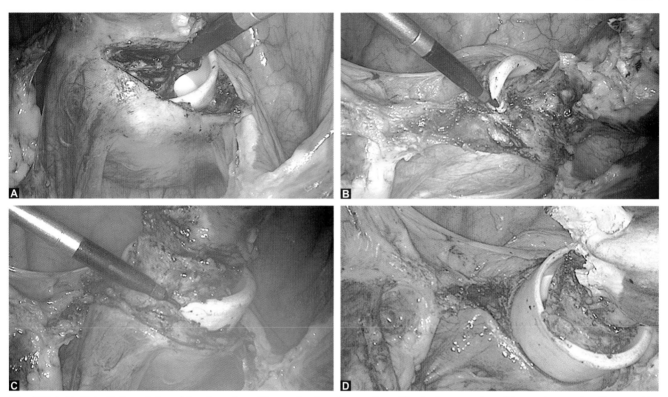

Figs 33A to D: (A to C) Completion of the dissection of the vagina from the cervix and beginning retraction of the uterine cervix still grasped by the manipulator forceps transvaginally; (D) The high amount of fog using monopolar current and the sharpness of the monopolar hook make precise preparation under complete sight necessary

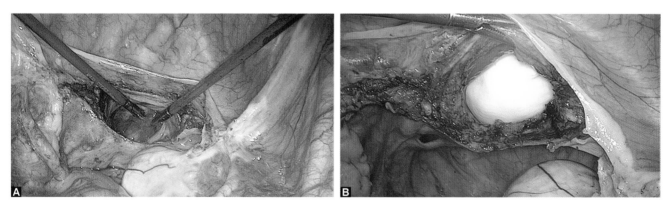

Figs 34A and B: (A) Retraction of uterus through the vagina; (B) Introduction of a cotton swab filled glove transvaginally to hinder the breakdown of CO_2 pneumoperitonium

Resection of the vagina from the cervix with the monopolar hook by stretching the manipulator firmly cranially, carefully performing an intrafacial dissection leaving the sacrouterine ligaments nearly completely in place (Figs 33A to D).

The uterus is retracted through the vagina while still fixed to the manipulator. If the uterus is too big, it has to be morcellated either intraabdominally or transvaginally.

While morcellating the cutting edge of the morcellator must be continuously visible (Figs 34A and B).

Closure of the vagina with 2 corner sutures and 1 or 2 sutures in between with both corner sutures. The sacrouterine ligaments and the middle portion of the vagina are stitched and elevated for prevention of vaginal prolapse or enterocele formation at a later time (Figs 35 to 44).

Final inspection as shown in Figures 45 and 46. Peritonealization and drainage is not required.

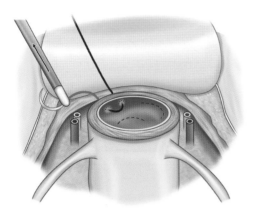

A vicryl CT 1 plus needle is passed through the endopelvic fascia and 1 cm below the cephaled edge of the vaginal epithelium

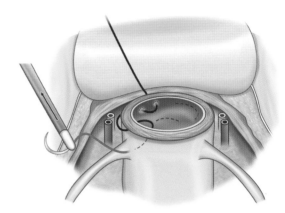

The needle is pushed from the vaginal lumen through the vaginal wall, passed between the uterine vessels (median part of the broad ligament) and brought back through the vaginal lumen

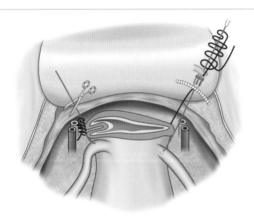

The sacrouterine ligament is identified before the suture is passed through. The needle is pushed from the vaginal lumen through the vaginal wall, rectovaginal septum and transpierces the sacrouterine ligament

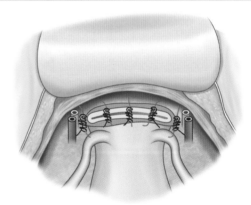

Closure of the vaginal vault with single stitches. Again, the stitch is drawn through the endopelvic fascia - vaginal wall - vaginal wall - rectovaginal septum

Fig. 35.1: Vaginal closure for descent prevention after retraction of the uterus

Posthysterectomy Inspection

Under a continuous irrigation with Ringer's lactate or Adept (Baxter), a careful inspection of pedicles, bladder, ureters and bowels has to be performed.

Postoperative Management

Retraction of urinary catheter, which only in specific cases remains. A postoperative cystoscopy is rarely performed in cases of severe endometriosis or adhesions that affect the upper part of the bladder. Early ambulation after a few hours postsurgically is a good practice. Clear liquids can be started 6 hours postsurgically followed by a light diet. The patient can be discharged after 8–12 hours, a postoperative ultrasound scan of the renal pelvis should be done and the

patient can perform normal light activities and can get back to work after 4–5 days.

Anticipated Problems

The vital symptoms, pain and temperature have to be meticulously controlled over the first 8 hours. A patient who is discharged early must have a phone number to call back in case of distress and pain.

Postoperative Management

Thromboprophylaxis (mechanical and medical) in appropriate cases must be applied. The urinary catheter is removed or may stay for 24 hours. Patients can be early ambulated and discharged on the same day or after 24–48 hours.

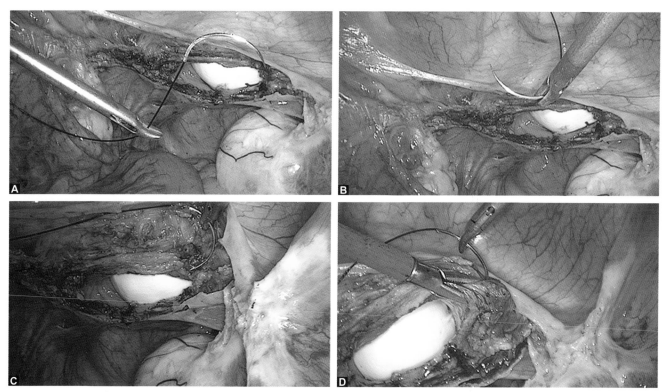

Figs 35.2A to D: LTH: Right corner suture uniting the vaginal anterior and posterior wall, and posterior peritoneum as well as right sacrouterine ligament. The bladder can be left out under sight. The forceps has to be sharp to definitely grab the vaginal epithelium. If only the vaginal wall is taken into the suture and the epithelium is left out, there is a high incidence of postoperative granulomas

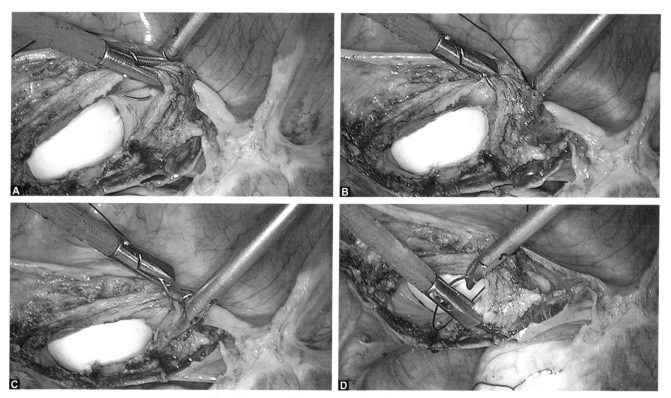

Figs 36A to D: LTH: Continuing the right corner suture

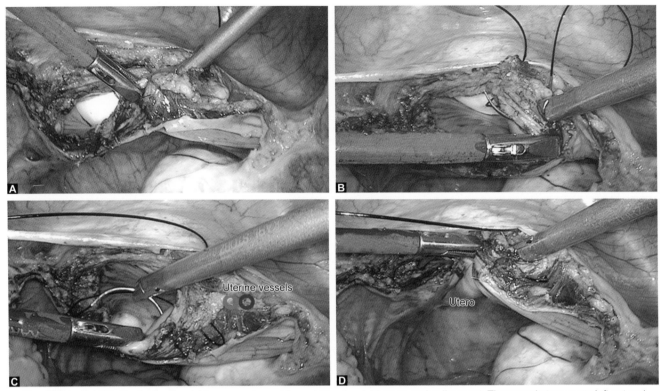

Figs 37A to D: LTH: Continuing the right corner suture while grabbing the right sacrouterine ligament. The vessel stumps are left out and lateralized. With this sort of suture, the vessels are mechanically compressed

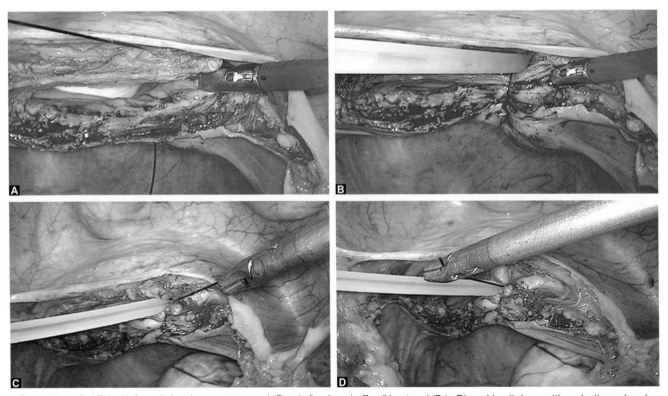

Figs 38A to D: LTH: (A) Completing the extracorporeal "Roeder" or "von Leffern" knot and (B to D) pushing it down with a plastic push rod. The edge is pulled into the abdomen to avoid the tissue disturbing the intravaginal sense

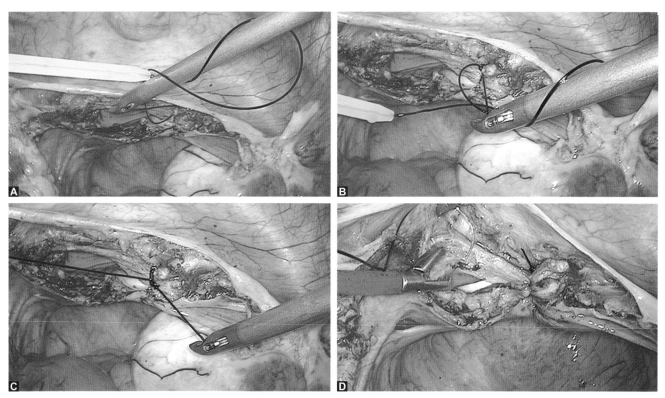

Figs 39A to D: LTH: Putting an intracorporeal security knot on the right corner stitch and cutting of the thread

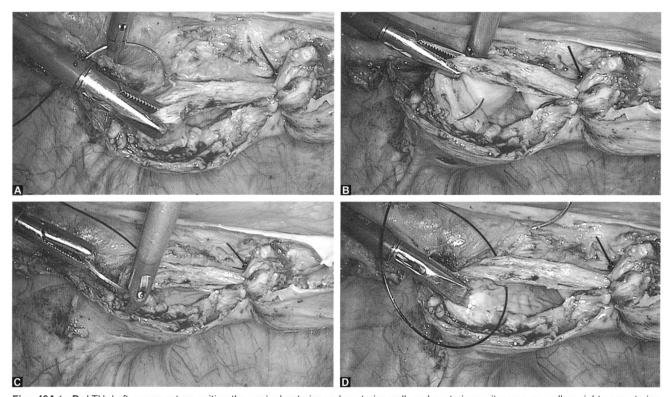

Figs 40A to D: LTH: Left corner suture uniting the vaginal anterior and posterior wall, and posterior peritoneum as well as right sacrouterine ligament. The bladder can be left out under sight. The forceps has to be sharp to definitely grab the vaginal epithelium. If only the vaginal wall is taken into the suture and the epithelium is left out, there is a high incidence of postoperative granulomas

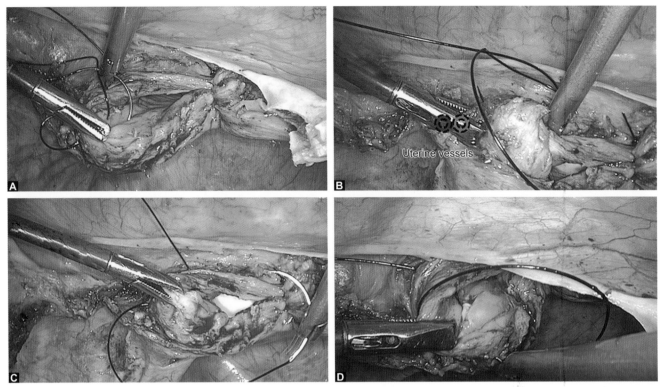

Figs 41A to D: LTH: Continuing the left corner suture. With this sort of suture, the vessels are mechanically compressed

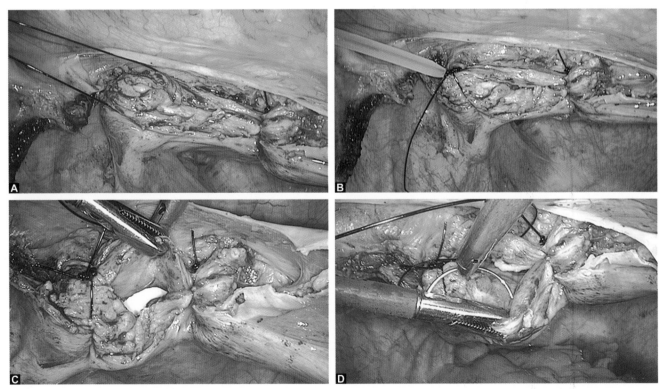

Figs 42A to D: LTH: (A to C) Completion of left corner suture and extracorporeal knot pushed down by the push rod; (D) Starting a U- or a Z-stitch in the middle. If the vaginal cuff is not 100% dry, it is easier to close the edges first. Therewith most of the bleeding stops automatically, and further coagulation can be avoided. Severe coagulation on the vaginal wall might increase the risk for vaginal stump infection or dehiscence

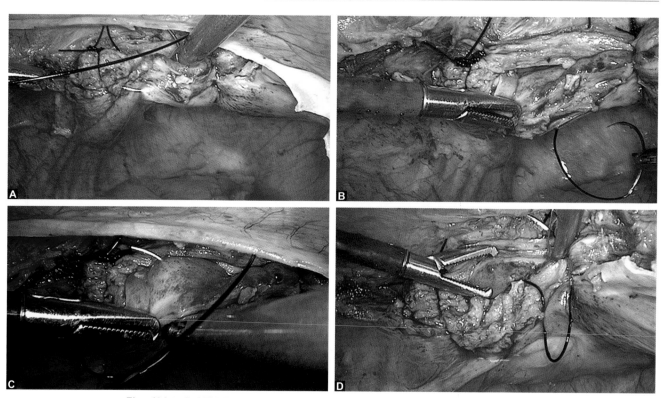

Figs 43A to D: LTH: Final closing of the remaining vaginal opening by figure of a U suture

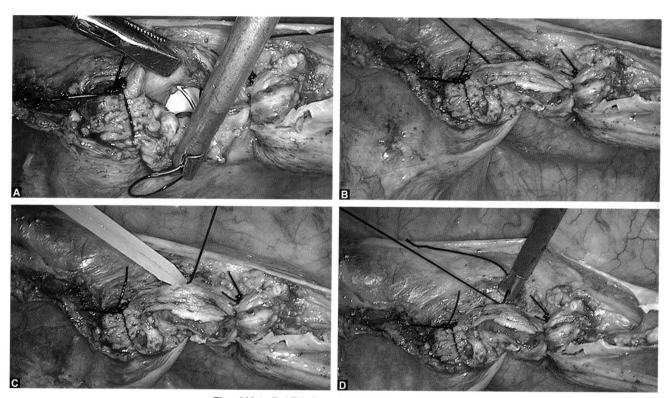

Figs 44A to D: LTH: Completion of the central suture

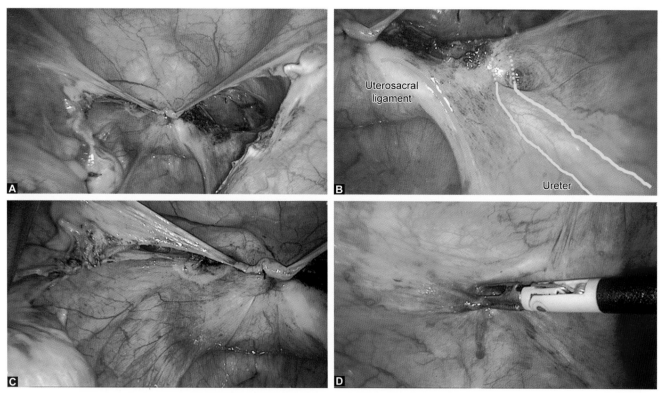

Figs 45A to D: LSH: Finishing picture after LSH procedure. The peritoneum is closing the cervical channel and there is possibility for draining from both sides. (A to C) Both sacrouterine ligaments are under light tension and therewith cervicosuspension is reached. Observation of ureteric integrity by observing the peristalsis; (D) Coagulation of the right trocar entry point after removal

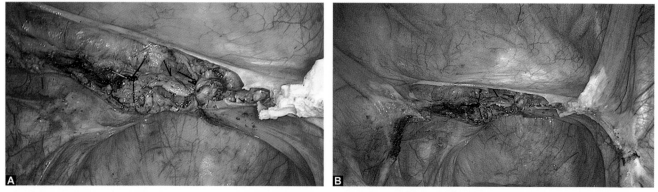

Figs 46A and B: LTH: Final sites after closure of vaginal stump and elevation of sacrouterine ligaments by 2 corner sutures. Both sacrouterine ligaments are under light tension and therewith colposuspension is reached. Reperitonealization will arise in between two weeks after operation. The PDS suture allows a safe closure and healing of the vaginal cuff as it is resorbable only after about 6 months

Anticipated Problems

Fever, early pain situations, abdominal distension, delirious situations, decreased urine output and shock index with hypotension, must be recognized and attended to immediately.

▌SUMMARY AND CONCLUSION

Besides the well known laparoscopic techniques for myomectomies as well as the hysteroscopic techniques for submucous fibroidectomy laparoscopic subtotal and total hysterectomy are surgical choices to be taken in a combined decision between patient and doctor for the treatment of multiple fibroids. The individual steps described in this chapter help to perform a satisfying surgery to finish the serious burden of multiple fibroids in a patient that has completed her family planning.

■ REFERENCES

1. Watson JD, Crick FH. Molecular structure of nucleic acids: A structure for deoxyribose nucleic acid. Nature. 1953;171(4356):737-8.

2. Watson JD, Crick FH. Genetical implications of the structure of deoxyribonucleic acid. Nature. 1953;171(4361):964-7.

3. Liebe Leserin, Lieber Leser. (2013). Seite nicht gefunden. Spektrum der Wissenschaft. [online] Available from http://spektrum.de/alias/2013.

4. Treloar SA, Martin NG, Dennerstein L, et al. Pathways to hysterectomy: Insights from longitudinal twin research. Am J Obstet Gynecol. 1992;167(1):82-8.

5. Snieder H, MacGregor AJ, Spector TD. Genes control the cessation of a woman's reproductive life: A twin study of hysterectomy and age at menopause. J Clin Endocrinol Metab. 1998;83(6):1875-80.

6. Vikhlyaeva EM, Khodzhaeva ZS, Fantschenko ND. Familial predisposition to uterine leiomyomas. Int J Gynaecol Obstet. 1995;51(2):127-31.

7. Van Voorhis BJ, Romitti PA, Jones MP. Family history as a risk factor for development of uterine leiomyomas. Results of a pilot study. J Reprod Med. 2002;47(8):663-9.

8. Al-Hendy A, Salama SA. Catechol-O-methyltransferase polymorphism is associated with increased uterine leiomyoma risk in different ethnic groups. J Soc Gynecol Investig. 2006;13(2):136-44.

9. Tsibris JC, Segars J, Coppola D, et al. Insights from gene arrays on the development and growth regulation of uterine leiomyomata. Fertil Steril. 2002;78(1):114-21.

10. Wang H, Mahadevappa M, Yamamoto K, et al. Distinctive proliferative phase differences in gene expression in human myometrium and leiomyomata. Fertil Steril. 2003;80(2):266-76.

11. Gross K, Morton C, Stewart E. Finding genes for uterine fibroids. Obstetrics and Gynecology. 2000;95(4):560.

12. Patterson-Keels LM, Selvaggi SM, Haefner HK, et al. Morphologic assessment of endometrium overlying sub-mucosal leiomyomas. J Reprod Med. 1994;39(8):579-84.

13. Flynn M, Jamison M, Datta S, et al. Health care resource use for uterine fibroid tumors in the United States. Am J Obstet Gynecol. 2006;195(4):955-64.

14. Hartmann KE, Birnbaum H, Ben-Hamadi R, et al. Annual costs associated with diagnosis of uterine leiomyomata. Obstet Gynecol. 2006;108(4):930-7.

15. Adashi EY. The climacteric ovary as a functional gonadotropin-driven androgen-producing gland. Fertil Steril. 1994;62(1):20-7.

16. Shifren JL. The role of androgens in female sexual dysfunction. Mayo Clin Proc. 2004;79(4):S19-24.

17. Buster JE, Kingsberg SA, Aguirre O, et al. Testosterone patch for low sexual desire in surgically menopausal woman: A randomized trial. Obstet Gynecol. 2005;105(5):944-52.

18. Nyunt A, Stephen G, Gibbin J, et al. Androgen status in healthy premenopausal women with loss of libido. J Sex Marital Ther. 2005;31(1):73-80.

19. Manson JE, Hsia J, Johnson KC, et al. Estrogen plus progestin and the risk of coronary heart disease. N Engl J Med. 2003;349(6):523-34.

20. Anderson GL, Limacher M, Assaf AR, et al. Effects of conjugated equine estrogen in postmenopausal women with hysterectomy: the Women's Health Initiative randomized controlled trial. JAMA. 2004;291(14):1701-12.

21. Parker WH, Broder MS, Liu Z, et al. Ovarian conservation at the time of hysterectomy for benign disease. Obstet Gynecol. 2005;106(2):219-26.

22. Dietl J, Wischhusen J, Häusler SF. The post-reproductive Fallopian tube: Better removed? Hum Reprod. 2011;26(11):2918-24.

23. Guldberg R, Wehberg S, Skovlund CW, et al. Salpingectomy as standard at hysterectomy? A Danish cohort study. 1977-2010. BMJ Open. 2013;20:3(6).

24. Palmer R. Safety in laparoscopy. J Reprod Med. 1974;13(1):1-5.

25. Nezhat F, Brill AI, Nezhat CH, et al. Laparoscopic appraisal of the anatomic relationship of the umbilicus to the aortic bifurcation. J Am Assoc Gynecol Laparosc. 1998;5(2):135-40.

26. Royal College of Obstetricians and Gynaecologists. "Preventing entry-related gynaecological laparoscopic injuries." RCOG Green-top Guideline. No. 49:1-10.

27. Pasic R. Creation of pneumoperitoneum and trocar insertion techniques. A Practical Manual of Laparoscopy and Minimally Invasive Gynecology: A Clinical Cookbook. Abingdon, UK: Informa Healthcare; 2007. pp. 57-74.

28. Schollmeyer T, Mettler L, Ruther D, et al. Practical Manual for Laparoscopic and Hysteroscopic Gynecological Surgery. New Delhi: Jaypee Brothers Medical Publishers (P) Ltd; 2013.

CHAPTER 16

Laparoscopy in Pregnancy

Pranay Shah

■ INTRODUCTION

Recent data show the safety and efficacy of laparoscopy during all trimesters for many surgical conditions with outcomes similar to conventional operations. Surgeons must be aware of the data regarding differences in techniques used for pregnant patients to optimize outcomes.

One in 500 women will require nonobstetrical abdominal surgery during their pregnancies.[1] The most common nonobstetrical surgical emergencies complicating pregnancy are acute appendicitis, cholecystitis, and intestinal obstruction. Other conditions requiring surgery during pregnancy include ovarian cysts, adnexal mass or torsion, heterotrophic pregnancy, abdominal cerclage, adrenal tumors, splenic disorders, obstructed hernias, complications of inflammatory bowel disease and abdominal pain of unknown etiology. During its infancy, laparoscopy was contraindicated during pregnancy due to concerns for uterine injury and fetal perfusion. As surgeons have gained more experience with laparoscopy, it has become the preferred treatment for many surgical diseases in the gravid patient.

■ PHYSIOLOGIC CHANGES IN PREGNANCY

The minute ventilation in pregnant women is 50% higher than in nonpregnant women. This change results in a marked decrease in carbon dioxide in the arterial concentration, and a mild respiratory alkalosis.[2] The fetus has a mild respiratory alkalosis in the normal state that may facilitate the delivery of oxygen. Many other changes in pregnancy occur including mild anemia, increased cardiac output, increased heart rate, and an increased oxygen consumption that allows the mother and fetus to be adequately oxygenated.

Often overlooked are the hematologic abnormalities in the pregnant patient. These changes include an increase in fibrinogen, factor VII, and factor XII, but a decrease in antithrombin III. All of these result in an increased risk of venous thromboembolism.[3]

■ DIAGNOSIS AND WORKUP

The clinical picture of acute abdomen in pregnancy is altered making diagnosis difficult. Nausea and vomiting are common. Leukocytosis is the norm. Low grade fever, mild hypotension, and anorexia are common. Gravid uterus pushes the abdominal contents cephalad, altering landmarks by displacing organs and possibly inhibiting the migration of the omentum. There is a decrease in gastric motility and an increase in the risk of gastroesophageal reflux, including aspiration (Mendelson's syndrome), a life-threatening issue feared by anesthesiologists and obstetricians alike.

The clinician must consider the risks and benefits of the diagnostic modalities and therapies to both the mother and the fetus. Sir Zachary Cope said in 1921, "Earlier diagnosis means better prognosis".[4] Fetal outcomes depend on the outcome of the mother. Optimal maternal outcome may require radiologic imaging, sometime ionizing radiation. A risk benefit discussion with the patient should occur prior to any diagnostic study.

Ultrasound

Ultrasound is considered safe, as no adverse effects to mother or fetus from ultrasound have been reported. It is the initial radiographic test of choice for most cases of abdominal pain in pregnancy. Gynecologic causes include adnexal mass, torsion, ectopic pregnancy, abruption, placenta previa, uterine rupture and fetal demise. Ultrasound is also useful for nongynecologic causes of abdominal pain, including symptomatic gallstones and appendicitis.

X-ray

Significant radiation exposure may lead to chromosomal mutations, neurologic abnormalities, mental retardation, and increased risk of childhood leukemia. The fetal age at exposure is important. Fetal mortality is greatest when exposure occurs within the first week of conception. The most sensitive time period for CNS teratogenesis is between 10 weeks and 17 weeks of gestation, and routine radiographs should be avoided during this time. In later pregnancy, the concern shifts from teratogenesis to increasing the risk of childhood hematologic malignancy. The background incidence of childhood cancer and leukemia is 0.2 –0.3%. Radiation may increase that incidence by 0.06% per 1 rad delivered to fetus.[5]

Exposure of the conceptus to 0.5 rad increases the risk of spontaneous abortion, major malformations, mental retardation, and childhood malignancy to one additional case in 6,000 above baseline risk.[6] The risk of teratogenesis is negligible at 5 rads and that risk significantly increases at doses above 15 rads.

Expeditious and accurate diagnosis should take precedence over concerns of ionizing radiation (Table 1). Cumulative radiation dosage should be limited to 5–10 rads during pregnancy. No single diagnostic study should exceed 5 rads.

Table 1: Radiation exposure to conceptus in common radiologic studies	
Study radiation	*Exposure (rads)*
Abdominal radiograph	0.1–0.3
Intraoperative cholangiography	0.2
Lumbar spine radiograph	0.6
Intravenous pyelogram	0.6
Barium enema	0.7
CT of pelvis	1–5
ERCP (without pelvic shielding)	2–12.5

CT Scan

Radiation exposure to the fetus may be as low as 2 rads for pelvic CT scans but can reach 5 rads when full scan of the abdomen and pelvis is performed. This radiation dose is considered safe but may affect teratogenesis and increase the risk of developing childhood hematologic malignancies.[7] CT scans may be used judiciously during pregnancy.

Magnetic Resonance Imaging

Magnetic resonance imaging (MRI) provides excellent soft tissue imaging without ionizing radiation and is safe to use in pregnant patients at any stage of pregnancy. Intravenous Gadolinium agents cross the placenta and may be detrimental; therefore their use during pregnancy should be confined to select cases where it is considered essential.

Nuclear Medicine

Administration of radionucleotides (including technetium-99m) for diagnostic studies is generally safe for mother and fetus.

Cholangiography

Radiation exposure during cholangiography is estimated to be 0.2–0.5 rads.[8] Intraoperative and endoscopic cholangiography exposes the mother and fetus to minimal radiation and may be used selectively during pregnancy. The lower abdomen should be shielded when performing cholangiography during pregnancy to decrease the radiation exposure to the fetus.

Endoscopic Retrograde Cholangiopancreatography

The radiation exposure during endoscopic retrograde cholangiopancreatography (ERCP) averages 2–12 rads, but can be substantially higher for long procedures. ERCP also carries a higher risk of bleeding and pancreatitis. Alternatives to fluoroscopy include intraoperative ultrasound and choledochoscopy. Magnetic resonance cholangiopancreatography (MRCP) is an alternative. It is a useful diagnostic tool but offers no therapeutic capability.

PATIENT SELECTION

Surgical treatment of acute abdominal disease has the same indications in pregnancy and nonpregnant patients. Once the decision to operate has been made, the surgical approach (laparotomy versus laparoscopy) should be determined based on the skills of the surgeon, availability of appropriate equipment and staff. A discussion with the patient regarding the risks and benefits of surgical intervention should be undertaken. Benefits of laparoscopy during pregnancy appear similar to those benefits in nonpregnant patients including postoperative pain, less postoperative ileus, decreased length of hospital stay and faster return to work.[9] Laparoscopy can be safely performed during any trimester of pregnancy.

Historical recommendations were to delay surgery until the second trimester in order to reduce the rates of spontaneous abortion and preterm labor. Recent literature has shown that pregnant patient may undergo laparoscopic surgery safely during any trimester without any increased risk to the mother or fetus.[10,11] Postponing necessary operations may in some cases, increase the rates of complications for both mother and fetus.

It has been suggested that the gestational age limit for successful completion of laparoscopic surgery during pregnancy is 26–28 weeks. This has been refuted by several studies in which laparoscopic appendectomy and cholecystectomy have been successfully performed late in third trimester.[12]

ANESTHESIA

General anesthesia with curarization and endotracheal intubation is essential for safely performing laparoscopy. The majority of anesthetic drugs, skeletal muscle relaxants and morphine-related drugs are nonteratogenic and nontoxic to fetus. They can be safely used during pregnancy.

PATIENT POSITIONING

When the pregnant patient is placed in a supine position, the gravid uterus places pressure on the inferior vena cava resulting in decreased venous return to the heart. The decrease in venous return results in significant reduction in cardiac output with concomitant maternal hypotension and decreased placental perfusion during surgery.

Gravid patients should be placed in the left lateral decubitus position to minimize compression of the vena cava.

A nasogastric tube is recommended in pregnant patients to decrease the risk of stomach injury and minimize the risk of aspiration of gastric contents.

INITIAL PORT PLACEMENT

There has been much debate regarding the best method of abdominal access in the pregnant patient, based on the concern for injury to the uterus or other intra-abdominal organs. Initial abdominal access can be safely accomplished with an open (Hasson) technique, Veress needle or optical trocar, if the location is adjusted according to fundal height, previous incisions and the abdominal wall is elevated during insertion. Initial access via a subcostal approach (Palmers point) has been recommended.[13]

INSUFFLATION PRESSURE

The potential for adverse consequences from CO_2 insufflation in the pregnant patient has led to apprehension over its use. Some authors advocate gasless laparoscopy, but this technique has not been widely adopted.

The pregnant patient's diaphragm is upwardly displaced by the growing fetus, which results in decreased residual lung volume and functional residual capacity. Some have recommended intra-abdominal pressures be maintained at less than 12 mm Hg to avoid worsening pulmonary physiology in gravid women.[14] Others argue that low pressures may not provide adequate visualization.[15]

Pressures of 15 mm Hg have been used during laparoscopy in pregnant patients without increasing adverse outcomes to the patient or her fetus.

There are no data showing detrimental effects to human fetuses from CO_2 pneumoperitoneum.[16] The risk of hypercapnia certainly does exist with CO_2 pneumoperitoneum.

Intra-operative CO_2 monitoring by capnography should be used during laparoscopy in pregnant patients. The goal should be end-tidal CO_2 of less than 35 mm Hg. Routine blood gas ($PaCO_2$) monitoring is unnecessary.

VENOUS THROMBOEMBOLIC PROPHYLAXIS

Pregnancy is a hypercoagulable state with 0.1–0.2% incidence of deep vein thrombosis (A100). Intraoperative and postoperative pneumatic compression devices and early postoperative ambulation are recommended.

There is no data regarding use of unfractionated or low molecular weight heparin for prophylaxis in pregnant patients undergoing laparoscopy. In patients who require anticoagulation, heparin has proven safe.[17]

■ HEMOSTATIC TECHNIQUES

Bipolar cautery is recommended for hemostasis to avoid 'sparking' phenomena associated with monopolar energy sources that may endanger the fetus or displace bowel. It is fair to extrapolate that newer energy sources that minimize the risk of thermal spread (Harmonic, Ligasure, Enseal, etc.) may be safer, although this has never been studied.

■ ADNEXAL MASSES

The incidence of adnexal masses is approximately 1 in 600 pregnancies. Only between 1% and 8% of adnexal masses in pregnant are found to be malignant.[18] Most are benign with an anechoic, simple cyst being the most common finding (and least risk of being malignant).[19] Among all adnexal masses in pregnancy, 30% are found to represent corpus luteum and between 25% and 40% represent dermoid cysts. Most adnexal masses discovered during the first trimester are functional cysts that resolve spontaneously by second trimester. Recent literature supports the safety of close observation in these patients when ultrasound findings are not suggestive of malignancy, tumor markers (CA125. LDH) are normal and the patient asymptomatic.

Traditional management has been to follow conservatively until 15–16 weeks of gestation. Waiting until 15–16 weeks gestation allows for the majority of cysts that are likely to regress to do so spontaneously, for the fetus to complete organogenesis and for spontaneous miscarriage to take place on its own. If the cysts persist beyond 15–16 weeks, they are surgically removed. However, unequivocal indications for surgical intervention in the first trimester do exist and operative laparoscopy in early pregnancy has been found to be both safe and feasible.[20] Ko reported a series of 11 patients undergoing successful laparoscopic surgery during the first trimester, the indications included persistent and enlarging cysts, torsion and rupture of cysts with internal bleeding.[21] A retrospective review of 88 pregnant women demonstrated equivalent maternal and fetal outcomes in adnexal masses managed laparoscopically and by laparotomy.[13]

Adnexal Torsion

Ten-to-fifteen percent of adnexal masses undergo torsion. Laparoscopy is the preferred method of both diagnosis and treatment in the gravid patient.[22] If diagnosed before tissue necrosis, adnexal torsion may be managed by simple laparoscopic detorsion.[23] Once detorsion is done and the ovary regains normal color, the cystectomy can be performed to prevent recurrence. Utero-ovarian ligament if elongated can be replicated and shortened. However, with late diagnosis of torsion, adnexal infarction may ensue, which can result in peritonitis, spontaneous abortion, preterm delivery and death. The gangrenous adnexa should be completely resected[24] and progesterone therapy initiated after removal of corpus luteum, if the gestation is less than 12 weeks.[23]

■ CERVICAL INCOMPETENCE

Traditionally, transvaginal cerclage placed during the first or early second trimester has been a common treatment for cervical incompetence. Unfortunately, in about 13% of women with cervical incompetence, the transvaginal approach to cerclage will not work.[25] Benson and Durfee first described the transabdominal approach to cerclage placement in 1965.[26] Placement of cerclage at the cervicoisthmic junction may be effective in decreasing the incidence of pregnancy loss in certain patients with cervical insufficiency. Generally accepted criteria for choosing the transabdominal approach to cerclage placement include:
- ❏ Congenitally short or amputated cervix
- ❏ Cervical scarring that would prevent a transvaginal approach; and
- ❏ Failure of prior vaginal cerclage.

Advantages of the transabdominal over the transvaginal approach include more proximal placement at the internal os. Furthermore, with a transabdominal cerclage, there is no vaginal foreign body, which theoretically may act as a nidus for infection. Additionally, transabdominal cerclage can be used in subsequent pregnancies, which is useful in patients desiring multiple future pregnancies.

Laparoscopic transcervical abdominal cerclage approach is safe and effective to pregnant patients between 11 weeks and 14 weeks, when abdominal cerclage is recommended and offers faster patient recovery.

■ HETEROTOPIC PREGNANCY

Heterotopic pregnancy is a condition on the rise. In 1948, just 1 in 30,000 gravidas presented with this disorder, in which uterine and extrauterine gestations exist concomitantly.[27] Today that rate is 1 in 3,800.[28] And for women undergoing in vitro fertilization (IVF), the number is a startling 1 in 100.[29] In fact, when more than 5 embryos are implanted, the risk of heterotopic pregnancy increases to 1 in 45.

Heterotopic pregnancy is extremely difficult to diagnose. More than 50% of these pregnancies are identified by sonography or laparoscopy; 2 weeks or more after the initial visualization of the intrauterine pregnancy,[30] though approximately 85% go undiagnosed before the rupture of the pregnancy.

Unfortunately, for women with heterotopic pregnancy who have undergone salpingectomy and whose pregnancy resides in the interstitial or cornual remnants of the Fallopian tube—a condition that occurs in 4% of heterotopic pregnancies[31]—an ultrasonic mass adjacent to the uterus is unlikely to raise suspicion of an ectopic pregnancy.

Any treatment of the ectopic pregnancy in a heterotopic pregnancy must consider the viability of the intrauterine pregnancy. It is important to note that one-third of intrauterine pregnancies accompanying heterotopic pregnancy miscarry in the first (89%) and second trimesters (8.5%). Miscarriage beyond the second trimester is rare; though preterm delivery may occur—particularly when heterotopic pregnancy is accompanied by multiple births. Still, a full two-thirds of intrauterine pregnancies accompanying heterotopic pregnancy do survive to term.

Early diagnosis is the key to successful treatment and delivery. Ultrasonographers must methodically examine the entire pelvic region, particularly in women who have had pelvic surgery, PID, or who are conceiving after a workup for fertility.

Treatment of choice is laparoscopic salpingectomy using bipolar or harmonic. Salpingotomy is not preferred. Medical treatment with injection of KCl has been attempted; however, methotrexate is contraindicated as it can harm the viable intrauterine pregnancy.

Once a woman has been treated for interstitial or cornual heterotopic pregnancy, close observation of the patient's hemodynamic status during labor is recommended, since the risk of uterine rupture is unknown.[29]

APPENDICITIS

Appendicitis is the most common acute general surgical condition during pregnancy. Approximately 0.05–0.1% of pregnant women will have appendicitis, which is evenly distributed through all three trimesters. Appendicitis in pregnancy presents a unique diagnostic challenge due to the anatomic and physiologic changes described previously. The preoperative diagnoses of appendicitis is correct in the first trimester 85% of time, but only correct 30–50% of the time in the second and third trimesters. When the diagnosis remains uncertain, prompt ultrasound or MRI are useful adjuncts to more accurate diagnosis. Accurate, timely diagnosis and treatment of appendicitis

in the gravid patient may minimize the risk of spontaneous miscarriage and preterm labor which increase greatly with perforation. It is recommended that the pregnant patient with acute appendicitis be treated in a manner identical to the nonpregnant patient with regard to rapid resuscitation with intravenous fluids, antibiotics and prompt surgical intervention. The laparoscopic approach is the preferred treatment for pregnant patients with presumed appendicitis, and the studies have shown the technique to be safe and effective.[32]

GALLBLADDER DISEASE

Pregnancy predisposes women to the formation of gallstones. While gallstones are found in 4–12% of all pregnant women, only 0.05% will suffer from symptomatic cholelithiasis.[33] Only 40% of these will require cholecystectomy. Until recently, symptomatic cholelithiasis in pregnancy was managed conservatively.[34] A review of 44 patients in 1987 with biliary colic showed that amongst the 26 patients managed conservatively, 58% had recurrent episodes with complications involving spontaneous abortion, preterm labor and pancreatitis. Of the 18 patients who underwent surgical treatment, none miscarried.[35]

At present, early surgical management is the treatment of choice. Laparoscopic cholecystectomy is the preferred method.[2] There have been no reports of fetal demise for laparoscopic cholecystectomy performed during the first and second trimesters. Furthermore, decreased rates of spontaneous abortion and preterm labor have been reported in laparoscopic cholecystectomy when compared to laparotomy.[34] Owing to the location of the gallbladder in the right upper quadrant, laparoscopic cholecystectomy appears feasible even at an advanced gestational age.

SOLID ORGAN RESECTION

Laparoscopic adrenalectomy during pregnancy has proven effective in management of primary hyperaldosteronism,[36] Cushing's syndrome,[37] and pheochromocytoma.[38] Laparoscopic splenectomy has been accepted in surgical treatment of hereditary spherocytosis[39] and autoimmune thrombocytopenic purpura.[40] Laparoscopic nephrectomy has been reported in first and second trimesters.[41]

PERIOPERATIVE CARE

No intraoperative fetal heart rate abnormalities have been reported during laparoscopic surgery. This has led some to recommend preoperative and postoperative monitoring of

FHR. Intraoperative monitoring is not needed.[11] Tocolytics should not be used prophylactically in pregnant women undergoing surgery but should be considered perioperative when signs of preterm labor are present. The specific agent and indications for the use of tocolysis should be individualized.

◼ CONCLUSION

Laparoscopic surgery in pregnancy is safe and feasible. It offers the patient all the benefits of minimal invasive surgery approach. The risks to the pregnancy appear smallest when surgery is performed in a nonemergent setting, in the second trimester and with careful monitoring of the special physiologic needs of the mother and fetus.

It is not acceptable to delay diagnosis and treatment of the surgical conditions in any patient owing to pregnancy status. Adnexal masses can be managed expectantly until they can be removed in the second trimester unless torsion, hemorrhage, suppuration, rapid enlargement or features of malignancy are evident. Pregnant patients with an acute abdomen, appendicitis or cholecystitis should be treated in a manner identical to the non pregnant patient with as little delay in surgical treatment as possible. Laparoscopic surgery will become the standard of care for management of surgical conditions during pregnancy.

◼ REFERENCES

1. Kammerer WS. Non-obstetric surgery during pregnancy. The Medical Clinic of North America. 1979;63:1157-64.
2. Barone JE, Bears S, Chen S, et al. Outcome study of cholecystectomy during pregnancy. Am J Surg. 1999;177:232-6.
3. Curet MJ. Special problems in laparoscopic surgery. Previous abdominal surgery, obesity and pregnancy. Surg Clin North Am. 2000;80:1093-110.
4. Baer J. Appendicitis in pregnancy with changes in position and axis of the normal appendix. JAMA. 1932;98:1359-64.
5. Karam PA. Determining and reporting fetal radiation exposure from diagnostic radiation. Health Phys. 2000;79:S85-90.
6. Chen MM, Coakley FV, Kaimal A, et al. Guidelines for CT and MRI use during pregnancy and lactation. Obstet Gynecol. 2008;112:333-40.
7. Hurwitz LM, Yoshizumi T, Reiman RE. Radiation dose to the fetus from body MDCT during early gestation. Am J Roentgenol. 2006;186:871-6.
8. Karthikesalingam A, Markar SR, Weerakkody R, et al. Radiation exposure during laparoscopic cholecystectomy with routine intraoperative cholangiography. Surg Endosc. 2009;23:1845-8.
9. Reedy MB, Galan HL, Richards WE, et al. Laparoscopy during pregnancy: A survey of Laparoendoscopic surgeons. J Reprod Med. 1997;42:338.
10. Reedy MB, Kallen B, Kuehl TJ. Laparoscopy during Pregnancy: A study of five fetal outcome parameters with use of Swedish Health Registry. Am J Obstet Gynecol. 1997;177:673-9.
11. Affleck DG, Handrahan DL, Egger MJ, et al. The laparoscopic management of appendicitis and cholelithiasis during pregnancy. Am J Surg. 1999;178:523-9.
12. Geisler JP, Rose SL, Mernitz CS, et al. Non-gynecologic laparoscopy in second and third trimester pregnancy: Obstetric implications. JSLS. 1998;2:235-8.
13. Soriano D, Yefet Y, Seidman DS, et al. Laparoscopy versus laparotomy in the management of adnexal masses during pregnancy. Fertil Steril. 1999;71:955-60.
14. Guidelines for laparoscopic surgery during pregnancy. Society of American Gastrointestinal Endoscopic Surgeons (SAGES). Surg Endosc. 1998;12:189-90.
15. Rollins MD, Chan KJ, Price RR. Laparoscopy for appendicitis and cholelithiasis during pregnancy: A new standard of care. Surg Endosc. 2004;18:237-41.
16. Fatum M, Rojansky N. Laparoscopic surgery during pregnancy. Obstet Gynecol Surv. 2001;56:50-9.
17. Casele HL. The use of unfractionated and LMW heparins in pregnancy. Clin Obstet Gynecol. 2006;49:895-905.
18. Nezhat FR, Tazuke S, Nezhat CH, et al. Laparoscopy during pregnancy: A literature review. JSLS. 1997;1:17-27.
19. Hogston P, Lilford RJ. Ultrasound study of ovarian cysts in pregnancy: prevalence and significance. Br J Obstet Gynecol. 1986;93:625-8.
20. Parker WH, Childers JM, Canis M, et al. Laparoscopic management of benign cystic teratomas during pregnancy. Am J Obstet Gynecol. 1996;174:1499-501.
21. Ko ML, Lai TH, Chen SC. Laparoscopic management of complicated adnexal masses in the first trimester of pregnancy. Fertil Steril. 2009;92:283-7.
22. Nichols DH, Julian PJ. Torsion of the adnexa. Clin Obstet Gynecol. 1985;28:375-80.
23. Argenta PA, Yeagley TJ, Ott G, et al. Torsion of the uterine adnexa: Pathologic correlations and current management trends. J Reprod Med. 2000;45:831-6.
24. Oelsner G, Bider D, Goldenberg M, et al. Long-term follow-up of the twisted ischemic adnexa managed by detorsion. Fertil Steril. 1993;60:976-9.
25. Harger JH. Cerclage and Cervical insufficiency: An evidence based analysis. Obstet Gynecol. 2002;100:1313-27.
26. Benson RC, Durfee RB. Transabdominal Cervicouterine cerclage during pregnancy for the treatment of cervical incompetency. Obstet Gynecol. 1965;25:145-55.
27. DeVOE RW, Pratt JH. Simultaneous intrauterine and extrauterine pregnancy. Am J Obstet Gynecol. 1948;56:1119-26.
28. Habana A, Dokras A, Giraldo JL, et al. Cornual heterotopic pregnancy: Contemporary management options. Am J Obstet Gynecol. 2000;182:1264-70.

29. Lau S, Tulandi T. Conservative medical and surgical management of interstitial ectopic pregnancy. Fertil Steril. 1999;72:207-15.

30. Tal J, Haddad S, Gordon N, et al. Heterotopic pregnancy after ovulation induction and assisted reproductive technologies: A literature review from 1971 to 1993. Fertil Steril. 1996;66:1-12.

31. Dumesic DA, Damario MA, Session DR. Interstitial heterotopic pregnancy in a woman conceiving by in vitro fertilization after bilateral salpingectomy. Mayo Clin Proc. 2001;76:90-2.

32. Korndorffer JR, Fellinger E, Reed W. SAGES Guidelines for Laparoscopic Appendectomy. Surg Endosc. 2010;24:757-61.

33. Graham G, Baxi L, Tharakan T. Laparoscopic cholecystectomy during pregnancy: A case series and review of the literature. Obstet Gynecol Surg. 1998;53:566-74.

34. Sharp HT. Gastrointestinal surgical conditions during pregnancy. Clin Obstet Gynecol. 1994;37:306-15.

35. Sen G, Nagabhushan JS, Joypaul V. Laparoscopic cholecystectomy in third trimester of pregnancy. J Obstet Gynaecol. 2002;22:556-7.

36. Shalhav AL, Landman J, Afane J, et al. Laparoscopic adrenalectomy for primary hyperaldosteronism during pregnancy. J Laparoendosc Adv Surg Tech A. 2000;10:169-71.

37. Lo CY, Lo CM, Lam KY. Cushing's syndrome secondary to adrenal adenoma during pregnancy. Surg Endosc. 2002;16:219-20.

38. Janetschek G, Finkenstedt G, Gasser R, et al. Laparoscopic surgery for pheochromocytoma: Adrenalectomy, partial resection, excision of paragangliomas. J Urol. 1998;160:330-4.

39. Allran CF Jr, Weiss CA 3rd, Park AE. Urgent laparoscopic splenectomy in a morbidly obese pregnant woman: Case report and literature review. J Laparoendosc Adv Surg Tech A. 2002;12:445-7.

40. Griffiths J, Sia W, Shapiro AM, et al. Laparoscopic splenectomy for the treatment of refractory immune thrombocytopenia in pregnancy. J Obstet Gynaecol Can. 2005;27:771-4.

41. O'Connor JP, Biyani CS, Taylor J, et al. Laparoscopic nephrectomy for renal-cell carcinoma during pregnancy. J Endourol. 2004;18:871-4.

CHAPTER 17

Non-Descent Vaginal Hysterectomy

JP Rath

▌ NATURAL ORIFICE HYSTERECTOMY

Much has been discussed and debated over the recent years about the preferred route for offering a woman who requires a hysterectomy. Training has been the essential decision maker, and not the ease, or ever if, the choice to patients on making the decision.

The fact remains that vaginal route is superior for most cases, if there is no gross deviation of anatomy. Indications have to be studied and a fair assessment of the patient before actually deciding to begin. Most gynecologists who have had practice in non descent vaginal hysterectomy (NDVH) do know that in any patient when difficulty is encountered can convert to either abdominal or laparoscopic (Lap) route.

The learning curve remains as in any case of surgical competence, and the mastery is easily achievable by most. The indications broaden as the horizon, with experience to do them, and an understanding in detecting and dealing with complications. Unfair to state that the complications are more in vaginal over abdominal as is the conventional teaching, or the time involved is more.

▌ INDICATIONS

Same as abdominal or laparoscopy with experience to do vaginal surgery.

▌ CONTRAINDICATIONS

❑ Too large uterus, usually 20 weeks or more, puckered abdominal wall with adherent uterus

❑ Previous sling wherein the uterus has moved up and not mobile
❑ Any impacted uterus in pelvis where lateral access is a challenge
❑ Severe endometriosis with dense adhesions
❑ Previous extensive Koch's disease.

▌ CAUTION

❑ Uterine size more than 16 weeks as in fibroids
❑ Beyond 14 weeks in adenoma of uterus
❑ Any uterus that is stuck to the abdominal wall due to previous surgery
❑ Repaired bladder fistula or bladder injury
❑ Previous three cesarean sections.

After careful assessment of patient, anesthetic fitness, medical fitness and counseling, patient is taken up for surgery. Preoperative enema till returning fluid is clear with antisepsis of vagina is done. The role of cleansing the bowel cannot but be over emphasized as the operative field remains clear during surgery.

> **Points to Remember**
> - Careful case selection
> - Patient counseling with advantages of surgery
> - Competency of surgeon in difficult cases

▌ ANESTHESIA

The preferred anesthesia is spinal using pencil point spinal needle of 27 gauge. Additive to bupivacaine like profentanyl or buprenorphine in small dosage makes postoperative period pain free and allows patient to be ambulated within 4 hours of surgery.

POSITION

Position of patient is paramount and an exaggerated lithotomy, with the pelvis thrust beyond the edge of the table and legs strung high or taken backward, opens the vagina making surgery easy. The lithotomy bars are inclined towards head end with an incline of 15° to achieve the exaggerated position. Padding may be given at pressure points. Thorough painting with Povidone-iodine is done, draping with only the introitus visible.

INSTRUMENTS

Same that one would use for abdominal, with addition of *2 single blade Sim's speculum,* this is a suitable replacement to bladder retractor (alternatively *Breisky* retractor may be used). Slender and long Sim's speculum may be used in cases of previous sections.

Ovarian clamps like those designed by various authors may also be used. Author uses curved *Satinsky* clamps or those designed by Professor Paily.

SUTURES

Usually prefer No. 1 vicryl (2347) for the pedicles and vicryl 2-0 (2317) for closure of vault. Suitable sutures may be used as per choice. Linen is not used. Plain loop suturing with adequate stump or transfixing sutures may be put depending on the comfort of the surgeon. Vicryl Rapide™ may be used for vaginal mucosa, as some patients do complain of discharge with dyed vicryl. Needle is held at an acute angle to the needle holder so as to occupy less space in the vagina and for easy movement.

METHOD

Assessment under anesthesia is vital before starting. Any one of the aforementioned caution should be assessed and size of uterus, its mobility, and palpation of any adnexal mass is done at this stage.

Bladder emptied, cervix held with two bulldog vulsellum, infiltration with diluted adrenalin solution is done on the anterior mucosa. Small quantity is used so as to raise the vaginal mucosa over bladder. This in itself demarcates the bladder extent, and a small U-shaped transverse incision is taken and the bladder pushed up using sharp dissection from the cervix. Gradually with

finger dissection on the lateral aspect, the entire bladder is pushed exposing the peritoneal fold, which is cut and the *anterior pouch*, thus, opened.

An Allice forceps holds the posterior mucosa at the junction of the uterosacral ligaments, and 3–5 mL of diluted adrenalin infiltrated. A bold cut is taken on the mucosa above the Allice catch, and often the *posterior pouch* is opened in this single cut. Sometimes only the mucosa and not the peritoneum is opened, simple dissection at this stage opens the pouch.

Both Sim's speculum is inserted into the respective pouch, and the mucosa need not be cut completely on the lateral aspect. Lateral clamps taken one at a time include the *cardinal ligaments* and the *uterosacral*. One clamp usually suffices for this, a cut is made leaving a generous stump, and this is sutured with vicryl, leaving a length of vicryl to

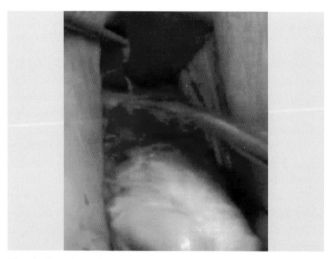

Fig. 1: Opening of anterior pouch: Tip: Adequate mobilization of bladder should to be done before careful opening of peritoneum. Often there is injury to bladder at this stage

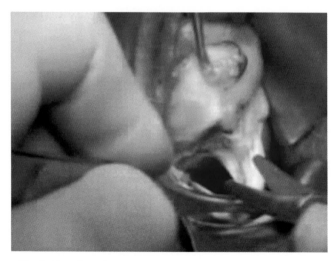

Fig. 2: Opening of posterior pouch: Tip: Stay close to uterus, as fat belongs to rectum

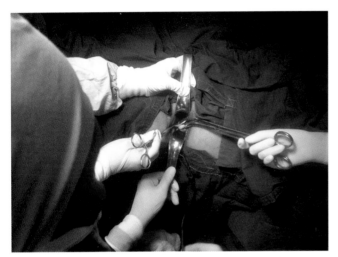

Fig. 3: Cardinal ligament and uterosacral: The lateral mucosa need not be denuded from the cervix, this reduces the oozing

manipulate the pedicle. While suturing the pedicle, the entire specimen is pushed into the pelvis cranially so as to create space for needle movement. The same repeated on the other side.

The next pedicle is that of the crucial *uterine artery*. Care is taken that both leaves of broad ligament are included in the clamp (i.e. anterior and posterior). Likewise the specimen is pushed in so as to make the ligature easy. The assistant holds the Sim's speculum at 1 and 5 O'clock position for the left pedicle and the 7 and 11 O'clock position for the right pedicle. It is wise to fix the uterine pedicle to the cardinal ligament pedicle, so the uterine if it slips may be accessed with pulling this pedicle and also the cardinal ligament is pulled up with the uterine pedicle, thus, strengthening the vault.

At this stage, a *bisection of uterus* is done and one part pushed deep into pelvis and the other pulled out. This gives ample space and also access to the *tubo-ovarian pedicle*. The round ligament is taken separately so that the infundibulopelvic ligament is seen, in case of adnexal removal. The infundibulopelvic ligament is severed at this stage with removal of ovary, ovarian clamp makes this step easier with its excessive curve. Long and slender Sim's speculum gives adequate exposure to these pedicles and after confirming that they are secure, closure may be affected. In case where the ovary is to be spared, the tube may be removed as mandated using the curved clamps.

After checking that the integrity and having achieved hemostasis, closure may be done. The potential *enterocele* may be dealt by passing a suture from the pedicles from right to left including the anterior part of the rectum high up, and held long for final suturing of vault. The lateral sutures held long of pedicles may be cut at this stage after ensuring hemostasis.

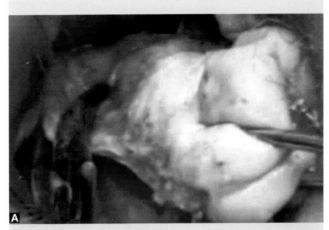

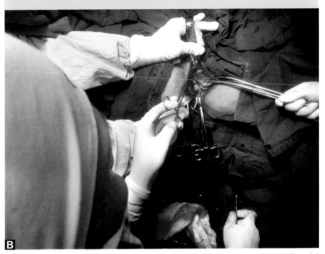

Figs 4A and B: Uterine pedicle ligation: (A) Tip: clamps should ideally be applied only when both pouches opened as the uterine artery lies in the leaves of the broad ligament. (B) While applying the clamp, it is advisable to pull the specimen onto the other side so that application is perfect

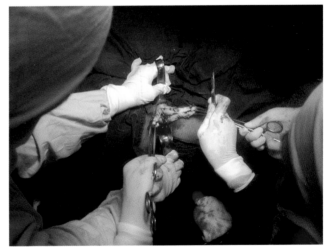

Fig. 5: Bisection of uterus: Bisection of uterus is done after both the uterine arteries are secured. This is completed with a gentle and continuous traction on the specimen. It reduces the space and by pushing in one-half the specimen, the contralateral tubo-ovarian pedicle is better accessed

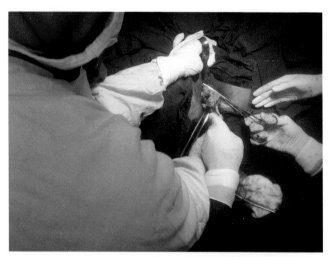

Fig. 6: The tubo-ovarian pedicle can be accessed easily after bisection of uterus

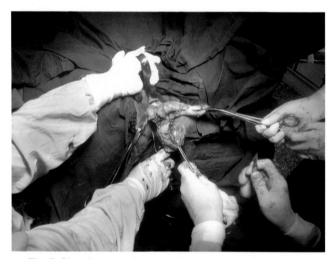

Fig. 7: Bisection, reveals the underlying fibroids which may be enucleated or removed as potato wedges depending on their sizes

Vault closure is done by using 2-0 vicryl, interrupted or mattress sutures with space on lateral aspect to facilitate drainage of collected blood. One set of sutures on either side and one mattress suture in the middle and the central suture place is fastened to the pedicle and thus pushing up the vault further up and help in preventing vault prolapse and also ensuring adequate length of vagina for future coitus.

In case of a *cystocele,* the mucosal flap is reflected and bladder is pushed and a repair is done as per the usual method. Thereafter the mucosa is closed.

Vagina is packed with gauze or simply with a sponge. The bladder catheterized and sanitization of perineum is done and legs are freed from its position.

> **Points to Remember**
> - Good position—better accessibility
> - Good illumination
> - Good assistance
> - Good instruments
> - Pushing-in of the specimen to expose the tip of Kocher's so as to tie the pedicle
> - Acute angle of needle to the holder for easy movement

POSTOPERATIVE CARE

Intravenous fluids and antibiotics should be given as desired, along with analgesics, if necessary. Patient's catheter and pack is removed after 4 hours and she is mobilized out of bed. Oral fluids may be given liberally, and after 8 hours soft diet is advised.

Patient may be discharged the following day or the next as per recovery with stool softeners, if desired.

ADVANTAGES

- ❑ Ease of surgery, well-defined tissue planes
- ❑ Less complication
- ❑ No gadgetry
- ❑ Early ambulation, feeding and discharge
- ❑ Less discomfort
- ❑ No visible sutures
- ❑ Least expensive with high patient satisfaction.

SPECIAL CASES

Previous Cesarean Section

This is essentially a mind block about the difficulty in accomplishing the surgery. The scar is seldom a problem, and can be dealt by raising the bladder from the cervix with a Babcock's forceps and by snipping with a metzenbaum or dissecting scissors the bladder is moved up. Bladder adhesions are very rarely seen in the lateral aspects and hence gentle tunneling may be done there. And rarely are they so very adherent that the planes are not identified, in such cases delivery of uterus is done posteriorly and fingers moved above the uterus and in the anterior pouch, and the pouch opened.

The chance of bladder injury is almost the same as with other routes, if restrain is exercised in the dissection. Small and midsized injuries may be managed on detection from the vaginal route itself, using 2-0 vicryl and the rent sutured in two layers. Major lacerations may need the assistance of a urological surgeon, and perhaps an abdominal approach. Cystoscope to study the extent of damage and also the integrity of the trigone, cannulation of ureter may be necessary.

Fibroids

Experience lets us define the limits in size of fibroid. Most literature tells us; comfortably up to 14 weeks, size may be attempted. The lateral space access is the defining limit, allowing a good ligaturing of the uterine pedicle. Slicing or bisection as needed can only be done once the uterine artery is well-secured. Slicing or coring at the uterus well within its boundary of serosa or capsule is safe. This is similar to morcellation and requires dexterity and patience. The constant traction on the cervix to pull out the uterus along with slicing like potato wedges causes the uterus to reduce in its transverse diameter and deliver out of the vagina with ease.

Multiple fibroids of varying sizes may be enucleated, or bisected and removed causing the shrinkage in the uterine size.

Adenomyoma

Adenomyomas have no defined boundary and hence difficult to slice, often the blood loss is more. These are dealt in similar ways as fibroids.

Endometriosis

The rectal endometriosis can pose a challenge in opening the posterior pouch, and for obvious reason the rectum is at risk of damage. The anterior pouch is opened and posteriorly the mucosa is pushed up and no attempt to open the pouch is made. The uterus is delivered through the anterior opened pouch and the serosal layer is sliced maintaining the integrity of the rectal wall. Chocolate cysts may be encountered; these are opened and drained, after the cyst collapses they are removed using clamps.

Adnexal Masses

These can be perplexing and removal requires competency. It is mandatory to rule out malignancy in these cases, and once sure they can be gently dissected and small pedicles taken to deliver them successfully.

Alternatively laparoscopically-assisted vaginal hysterectomy (LAVH) may be done for the less accessible masses.

Slipped Ligature

Especially the uterine pedicle, if detected on table, it may be successfully dealt with from vaginal route itself. Quick removal of the specimen yields enough space for visualization coupled with traction of the cardinal ligament pedicle, exposes the spurting vessel. In spite of efforts, one cannot trace the vessel origin, packing with a sponge is done and then convert into abdominal route, and tackle the bleeding vessel.

> **Points to Remember**
> - Competency of surgeon is paramount in dealing with difficult cases
> - Like in any pelvic surgery, knowledge of anatomy should be perfect
> - Nothing is bigger than ego, so let go off it
> - Call for expert help, when needed

■ COMPLICATIONS

❑ Bladder injuries
❑ Slipped ligature and hemorrhage
❑ Pelvic hematoma and or pelvic abscess
❑ Long operating time may cause hyperesthesia or pain in legs of patient due to tying.

Changing over from vaginal to abdominal: Care should be taken in catheterization, sponge count and tie on anterior and posterior flap of mucosa are kept long, so that closure of vault is easy.

It is for us to rue the fact, that the most preferred route is seldom the choice. Vaginal hysterectomy should be encouraged by all gynecologists as the first option, and spare the patient of a large wound, expense, gadgetry, and prolonged risk of anesthesia and surgery.

Section 5

COMPLICATIONS

- Diagnosis and Management of Laparoscopic Complications
- Medicolegal Cases

"At his best, man is the noblest of all animals; separated from law and justice he is the worst."

Aristotle

CHAPTER 18

Diagnosis and Management of Laparoscopic Complications

Shailesh Puntambekar, Seema Puntambekar, Geetanjali Joshi, Nandan Purandare

■ COMPLICATIONS

Complications are an integral part of advanced laparoscopic surgeries. Many of these are iatrogenic and hence avoidable. These are either due to faulty technique or inadvertent use of energy sources. These complications are, therefore ,divided into:

❑ Intraoperative
❑ Postoperative.

Intraoperative

They are further subclassified as: Vascular, urological injuries, organ injury and general.

Vascular Complications

❑ Arterial
❑ Venous.

Arterial bleeding: Arterial bleeding is easily tackled than venous bleeding. The source is easily identified and hence can be controlled by various measures like:

❑ Clips
❑ Vessel sealing devices like Ligasure or gyrus
❑ Suture.

The bleeding needs to be tackled immediately as the blood loss can be life-threatening.

Whenever there is arterial bleeding, there can be spurting of the blood on the telescope, thereby obscuring the vision. The main task is to avoid this blood spurting. This can be done by withdrawing the telescope into the trocars (Fig. 1).

The next step is to identify and catch the bleeding point. It is always advisable to keep the left hand grasper free. The left hand grasper should immediately catch the bleeding point (Fig. 2). If the left hand grasper is not free, an additional trocar can be inserted and a grasper is passed through that to hold the bleeder. Once the bleeder is caught, the choice is between applying clips or sealing the vessels. If either of this is not successful then a suture can be passed and the vessel can be ligated. It is not advisable to use compression for arterial bleeding. The commonest site of arterial bleeding is near the uterus. Very often the cut uterine stump cannot be seen, and thus, ligation has to be done.

Venous bleeding: Venous bleeding is difficult to tackle due to the following reasons:

❑ No identifiable bleeding point

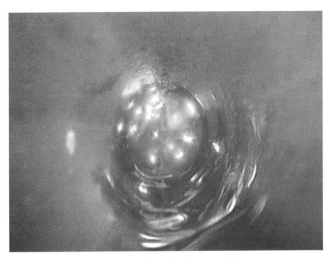

Fig. 1: Withdrawing of telescope in trocar

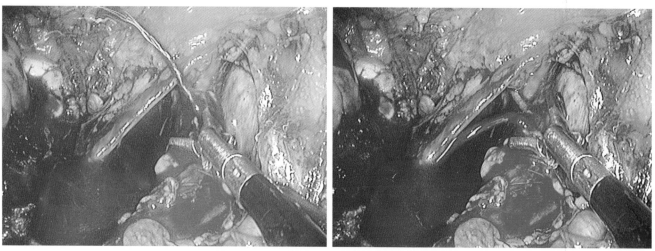

Fig. 2: Left hand grasper catching the bleeding point

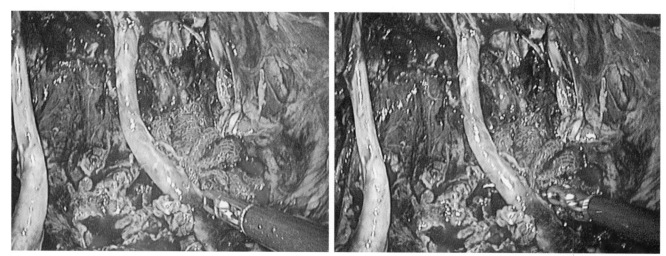

Fig. 3: Packing with gauze

❏ Smaller caliber of the vessels
❏ Lack of adventitia, hence, sealing devices not very useful.

There are various ways of tackling the venous bleeding (Table 1). It depends on the size of the vessel and the site of injury. Packing with gauze is the best way to manage venous bleeds. Multiple gauze pieces may be used for compression. Small venous bleeding during lymphadenectomy and bleeding from the presacral veins can be easily dealt with this method (Fig. 3).

Gauze compression can be combined with desufflation to enhance coagulation. One should stop CO_2 insufflation and wait for 7–10 minutes, so as to allow clotting. This achieves immediate hemostasis.

The next method of controlling venous bleeding is using bipolar energy sources. Due to the lack of adventitia of the vein, vessel sealing devices cannot effectively seal the vessels. The bipolar energy source is the best method

Table 1: Tricks to control venous bleeding
• Packing
• Desufflation
• Clips
• Bipolar energy sources
• Ligation
• Occasionally vessel sealing devices

of vessel coagulation. Care should be taken to avoid using bipolar at high current as the jaws stick to the tissues (Fig. 4).

The clipping of the vein can be done, if enough stump is available (Fig. 5).

If all these measures fail to achieve hemostasis, then suturing should be done (Fig. 6). This is a reliable method of controlling bleeding.

The greatest danger of the venous bleeding is CO_2 embolism. Therefore in an event of a major venous bleeding, one should also monitor the end titled (ET) CO_2 levels.

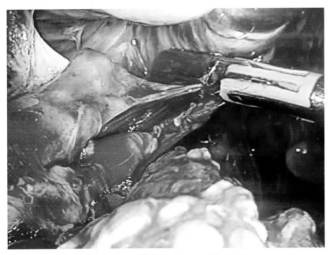

Fig. 4: Coagulation of vein with bipolar

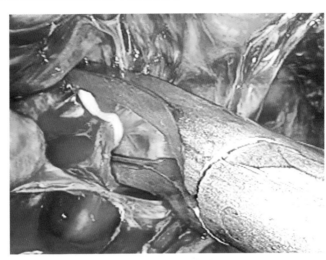

Fig. 5: Clipping of vein

Table 2: Control of vascular complications	
Arterial bleeding	*Venous bleeding*
• Keep the left hand free to grasp	• Packing
• Additional port placement	• Desufflate
• Use clips/vessel sealing devices	• Bipolar energy
• Suturing	• Suturing
	• Vessel sealing devices

In case the ET CO$_2$ level is falling, the measures to be taken are:
❏ Stop insufflation
❏ Hyperventilate the patient.
    The ways to control arterial and venous bleeding are given in Table 2.

Urological Injuries

As the limits of laparoscopy have widened to include advanced pelvic surgeries, injuries to the genitourinary tract are increasing. Anticipation of injuries in difficult cases and efforts to recognize injuries help in decreasing postoperative morbidity. Bladder pathology, adhesions, previous surgery, inflammation, or endometriosis increase the risk of bladder and ureteric injuries. These injuries can be managed laparoscopically and conversion to laparotomy is not required.
    These injuries are divided into:
❏ *Bladder*
  ❖ Immediate
  ❖ Delayed
❏ *Ureteric*
  ❖ Immediate
  ❖ Delayed.

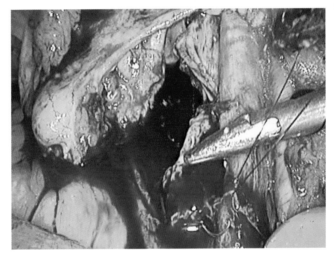

Fig. 6: Suturing of external iliac vein

Bladder Injuries

❏ *Immediate bladder injury*: The commonest causes of bladder injuries are: (a) Previous surgical, cesarean section; (b) Involvement by tumor (Fig. 7). Bladder injuries are fairly easy to tackle. The bladder has to be sutured with an absorbable suture (Fig. 8). This can be done in one or two layers. The best method to identify the bladder injury is to fill the bladder with a colored fluid (methylene blue or betadine). The borderline bladder injuries can be identified.
Bladder is a surgeon friendly organ. Suturing followed by prolonged bladder drainage with Foley's catheter is the best way to tackle bladder injuries.
❏ *Delayed bladder injury*: These are due to avascular necrosis of the bladder wall. This is caused by the

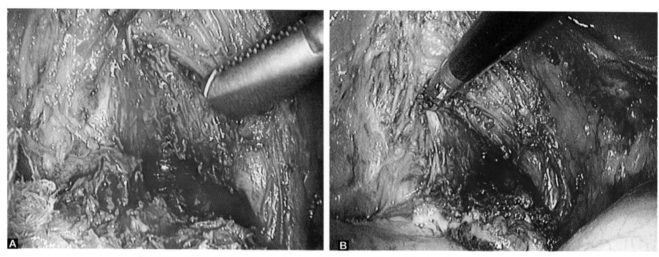

Figs 7A and B: (A) Bladder involvement by tumor; (B) Bladder involvement by tumor

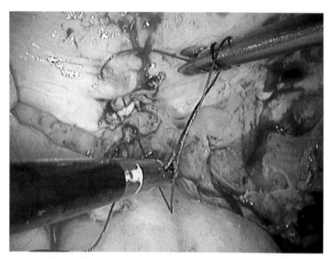

Fig. 8: Bladder suturing by absorbable suture (vicryl)

excessive use of energy sources near the bladder base. They present as vesicovaginal fistula (VVF) and decrease in urine output. This is a difficult situation to manage. If the leak is intraperitoneal, there will be abdominal distention, ileus or fever. An immediate computerized tomography or an ultrasound should be done. If there is a small leak, it can be closed primarily. The VVF should be repaired 3–6 weeks after its presentation. This allows the fistula tract to mature with good fibrosis. The VVF repair can be done either by laparotomy, vaginally or laparoscopy. We have successfully managed more than 20 cases of VVF laparoscopically with the need for laparotomy. The ways to control arterial and venous bleeding is given in Table 2.

Laparoscopic transvesical approach for VVF repair: The three main principles of fistula repair are:

1. Excision
2. Exclusion
3. Reconstruction.

The bladder is mobilized anteriorly. It can be done with sharp dissection or with a monopolar hook. The fistula is recognized. For a transvesical repair, the bladder is opened on the anterior wall. The ureteric orifices are cannulated with infant feeding tube. This delineated the ureters and helped to prevent the damage. The next step is to cut the posterior wall up to the fistulous tract. The fistula is isolated and the bladder wall is separated from the vaginal wall. Excision of the entire fistulous tract is done. It is advisable to use harmonic for this dissection as this dissection can be difficult and bloody. One should be very careful not to damage the trigonal area and the urethra. The vaginal margins are refreshed for better closure and healing. Vaginal closure is done with 2-0 vicryl. The omentum is now brought down from the left paracolic gutter. It is sutured to the vagina with a few sutures so as to prevent slippage. This forms the posterior basis of the wall of the bladder, which is to be reconstructed. The bladder reconstruction is done by bringing the anterior layer close to the posterior wall. Thus, one is approximating the two cut edges by reinserting healthy bladder mucosa, over the fistulous area and not just joining the two cut edges. One side of the bladder flap is turned inwards and brought close to the fistulous area and sutured with 2-0 vicryl. Barbed sutures can also be used to avoid the knotting. The posterior bladder wall is reconstructed by placing healthy bladder mucosa from the other cut flap of the bladder. Anterior wall of the bladder is closed by continuous suturing. Catheter is kept in situ for three weeks.

Bladder injuries can be prevented by:
- Carry out the dissection close to the cervix
- Remember the dictum "fat always belongs to bladder"
- Begin the dissection laterally than from the center
- Use combination of scissors and gauze
- Anticipate injuries in difficult cases

Flow chart 1: Clinical management of ureteral injury

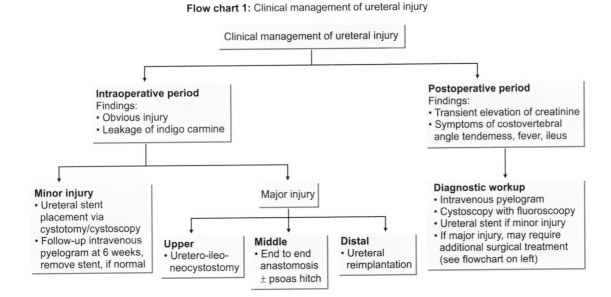

Clinical management of ureteral injury

Intraoperative period
Findings:
• Obvious injury
• Leakage of indigo carmine

Postoperative period
Findings:
• Transient elevation of creatinine
• Symptoms of costovertebral angle tendemess, fever, ileus

Minor injury
• Ureteral stent placement via cystotomy/cystoscopy
• Follow-up intravenous pyelogram at 6 weeks, remove stent, if normal

Major injury

Upper
• Uretero-ileo-neocystostomy

Middle
• End to end anastomosis ± psoas hitch

Distal
• Ureteral reimplantation

Diagnostic workup
• Intravenous pyelogram
• Cystoscopy with fluoroscoopy
• Ureteral stent if minor injury
• If major injury, may require additional surgical treatment (see flowchart on left)

No loss of length

Minimal loss of length

Significant loss of length

Fig. 9: Common site of ureteric injury

Ureteric injury: Ureteric injuries are common in oncological surgeries, especially in postchemotherapy or postradiation patients. Injuries can also be attributed to poor anatomical knowledge and callous use of energy sources (Fig. 9). It is pertinent to anticipate ureteric injuries in such cases. The injury needs to be detected and treated at the earliest. A leakage of urine or an obvious injury can be detected intraoperatively. Postoperatively, the patient can present with ureterovesical fistula.

Investigations to be done are intravenous pyelography and cystogram.

Once the injury is detected, the treatment depends on the site of injury. Not every injury needs to be reimplanted (Flow chart 1).

In cases of small injuries, a double J stent can be placed. In cases of small and single wall injury, a primary closure can be attempted. First a double J stent insertion should be done. The guide wire can also be guided laparoscopically. The injury is then sutured (Fig. 10).

Ureteroneocystostomy

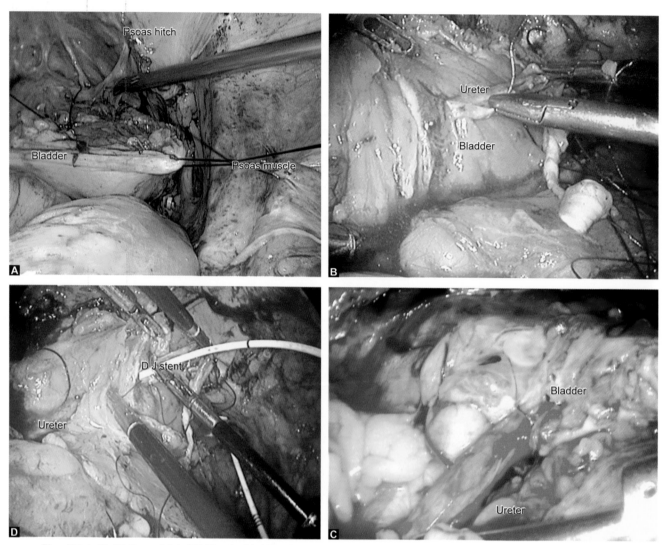

Figs 10A to D: (A) Psoas hitch (Hitching the bladder with psoas muscle); (B) Suturing of ureter with bladder after making tunnel; (C) Laparoscopic placement of DJ stent in ureter; (D) Final picture of ureteroneocystostomy

CHAPTER 19

Medicolegal Cases

Dilip Walke

"There have been several cases in Indian Courts involving gynecological laparoscopy and hysteroscopy surgeries. The present chapter describes some of the cases which offer carry home messages for safe practice."

▌CASE NO. 1

The first case is important because it describes the concept of consent in Indian context for all surgeries and procedures in general and laparoscopic surgeries in particular.

Samira Kohli v/s Dr Prabha Manchanda & Another Decided on 06-01-2008 at the Supreme Court of India by Hon Justice BN Agarwal, Hon Justice PP Naolekar and Hon Justice RV Raveendran

Judgment

Raveendran, J

This appeal is filed against the order dated 19.11.2003 passed by the National forum.

1. On 9.5.1995, Samira Kohli aged 44-year-old unmarried woman approached with 9 days per vaginum. USG was done on the same day and she was advised to get laparoscopy done on the next day under general anesthesia for affirmative diagnosis.

2. Accordingly, on 10.5.1995, the appellant went to the respondent's clinic with her mother. On admission, the appellant's signatures were taken on (i) admission and discharge card; (ii) consent form for hospital admission and medical treatment; and (iii) consent form for surgery. The Admission Card showed that admission was for diagnostic and operative laparoscopy on 10.5.1995. The consent form for surgery filled by Dr Lata Rangan (respondent's assistant) described the procedure to be undergone by the appellant as "diagnostic and operative laparoscopy. Laparotomy may be needed". Thereafter, appellant was put under general anesthesia and subjected to a laparoscopic examination.

3. When the appellant was still unconscious, Dr Lata Rangan, who was assisting the respondent, came out of the Operation Theater and took the consent of appellant's mother, who was waiting outside, for performing hysterectomy under general anesthesia. Thereafter, the respondent performed an abdominal hysterectomy (removal of uterus) and bilateral salpingo-oophorectomy (removal of ovaries and fallopian tubes). The appellant left the respondent's clinic on 15.5.1995 without settling the bill.

4. On 23.5.1995, the respondent lodged a complaint with the Police alleging that on 15.5.1995, the appellant's friend (Commander Zutshi) had abused and threatened her (respondent) and that against medical advice, he

got the appellant discharged without clearing the bill. The appellant also lodged a complaint against the respondent on 31.5.1995, alleging negligence and unauthorized removal of her reproductive organs. The first respondent issued a legal notice dated 5.6.1995 demanding ₹ 39,325/- for professional services. The appellant sent a reply dated 12.7.1995. There was a rejoinder dated 18.7.1995 from the respondent and a further reply dated 11.9.1995 from the appellant. On 19.1.1996, the appellant filed a complaint before the Commission claiming a compensation of ₹ 25 lakhs from the respondent. The appellant alleged that respondent was negligent in treating her; that the radical surgery by which her uterus, ovaries and fallopian tubes were removed without her consent, when she was under general anesthesia for a laparoscopic test, was unlawful, unauthorized and unwarranted; that on account of the removal of her reproductive organs, she had suffered premature menopause necessitating a prolonged medical treatment and a hormone replacement therapy (HRT) course, apart from making her vulnerable to health problems by way of side effects. The compensation claimed was for the loss of reproductive organs and consequential loss of opportunity to become a mother, for diminished matrimonial prospects, for physical injury resulting in the loss of vital body organs and irreversible permanent damage, for pain, suffering emotional stress and trauma, and for decline in the health and increasing vulnerability to health hazards.

5. During the pendency of the complaint, at the instance of the respondent, her insurer—New India Assurance Co. Ltd., was impleaded as the second respondent. Parties led evidence—both oral and documentary, appellant examined an expert witness (Dr Puneet Bedi, Obstetrician & Gynecologist), her mother (Sumi Kohli) and herself. The respondent examined herself, an expert witness (Dr Sudha Salhan, Professor of Obstetrics & Gynecology and President of Association of Obstetricians and Gynaecologists of Delhi), Dr Lata Rangan (Doctor who assisted the respondent) and Dr Shiela Mehra (anesthetist for the surgery). The medical records and notices exchanged were produced as evidence. After hearing arguments, the Commission dismissed the complaint by order dated 19.11.2003. The Commission held: (i) the appellant voluntarily visited the respondent's clinic for treatment and consented for diagnostic procedures and operative surgery; (ii) the hysterectomy and other surgical procedures were done with adequate care and caution; and (iii) the surgical removal of uterus, ovaries, etc. was necessitated as the

appellant was found to be suffering from endometriosis (Grade IV), and if they had not been removed, there was likelihood of the lesion extending to the intestines and bladder and damaging them. Feeling aggrieved, the appellant has filed this appeal.

The appellant's version:

6. The appellant consulted respondent on 9.5.1995. Respondent wanted an ultrasound test to be done on the same day. In the evening, after seeing the ultrasound report, the respondent informed her that she was suffering from fibroids and that to make a firm diagnosis, she had to undergo a laparoscopic test the next day. The respondent informed her that the test was a minor procedure involving a small puncture for examination under general anesthesia. The respondent informed her that the costs of laparoscopic test, hospitalization and anesthetists charges would be around ₹ 8,000/- to 9,000/-. Respondent spent hardly 4 to 5 minutes with her and there was no discussion about the nature of treatment. Respondent merely told her that she will discuss the line of treatment, after the laparoscopic test. On 10.5.1995, she went to the clinic only for a diagnostic laparoscopy. Her signature was taken on some blank printed forms without giving her an opportunity to read the contents. As only a diagnostic procedure by way of a laparoscopic test was to be conducted, there was no discussion, even on 10.5.1995, with regard to any proposed treatment. As she was intending to marry within a month and start a family, she would have refused consent for removal of her reproductive organs and would have opted for conservative treatment, had she been informed about any proposed surgery for removal of her reproductive organs.

7. When the appellant was under general anesthesia, respondent rushed out of the operation theater and told appellant's mother that she had started bleeding profusely and gave an impression that the only way to save her life was by performing an extensive surgery. Appellant's aged mother was made to believe that there was a life-threatening situation, and her signature was taken to some paper. Respondent did not choose to wait till appellant regained consciousness, to discuss about the findings of the laparoscopic test and take her consent for treatment. The appellant was kept in the dark about the radical surgery performed on her. She came to know about it, only on 14.5.1995 when respondent's son casually informed her about the removal of her reproductive organs. When she asked the respondent as to why there should be profuse

bleeding during a laparoscopic test (as informed to appellant's mother) and why her reproductive organs were removed in such haste without informing her, without her consent, and without affording her an opportunity to consider other options or seek other opinion, the respondent answered rudely that due to her age, conception was not possible, and therefore, the removal of her reproductive organs did not make any difference.

8. As she was admitted only for a diagnostic procedure, namely a laparoscopy test, and as she had given consent only for a laparoscopy test and as her mother's consent for conducting hysterectomy had been obtained by misrepresentation, there was no valid consent for the radical surgery. The respondent also tried to cover-up her unwarranted/negligent act by falsely alleging that the appellant was suffering from endometriosis. The respondent was guilty of two distinct acts of negligence: the first was the failure to take her consent, much less an informed consent, for the radical surgery involving removal of reproductive organs; and the second was the failure to exhaust conservative treatment before resorting to radical surgery, particularly when such drastic irreversible surgical procedure was not warranted in her case. The respondent did not inform the appellant, of the possible risks, side effects and complications associated with such surgery, before undertaking the surgical procedure. Such surgery without her consent was also in violation of medical rules and ethics. Removal of her reproductive organs also resulted in a severe physical impairment, and necessitated prolonged further treatment. The respondent was also not qualified to claim to be a specialist in obstetrics and gynecology and therefore could not have performed the surgery which only a qualified gynecologist could perform.

The respondent's version:

9. The appellant had an emergency consultation with the respondent on 9.5.1995, complaining that she had heavy vaginal bleeding from 30.4.1995, that her periods were irregular, and that she was suffering from excessive, irregular and painful menstruation (menorrhagia and dysmenorrhea) for a few months. On a clinical examination, the respondent found a huge mass in the pelvic region and tenderness in the whole area. In view of the severe condition, respondent advised an ultrasound examination on the same evening. Such examination showed fibroids in the uterus, a large chocolate cyst (also known as endometrial cyst) on the right side and small cysts on the left side. On the basis of clinical and ultrasound examination, she made a provisional diagnosis of endometriosis and informed the appellant about the nature of the ailment, the anticipated extent of severity, and the modality of treatment. She further informed the appellant that a laparoscopic examination was needed to confirm the diagnosis; that if on such examination, she found that the condition was manageable with conservative surgery, she would only remove the chocolate cyst and fulgurate the endometrial areas and follow it by medical therapy; and that if the lesion was extensive, then considering her age and likelihood of destruction of the function of the tubes, she will perform hysterectomy. She also explained the surgical procedure involved, and answered appellant's queries. The appellant stated that she was in acute discomfort and wanted a permanent cure and, therefore, whatever was considered necessary, including a hysterectomy may be performed. When appellant's mother called on her on the same evening, the respondent explained to her also about the nature of disease and the proposed treatment, and appellant's mother stated that she may do whatever was best for her daughter. According to the accepted medical practice, if endometriosis is widespread in the pelvis causing adhesions, and if the woman is over 40 years of age, the best and safest form of cure was to remove the uterus and the ovaries. As there is a decline in fecundity for most women in the fourth decade and a further decline in women in their forties, hysterectomy is always considered as a reasonable and favored option. Further, endometriosis itself affected fertility adversely. All these were made known to the appellant before she authorized the removal of uterus and ovaries, if found necessary on laparoscopic examination.

10. On 10.5.1995, the appellant's consent was formally recorded in the consent form by Dr Lata Rangan—respondent's assistant. Dr Lata Rangan informed the appellant about the consequences of such consent and explained the procedure that was proposed. The appellant signed the consent forms only after she read the duly filled up forms and understood their contents. All the requisite tests to be conducted mandatorily before the surgery were performed including blood grouping, HIV, hemoglobin, PCV, BT, CT and ECG. The laparoscopic examination of the uterus surface confirmed the provisional diagnosis of endometriosis. The right ovary was enlarged and showed a chocolate cyst stuck to the bowel. Right tube was also involved in the lesion. The left ovary and tube were also stuck to the bowel near the cervix. A few small cysts were

seen on the left ovary. The pelvic organs were thick and difficult to mobilize. Having regard to the extent of the lesion and the condition of appellant's uterus and ovaries, she decided that conservative surgery would not be sufficient and the appellant's problem required removal of uterus and ovaries. The respondent sent her assistant, Dr Lata Rangan to explain to appellant's mother that the lesion would not respond to conservative surgery and a hysterectomy had to be performed and took her consent. The surgery was extremely difficult due to adhesions and vascularity of surface. A subtotal hysterectomy was done followed by the removal of rest of the stump of cervix. As the right ovary was completely stuck down to bowel, pouch of Douglas, post surface and tube, it had to be removed piecemeal. When appellant regained consciousness, she was informed about the surgery. The appellant felt assured that heavy bleeding and pain would not recur. There was no protest either from the appellant or her mother, in regard to the removal of the ovaries and uterus.

11. However, on 15.5.1995, Commander Zutshi to whom appellant was said to have been engaged, created a scene and got her discharged. At the time of discharge, the summary of procedure and prescription of medicines were given to her. As the bill was not paid, the respondent filed Suit No. 469/1995 for recovery of the bill amount and the said suit was decreed in due course.

12. Respondent performed the proper surgical procedure in pursuance of the consent given by the appellant and there was no negligence, illegality, impropriety or professional misconduct. There was real and informed consent by the appellant for the removal of her reproductive organs. The surgery (removal of uterus and ovaries), not only cured the appellant of her disease but also saved her intestines, bladder and ureter from possible damage. But for the surgical removal, there was likelihood of the intestines being damaged due to extension of lesion thereby causing bleeding, fibrosis and narrowing of the gut; there was also likelihood of the lesion going to the surface of the bladder penetrating the wall and causing hematuria and the ureter being damaged due to fibrosis and leading to damage of the kidney, with a reasonable real chance of developing cancer. As the complainant was already on the wrong side of 40 years which is a perimenopausal age and as the appellant had menorrhagia which prevented her from ovulating regularly and giving her regular cycle necessary for pregnancy and as endometriosis prevented fertilization

and also produced reaction in the pelvis which increased the lymphocytes and macrophages which destroyed the ova and sperm, there was no chance of appellant conceiving, even if the surgery had not been performed. The removal of her uterus and ovaries was proper and necessary and there was no negligence on the part of the respondent in performing the surgery. A doctor who has acted in accordance with a practice accepted as proper by medical fraternity cannot be said to have acted negligently. In the realm of diagnosis and treatment, there is ample scope for genuine differences of opinion and no doctor can be said to have acted negligently merely because his or her opinion differs from that of other doctors or because he or she has displayed lesser skill or knowledge when compared to others. There was thus no negligence on her part.

Questions for consideration:

13. On the contentions raised, the following questions arise for our consideration:
    i. Whether informed consent of a patient is necessary for surgical procedure involving removal of reproductive organs. If so what is the nature of such consent.
    ii. When a patient consults a medical practitioner, whether consent given for diagnostic surgery, can be construed as consent for performing additional or further surgical procedure—either as conservative treatment or as radical treatment—without the specific consent for such additional or further surgery.
    iii. Whether there was consent by the appellant, for the abdominal hysterectomy and bilateral salpingo-oophorectomy (AH-BSO) performed by the respondent.
    iv. Whether the respondent had falsely invented a case that appellant was suffering from endometriosis to explain the unauthorized and unwarranted removal of uterus and ovaries, and whether such radical surgery was either to cover-up negligence in conducting diagnostic laparoscopy or to claim a higher fee.
    v. Even if appellant was suffering from endometriosis, the respondent ought to have resorted to conservative treatment/surgery instead of performing radical surgery.
    vi. Whether the respondent is guilty of the tortious act of negligence/battery amounting to deficiency in service, and consequently liable to pay damages to the appellant.

Re: Question No. (i) and (ii)

14. Consent in the context of a doctor-patient relationship, means the grant of permission by the patient for an act to be carried out by the doctor, such as a diagnostic, surgical or therapeutic procedure. Consent can be implied in some circumstances from the action of the patient. For example, when a patient enters a Dentist's clinic and sits in the Dental chair, his consent is implied for examination, diagnosis and consultation. Except where consent can be clearly and obviously implied, there should be expressed consent. There is, however, a significant difference in the nature of express consent of the patient, known as "real consent" in UK and as "informed consent" in America. In UK, the elements of consent are defined with reference to the patient and a consent is considered to be valid and "real' when (i) the patient gives it voluntarily without any coercion; (ii) the patient has the capacity and competence to give consent; and (iii) the patient has the minimum of adequate level of information about the nature of the procedure to which he is consenting to. On the other hand, the concept of "informed consent" developed by American courts, while retaining the basic requirements consent, shifts the emphasis to the doctor's duty to disclose the necessary information to the patient to secure his consent. "Informed consent" is defined in Taber's Cyclopedic Medical Dictionary thus:

"Consent that is given by a person after receipt of the following information: the nature and purpose of the proposed procedure or treatment; the expected outcome and the likelihood of success; the risks; the alternatives to the procedure and supporting information regarding those alternatives; and the effect of no treatment or procedure, including the effect on the prognosis and the material risks associated with no treatment. Also included are instructions concerning what should be done if the procedure turns out to be harmful or unsuccessful."

In Canterbury vs. Spence—1972 [464] Federal Reporter 2d. 772, the United States Courts of Appeals, District of Columbia Circuit, emphasized the element of Doctor's duty in "informed consent" thus:

"It is well established that the physician must seek and secure his patient's consent before commencing an operation or other course of treatment. It is also clear that the consent, to be efficacious, must be free from imposition upon the patient. It is the settled rule that therapy not authorized by the patient may amount to a tort—a common law battery—by the physician. And it is evident that it is normally impossible to obtain a consent worthy of the name unless the physician first elucidates the options and the perils for the patient's edification. Thus, the physician has long borne a duty, on pain of liability for unauthorized treatment, to make adequate disclosure to the patient."

[Emphasis supplied]

15. The basic principle in regard to patient's consent may be traced to the following classic statement by Justice Cardozo in Schoendorff vs. Society of New York Hospital—(1914) 211 NY 125:

"Every human being of adult years and sound mind has a right to determine what should be done with his body; and a surgeon who performs the operation without his patient's consent, commits an assault for which he is liable in damages."

This principle has been accepted by English court also. In Re: F. 1989(2) All ER 545, the House of Lords while dealing with a case of sterilization of a mental patient reiterated the fundamental principle that every person's body is inviolate and performance of a medical operation on a person without his or her consent is unlawful. The English law on this aspect is summarized thus in Principles of Medical Law (published by Oxford University Press—Second Edition, edited by Andrew Grubb, Para 3.04, Page 133):

"Any intentional touching of a person is unlawful and amounts to the tort of battery unless it is justified by consent or other lawful authority. In medical law, this means that a doctor may only carry out a medical treatment or procedure which involves contact with a patient if there exists a valid consent by the patient (or another person authorized by law to consent on his behalf) or if the touching is permitted notwithstanding the absence of consent."

16. The next question is whether in an action for negligence/battery for performance of an unauthorized surgical procedure, the Doctor can put forth as defense the consent given for a particular operative procedure, as consent for any additional or further operative procedures performed in the interests of the patient. In Murray vs. McMurchy—1949 (2) DLR 442, the Supreme Court of BC, Canada, was considering a claim for battery by a patient who underwent a cesarean section. During the course of cesarean section, the doctor found fibroid tumors in the patient's uterus. Being of the view that such tumors would be a danger in case of future pregnancy, he performed a sterilization operation. The court upheld the claim for damages for battery. It held that sterilization could not be justified under the principle of necessity, as there was no immediate threat or danger to the patient's health or life and it would not

have been unreasonable to postpone the operation to secure the patient's consent. The fact that the doctor found it convenient to perform the sterilization operation without consent as the patient was already under general anesthetic, was held to be not a valid defense. A somewhat similar view was expressed by Court of Appeal in England in Re: F. (supra). It was held that the additional or further treatment which can be given (outside the consented procedure) should be confined to only such treatment as is necessary to meet the emergency, and as such needs to be carried out at once and before the patient is likely to be in a position to make a decision for himself. Lord Goff observed:

"Where, for example, a surgeon performs an operation without his consent on a patient temporarily rendered unconscious in an accident, he should do no more than is reasonably required, in the best interests of the patient, before he recovers consciousness. I can see no practical difficulty arising from this requirement, which derives from the fact that the patient is expected before long to regain consciousness and can then be consulted about longer term measures."

The decision in Marshell vs. Curry—1933 (3) DLR 260 decided by the Supreme Court of NS, Canada, illustrates the exception to the rule, that an unauthorized procedure may be justified if the patient's medical condition brooks no delay and warrants immediate action without waiting for the patient to regain consciousness and take a decision for himself. In that case, the doctor discovered a grossly diseased testicle while performing a hernia operation. As the doctor considered it to be gangrenous, posing a threat to patient's life and health, the doctor removed it without consent, as a part of the hernia operation. An action for battery was brought on the ground that the consent was for a hernia operation and removal of testicle was not consent. The claim was dismissed. The court was of the view that the doctor can act without the consent of the patient where it is necessary to save the life or preserve the health of the patient. Thus, the principle of necessity by which the doctor is permitted to perform further or additional procedure (unauthorized) is restricted to cases where the patient is temporarily incompetent (being unconscious), to permit the procedure delaying of which would be unreasonable because of the imminent danger to the life or health of the patient.

17. It is quite possible that if the patient been conscious, and informed about the need for the additional procedure, the patient might have agreed to it. It may be that the additional procedure is beneficial and in the interests of the patient. It may be that postponement of the additional procedure (say removal of an organ) may require another surgery, whereas removal of the affected organ during the initial diagnostic or exploratory surgery, would save the patient from the pain and cost of a second operation. Howsoever practical or convenient the reasons may be, they are not relevant. What is relevant and of importance is the inviolable nature of the patient's right in regard to his body and his right to decide whether he should undergo the particular treatment or surgery or not. Therefore at the risk of repetition, we may add that unless the unauthorized additional or further procedure is necessary in order to save the life or preserve the health of the patient and it would be unreasonable (as contrasted from being merely inconvenient) to delay the further procedure until the patient regains consciousness and takes a decision, a doctor cannot perform such procedure without the consent of the patient.

18. We may also refer to the code of medical ethics laid down by the Medical Council of India (approved by the Central Government under section 33 of Indian Medical Council Act, 1956). It contains a chapter relating to disciplinary action which enumerates a list of responsibilities, violation of which will be professional misconduct. Clause 13 of the said chapter places the following responsibility on a doctor:

"13. Before performing an operation, the physician should obtain in writing the consent from the husband or wife, parent or guardian in the case of a minor, or the patient himself as the case may be. In an operation which may result in sterility the consent of both husband and wife is needed."

We may also refer to the following guidelines to doctors, issued by the General Medical Council of UK in seeking consent of the patient for investigation and treatment:

"Patients have a right to information about their condition and the treatment options available to them. The amount of information you give each patient will vary, according to factors such as the nature of the condition, the complexity of the treatment, the risks associated with the treatment or procedure, and the patient's own wishes. For example, patients may need more information to make an informed decision about the procedure which carries a high risk of failure or adverse side effects; or about an investigation for a condition which, if present, could have serious implications for the patient's employment, social or personal life.

You should raise with patients the possibility of additional problems coming to light during a procedure when the patient is unconscious or otherwise unable to make a decision. You should seek consent to treat any problems which you think may arise and ascertain whether there are any procedures to which the patient would object, or prefer to give further thought before you proceed."

The Consent form for Hospital admission and medical treatment, to which appellant's signature was obtained by the respondent on 10.5.1995, which can safely be presumed to constitute the contract between the parties, specifically states:

"(A) It is customary, except in emergency or extraordinary circumstances, that no substantial procedures are performed upon a patient unless and until he or she has had an opportunity to discuss them with the physician or other health professional to the patient's satisfaction.

(B) Each patient has right to consent, or to refuse consent, to any proposed procedure of therapeutic course."

19. We therefore hold that in Medical Law, where a surgeon is consulted by a patient, and consent of the patient is taken for diagnostic procedure/surgery, such consent cannot be considered as authorization or permission to perform therapeutic surgery either conservative or radical (except in life-threatening or emergent situations). Similarly, where the consent by the patient is for a particular operative surgery, it cannot be treated as consent for an unauthorized additional procedure involving removal of an organ, only on the ground that such removal is beneficial to the patient or is likely to prevent some danger developing in future, where there is no imminent danger to the life or health of the patient.

20. We may next consider the nature of information that is required to be furnished by a doctor to secure a valid or real consent. In Bowater vs. Rowley Regis Corporation— [1944] 1 KB 476, Scott L.J. observed: "A man cannot be said to be truly 'willing' unless he is in a position to choose freely, and freedom of choice predicates, not only full knowledge of the circumstances on which the exercise of choice is conditioned, so that he may be able to choose wisely, but the absence from his mind of any feeling of constraint so that nothing shall interfere with the freedom of his will."

In Salgo vs. Leland Stanford [154 Cal. App. 2d. 560 (1957)], it was held that a physician violates his duty to his patient and subjects himself to liability if he withholds any facts which are necessary to form the basis of an intelligent consent by the patient to the proposed treatment.

21. Canterbury (supra) explored the rationale of a doctor's duty to reasonably inform a patient as to the treatment alternatives available and the risk incidental to them, as also the scope of the disclosure requirement and the physician's privileges not to disclose. It laid down the "reasonably prudent patient test" which required the doctor to disclose all material risks to a patient, to show an "informed consent". It was held:

"True consent to what happens to one's self is the informed exercise of a choice, and that entails an opportunity to evaluate knowledgeably the options available and the risks attendant upon each. The average patient has little or no understanding of the medical arts, and ordinarily has only his physician to whom he can look for enlightenment with which to reach an intelligent decision. From these almost axiomatic considerations springs the need, and in turn the requirement, of a reasonable divulgence by physician to patient to make such a decision possible. Just as plainly, due care normally demands that the physician warn the patient of any risks to his well-being which contemplated therapy may involve. The context in which the duty of risk disclosure arises is invariably the occasion for decision as to whether a particular treatment procedure is to be undertaken. To the physician, whose training enables a self-satisfying evaluation, the answer may seem clear, but it is the prerogative of the patient, not the physician, to determine for himself the direction in which his interests seem to lie. To enable the patient to chart his course understandably, some familiarity with the therapeutic alternatives and their hazards become essential. A reasonable revelation in these respects is not only a necessity but, as we see it, is as much a matter of the physician's duty. It is a duty to warn of the dangers lurking in the proposed treatment, and that is surely a facet of due care. It is, too, a duty to impart information which the patient has every right to expect. The patient's reliance upon the physician is a trust of the kind which traditionally has exacted obligations beyond those associated with arm's length transactions. His dependence upon the physician for information affecting his well-being, in terms of contemplated treatment, is well-nigh abject. We ourselves have found "in the fiducial qualities of (the physician-patient) relationship the physician's duty to reveal to the patient that which in his best interests it is important that he should know". We now find, as a part of the physician's overall obligation to the patient, a similar duty of reasonable disclosure of the choices with respect to proposed therapy and the dangers inherently and potentially involve. In our view, the patient's right of self-decision shapes the boundaries of the duty to reveal. That right can be effectively exercised only if the patient possesses enough information to enable an intelligent choice. The scope of the physician's communications to the patient, then, must be measured by the patient's need, and that need is the information material to the decision. Thus, the test for determining whether a particular peril must be divulged is its materially to the patient's decision: all risks potentially affecting the decision must be unmasked."

It was further held that a risk is material "when a reasonable person, in what the physician knows or should know to be the patient's position, would be likely to attach significance to the risk or cluster of risks in deciding whether or not to forego the proposed therapy". The doctor, therefore, is required to communicate all inherent and potential hazards of the proposed treatment, the alternatives to that treatment, if any, and the likely effect if the patient remained untreated. This stringent standard of disclosure was subjected to only two exceptions: (i) where there was a genuine emergency, e.g. the patient was unconscious; and (ii) where the information would be harmful to the patient, e.g. where it might cause psychological damage, or where the patient would become so emotionally distraught as to prevent a rational decision. It, however, appears that several States in USA have chosen to avoid the decision in Canterbury by enacting legislation which severely curtails operation of the doctrine of informed consent.

22. The stringent standards regarding disclosure laid down in Canterbury, as necessary to secure an informed consent of the patient, was not accepted in the English courts. In England, standard applicable is popularly known as the Bolam test, first laid down in Bolam vs. Friern Hospital Management Committee—[1957] 2 All ER 118. McNair J., in a trial relating to negligence of a medical practitioner, while instructing the Jury, stated thus:

   i. A doctor is not negligent, if he has acted in accordance with a practice accepted as proper by a responsible body of medical men skilled in that particular art. Putting it the other way round, a doctor is not negligent, if he is acting in accordance with such a practice, merely because there is a body of opinion that takes a contrary view. At the same time, that does not mean that a medical man can obstinately and pig-headedly carry on with some old technique if it has been proved to be contrary to what is really substantially the whole of informed medical opinion.

   ii. When a doctor dealing with a sick man strongly believed that the only hope of cure was submission to a particular therapy, he could not be criticized if, believing the danger involved in the treatment to be minimal, did not stress them to the patient.

   iii. In order to recover damages for failure to give warning the plaintiff must show not only that the failure was negligent but also that if he had been warned he would not have consented to the treatment.

23. Hunter vs. Hanley (1955 SC 200), a Scottish case is also worth noticing. In that decision, Lord President Clyde held:

   "In the realm of diagnosis and treatment, there is ample scope for genuine difference of opinion and one man clearly is not negligent merely because his conclusion differs from that of other professional men, nor because he has displayed less skill or knowledge than others would have shown. The true test for establishing negligence in diagnosis or treatment on the part of a doctor is whether he has been proved to be guilty of such failure as no doctor of ordinary skill would be guilty of if acting with ordinary care."

   He also laid down the following requirements to be established by a patient to fasten liability on the ground of want of care or negligence on the part of the doctor: "To establish liability by a doctor where deviation from normal practice is alleged, three facts require to be established. First of all it must be proved that there is a usual and normal practice; secondly, it must be proved that the defender has not adopted that practice; and thirdly (and this is of crucial importance), it must be established that the course the doctor adopted is one which no professional man of ordinary skill would have taken if he had been acting with ordinary care."

24. In Sidaway vs. Bethlem Royal Hospital Governors & Ors. [1985] 1 All ER 643, the House of Lords, per majority, adopted the Bolam test, as the measure of doctor's duty to disclose information about the potential consequences and risks of proposed medical treatment. In that case, the defendant, a surgeon, warned the plaintiff of the possibility of disturbing a nerve root while advising an operation on the spinal column to relieve shoulder and neck pain. He did not however mention the possibility of damage to the

spinal cord. Though the operation was performed without negligence, the plaintiff sustained damage to spinal cord resulting in partial paralysis. The plaintiff alleged that defendant was negligent in failing to inform her about the said risk and that had she known the true position, she would not have accepted the treatment. The trial Judge and Court of Appeal applied the Bolam test and concluded that the defendant had acted in accordance with a practice accepted as proper by a responsible body of medical opinion, in not informing the plaintiff of the risk of damage to spinal cord. Consequently, the claim for damages was rejected. The House of Lords upheld the decision of the Court of Appeal that the doctrine of informed consent based on full disclosure of all the facts to the patient, was not the appropriate test of liability for negligence, under English law. The majority were of the view that the test of liability in respect of a doctor's duty to warn his patient of risks inherent in treatment recommended by him was the same as the test applicable to diagnosis and treatment, namely, that the doctor was required to act in accordance with the practice accepted at the time as proper by a responsible body of medical opinion.

Lord Diplock stated:

"In English jurisprudence, the doctor's relationship with his patient which gives rise to the normal duty of care to exercise his skill and judgment to improve the patient's health in any particular respect in which the patient has sought his aid has hitherto been treated as a single comprehensive duty covering all the ways in which a doctor is called on to exercise his skill and judgment in the improvement of the physical or mental condition of the patient for which his services either as a general practitioner or as a specialist have been engaged. This general duty is not subject to dissection into a number of component parts to which different criteria of what satisfy the duty of care apply, such as diagnosis, treatment and advice (including warning of any risks of something going wrong however skillfully the treatment advised is carried out). The Bolam case itself embraced failure to advise the patient of the risk involved in the electric shock treatment as one of the allegations of negligence against the surgeon as well as negligence in the actual carrying out of treatment in which that risk did result in injury to the patient. The same criteria were applied to both these aspects of the surgeon's duty of care. In modern medicine and surgery such dissection of the various things, a doctor has to do in the exercise of his whole duty of care owed to his patient is neither legally meaningful nor medically practicable. To decide what risks the existence of which

a patient should be voluntarily warned and the terms in which such warning, if any, should be given, having regard to the effect that the warning may have, is as much an exercise of professional skill and judgment as any other part of the doctor's comprehensive duty of care to the individual patient, and expert medical evidence on this matter should be treated in just the same way. The Bolam test should be applied."

Lord Bridge stated:

"I recognize the logical force of the Canterbury doctrine, proceeding from the premise that the patient's right to make his own decision must at all costs be safeguarded against the kind of medical paternalism which assumes that "doctor knows best". But, with all respect, I regard the doctrine as quite impractical in application for three principal reasons. First, it gives insufficient weight to the realities of the doctor/patient relationship. A very wide variety of factors must enter into a doctor's clinical judgment not only as to what treatment is appropriate for a particular patient, but also as to how best to communicate to the patient the significant factors necessary to enable the patient to make an informed decision whether to undergo the treatment. The doctor cannot set out to educate the patient to his own standard of medical knowledge of all the relevant factors involved. He may take the view, certainly with some patients, that the very fact of his volunteering, without being asked, information of some remote risk involved in the treatment proposed, even though he described it as remote, may lead to that risk assuming an undue significance in the patient's calculations. Second, it would seem to me quite unrealistic in any medical negligence action to confine the expert medical evidence to an explanation of the primary medical factors involved and to deny the court the benefit of evidence of medical opinion and practice on the particular issue of disclosure which is under consideration. Third, the objective test which Canterbury propounds seems to me to be so imprecise as to be almost meaningless. If it is to be left to individual judges to decide for themselves what "a reasonable person in the patient's position" would consider a risk of sufficient significance that he should be told about it, the outcome of litigation in this field is likely to be quite unpredictable."

Lord Bridge however made it clear that when questioned specifically by the patient about the risks involved in a particular treatment proposed, the doctor's duty is to answer truthfully and as fully as the questioner requires. He further held that remote risk of damage (referred to as risk at 1% or 2%) need not be disclosed but if the risk of damage is substantial (referred to as 10% risk), it may have to be disclosed. Lord Scarman, in minority, was inclined to adopt the more stringent test laid down in Canterbury.

25. In India, Bolam test has broadly been accepted as the general rule. We may refer three cases of this Court. In Achutrao Haribhau Khodwa vs. State of Maharastra—1996 (2) SCC 634, this Court held:
"The skill of medical practitioners differs from doctor to doctor. The nature of the profession is such that there may be more than one course of treatment which may be advisable for treating a patient. Courts would indeed be slow in attributing negligence on the part of a doctor if he has performed his duties to the best of his ability and with due care and caution. Medical opinion may differ with regard to the course of action to be taken by a doctor treating a patient, but as long as a doctor acts in a manner which is acceptable to the medical profession and the Court finds that he has attended on the patient with due care skill and diligence and if the patient still does not survive or suffers a permanent ailment, it would be difficult to hold the doctor to be guilty of negligence. In cases where the doctors act carelessly and in a manner which is not expected of a medical practitioner, then in such a case an action in torts would be maintainable."
In Vinitha Ashok vs. Lakshmi Hospital—2001 (8) SCC 731, this Court after referring to Bolam, Sidaway and Achutrao, clarified: "A doctor will be liable for negligence in respect of diagnosis and treatment in spite of a body of professional opinion approving his conduct where it has not been established to the court's satisfaction that such opinion relied on is reasonable or responsible. If it can be demonstrated that the professional opinion is not capable of withstanding the logical analysis, the court would be entitled to hold that the body of opinion is not reasonable or responsible. In Indian Medical Association vs. V.P. Shantha—1995 (6) SCC 651, this Court held:
"The approach of the courts is to require that professional men should possess a certain minimum degree of competence and that they should exercise reasonable care in the discharge of their duties. In general, a professional man owes to his client a duty in tort as well as in contract to exercise reasonable care in giving advice or performing services."
Neither Achutrao nor Vinitha Ashok referred to the American view expressed in Canterbury.

26. In India, majority of citizens requiring medical care and treatment fall below the poverty line. Most of them are illiterate or semiliterate. They cannot comprehend medical terms, concepts and treatment procedures. They cannot understand the functions of various organs or the effect of removal of such organs. They do not have access to effective but costly diagnostic procedures. Poor patients lying in the corridors of hospitals after admission for want of beds or patients waiting for days on the roadside for an admission or a mere examination, is a common sight. For them, any treatment with reference to rough and ready diagnosis based on their outward symptoms and doctor's experience or intuition is acceptable and welcome so long as it is free or cheap; and whatever the doctor decides as being in their interest, is usually unquestioningly accepted. They are a passive, ignorant and uninvolved in treatment procedures. The poor and needy face a hostile medical environment—inadequacy in the number of hospitals and beds, nonavailability of adequate treatment facilities, utter lack of qualitative treatment, corruption, callousness and apathy. Many poor patients with serious ailments (e.g. heart patients and cancer patients) have to wait for months for their turn even for diagnosis, and due to limited treatment facilities, many die even before their turn comes for treatment. What choice do these poor patients have? Any treatment of whatever degree is a boon or a favor for them. The stark reality is that for a vast majority in the country, the concepts of informed consent or any form of consent, and choice in treatment, have no meaning or relevance. The position of doctors in Government and charitable hospitals, who treat them, is also unenviable. They are overworked, understaffed, with little or no diagnostic or surgical facilities and limited choice of medicines and treatment procedures. They have to improvise with virtual nonexistent facilities and limited dubious medicines. They are required to be committed, service oriented and noncommercial in outlook. What choice of treatment can these doctors give to the poor patients? What informed consent they can take from them?

27. On the other hand, we have the doctors, hospitals, nursing homes and clinics in the private commercial sector. There is a general perception among the middle class public that these private hospitals and doctors prescribe avoidable costly diagnostic procedures and medicines, and subject them to unwanted surgical procedures, for financial gain. The public feel that many doctors who have spent a crore or more for becoming a specialist, or nursing homes which have invested several crores on diagnostic and infrastructure facilities, would necessarily operate with a purely

commercial and not service motive; that such doctors and hospitals would advise extensive costly treatment procedures and surgeries, where conservative or simple treatment may meet the need; and that what used to be a noble service oriented profession is slowly but steadily converting into a purely business.

28. But unfortunately not all doctors in government hospitals are paragons of service, nor fortunately, all private hospitals/doctors are commercial minded. There are many doctors in government hospitals who do not care about patients and unscrupulously insist upon "unofficial" payment for free treatment or insist upon private consultations. On the other hand, many private hospitals and doctors give the best of treatment without exploitation, at a reasonable cost, charging a fee, which is reasonable recompense for the service rendered. Of course, some doctors, both in private practice or in government service, look at patients not as persons who should be relieved from pain and suffering by prompt and proper treatment at an affordable cost, but as potential income-providers/customers who can be exploited by prolonged or radical diagnostic and treatment procedures. It is this minority who bring a bad name to the entire profession.

29. Health care (like education) can thrive in the hands of charitable institutions. It also requires more serious attention from the State. In a developing country like ours where teeming millions of poor, downtrodden and illiterate cry out for health care, there is a desperate need for making health care easily accessible and affordable. Remarkable developments in the field of medicine might have revolutionized health care. But they cannot be afforded by the common man. The woes of non-affording patients have in no way decreased. Gone are the days when any patient could go to a neighborhood general practitioner or a family doctor and get affordable treatment at a very reasonable cost, with affection, care and concern. Their noble tribe is dwindling. Every doctor wants to be a specialist. The proliferation of specialists and super specialists have exhausted many a patient both financially and physically, by having to move from doctor to doctor, in search of the appropriate specialist who can identify the problem and provide treatment. What used to be competent treatment by one General Practitioner has now become multipronged treatment by several specialists. Law stepping in to provide remedy for negligence or deficiency in service by medical practitioners has its own twin adverse effects. More and more private doctors and hospitals have, of necessity, started playing it safe, by subjecting or requiring the patients to undergo various costly diagnostic procedures and tests to avoid any allegations of negligence, even though they might have already identified the ailment with reference to the symptoms and medical history with 90% certainly, by their knowledge and experience. Secondly more and more doctors particularly surgeons in private practice are forced to cover themselves by taking out insurance, the cost of which is also ultimately passed on to the patient, by way of a higher fee. As a consequence, it is now common that a comparatively simple ailment, which earlier used to be treated at the cost of a few rupees by consulting a single doctor, requires an expense of several hundred or thousands on account of four factors: (i) commercialization of medical treatment; (ii) increase in specialists as contrasted from general practitioners and the need for consulting more than one doctor; (iii) varied diagnostic and treatment procedures at high cost; and (iv) need for doctors to have insurance cover. The obvious, may be now, answer to unwarranted diagnostic procedures and treatment and prohibitive cost of treatment, is an increase in the participation of health care by the state and charitable institutions. An enlightened and committed medical profession can also provide a better alternative. Be that as it may. We are not trying to intrude on matters of policy, nor are we against proper diagnosis or specialization. We are only worried about the enormous hardship and expense to which the common man is subjected, and are merely voicing the concern of those who are not able to fend for themselves. We will be too happy if what we have observed is an overstatement, but our intuition tells us that it is an understatement.

30. What we are considering in this case, is not the duties or obligations of doctors in government charitable hospitals where treatment is free or on actual cost basis. We are concerned with doctors in private practice and hospitals and nursing homes run commercially, where the relationship of doctors and patients are contractual in origin, the service is in consideration of a fee paid by the patient, where the contract implies that the professional men possessing a minimum degree of competence would exercise reasonable care in the discharge of their duties while giving advice or treatment.

31. There is a need to keep the cost of treatment within affordable limits. Bringing in the American concepts and standards of treatment procedures and disclosure of risks, consequences and choices will inevitably bring in higher cost-structure of American medical

care. Patients in India cannot afford them. People in India still have great regard and respect for Doctors. The Members of medical profession have also, by and large, shown care and concern for the patients. There is an atmosphere of trust and implicit faith in the advice given by the Doctor. The Indian psyche rarely questions or challenges the medical advice. Having regard to the conditions obtaining in India, as also the settled and recognized practices of medical fraternity in India, we are of the view that to nurture the doctor-patient relationship on the basis of trust, the extent and nature of information required to be given by doctors should continue to be governed by the Bolam test rather than the "reasonably prudential patient" test evolved in Canterbury. It is for the doctor to decide, with reference to the condition of the patient, nature of illness, and the prevailing established practices, how much information regarding risks and consequences should be given to the patients, and how they should be couched, having the best interests of the patient. A doctor cannot be held negligent either in regard to diagnosis or treatment or in disclosing the risks involved in a particular surgical procedure or treatment, if the doctor has acted with normal care, in accordance with a recognized practices accepted as proper by a responsible body of medical men skilled in that particular field, even though there may be a body of opinion that takes a contrary view. Where there are more than one recognized school of established medical practice, it is not negligence for a doctor to follow any one of those practices, in preference to the others.

32. We may now summarize principles relating to consent as follows:

    i. A doctor has to seek and secure the consent of the patient before commencing a "treatment" (the term "treatment" includes surgery also). The consent so obtained should be real and valid, which means that: the patient should have the capacity and competence to consent; his consent should be voluntary; and his consent should be on the basis of adequate information concerning the nature of the treatment procedure, so that he knows what is consenting to.

    ii. The "adequate information" to be furnished by the doctor (or a member of his team) who treats the patient, should enable the patient to make a balanced judgment as to whether he should submit himself to the particular treatment or not. This means that the Doctor should disclose (a) nature and procedure of the treatment and its purpose, benefits and effect; (b) alternatives if any available; (c) an outline of the substantial risks; and (d) adverse consequences of refusing treatment. But there is no need to explain remote or theoretical risks involved, which may frighten or confuse a patient and result in refusal of consent for the necessary treatment. Similarly, there is no need to explain the remote or theoretical risks of refusal to take treatment which may persuade a patient to undergo a fanciful or unnecessary treatment. A balance should be achieved between the need for disclosing necessary and adequate information and at the same time avoid the possibility of the patient being deterred from agreeing to a necessary treatment or offering to undergo an unnecessary treatment.

    iii. Consent given only for a diagnostic procedure, cannot be considered as consent for therapeutic treatment. Consent given for a specific treatment procedure will not be valid for conducting some other treatment procedure. The fact that the unauthorized additional surgery is beneficial to the patient, or that it would save considerable time and expense to the patient, or would relieve the patient from pain and suffering in future, are not grounds of defense in an action in tort for negligence or assault and battery. The only exception to this rule is where the additional procedure though unauthorized, is necessary in order to save the life or preserve the health of the patient and it would be unreasonable to delay such unauthorized procedure until patient regains consciousness and takes a decision.

    iv. There can be a common consent for diagnostic and operative procedures where they are contemplated. There can also be a common consent for a particular surgical procedure and an additional or further procedure that may become necessary during the course of surgery.

    v. The nature and extent of information to be furnished by the doctor to the patient to secure the consent need not be of the stringent and high degree mentioned in Canterbury but should be of the extent which is accepted as normal and proper by a body of medical men skilled and experienced in the particular field. It will depend upon the physical and mental condition of the patient, the nature of treatment, and the risk and consequences attached to the treatment.

33. We may note here that courts in Canada and Australia have moved towards Canterbury standard of disclosure and informed consent—vide Reibl vs. Hughes (1980) 114 DLR (3d.) 1 decided by the Canadian Supreme Court and Rogers vs. Whittaker—1992 (109) ALR 625 decided by the High Court of Australia. Even in England there is a tendency to make the doctor's duty to inform more stringent than Bolam's test adopted in Sidaway. Lord Scarman's minority view in Sidaway favoring Canterbury, in course of time, may ultimately become the law in England. A beginning has been made in Bolitho vs. City and Hackney HA—1998 1 AC 232 and Pearce vs. United Bristol Healthcare NHS Trust 1998 (48) BMLR 118. We have however consciously preferred the "real consent" concept evolved in Bolam and Sidaway in preference to the "reasonably prudent patient test" in Canterbury, having regard to the ground realities in medical and health care in India. But if medical practitioners and private hospitals become more and more commercialized, and if there is a corresponding increase in the awareness of patient's rights among the public, inevitably, a day may come when we may have to move towards Canterbury. But not for the present.

Re: Question No. (iii)

34. "Gynaecology" (second edition) edited by Robert W. Shah, describes "real consent" with reference to Gynaecologists (page 867 et seq) as follows:

"An increasingly important risk area for all doctors is the question of consent. No one may lay hands on another against their will without running the risk of criminal prosecution for assault and, if injury results, a civil action for damages for trespass or negligence. In the case of a doctor, consent to any physical interference will readily be implied; a woman must be assumed to consent to a normal physical examination if she consults a gynecologist, in the absence of clear evidence of her refusal or restriction of such examination. The problems arise when the gynecologist's intervention results in unfortunate side effects or permanent interference with a function, whether or not any part of the body is removed. For example, if the gynecologist agrees with the patient to perform a hysterectomy and removes the ovaries without her specific consent, that will be a trespass and an act of negligence. The only available defense will be that it was necessary for the life of the patient to proceed at once to remove the ovaries because of some perceived pathology in them. What is meant by consent? The term "informed consent" is often used, but there is no such concept in English law. The consent must be real: that is to say, the patient must have been given sufficient information for her to understand the nature of the operation, its likely effects, and any complications which may arise and which the surgeon in the exercise of his duty to the patient considers she should be made aware of; only then can she reach a proper decision. But the surgeon need not warn the patient of remote risks, any more than an anesthetist need warn the patient that a certain small number of those anesthetized will suffer cardiac arrest or never recover consciousness. Only where there is a recognized risk, rather than a rare complication, is the surgeon under an obligation to warn the patient of that risk. He is not under a duty to warn the patient of the possible results of hypothetical negligent surgery.

In advising an operation, therefore, the doctor must do so in the way in which a competent gynecologist exercising reasonable skill and care in similar circumstances would have done. In doing this he will take into account the personality of the patient and the importance of the operation to her future well-being. It may be good practice not to warn a very nervous patient of any possible complications if she requires immediate surgery for, say, a malignant condition. The doctor must decide how much to say to her taking into account his assessment of her personality, the questions she asks and his view of how much she understands. If the patient asks a direct question, she must be given a truthful answer. To take the example of hysterectomy: although the surgeon will tell the patient that it is proposed to remove her uterus and perhaps her ovaries, and describe what that will mean for her future well-being (sterility, premature menopause), she will not be warned of the possibility of damage to the ureter, vesicovaginal fistula, fatal hemorrhage or anesthetic death."

35. The specific case of the appellant was that she got herself admitted on 10.5.1995 only for a diagnostic laparoscopy; that she was not informed either on 9th or 10th that she was suffering from endometriosis or that her reproductive organs had to be removed to cure her from the said disease; that her consent was not obtained for the removal of her reproductive organs; and that when she was under general anesthesia for diagnostic laparoscopy, respondent came out of the operation theater and informed her aged mother that the patient was bleeding profusely which might endanger her life and hysterectomy was the only option to save her life, and took her consent.

36. The respondent on the other hand contends that on the basis of clinical and ultrasound examination on 9.5.1995, she had made a provisional diagnosis of endometriosis; that on same day, she informed the complainant and her mother separately, that she would do a diagnostic laparoscopy on the next day and if the endometrial lesion was found to be mild or moderate, she will adopt a conservative treatment by operative laparoscopy, but if the lesion was extensive then considering her age and extent of lesion and likelihood of destruction of the functions of the tube, a laparotomy would be done; that the appellant was admitted to the hospital for diagnostic and operative laparoscopy and laparotomy and appellant's consent was obtained for such procedures; that the decision to operate and remove the uterus and ovaries was not sudden, nor on account of any emergent situation developing during laparoscopy; and that the radical surgery was authorized, as it was preceded by a valid consent. She also contends that as the appellant wanted a permanent cure, the decision to conduct a hysterectomy was medically correct and the surgical procedure in fact cured the appellant and saved her intestines, bladder and ureter being damaged due to extension of the lesion. She had also tried to justify the surgical removal of the uterus and ovaries, with reference to the age and medical condition of the complainant.

37. The summary of the surgical procedure (dictated by respondent and handwritten by her assistant Dr Lata Rangan) furnished to the appellant also confirms that no emergency or life-threatening situation developed during laparoscopy. This is reiterated in the evidence of respondent and Dr Lata Rangan. In her affidavit dated 16.2.2002 filed by way of examination-in-chief, the respondent stated:

"15. The laparoscopic examination revealed a frozen pelvis and considering the extent of the lesion it was decided that conservative surgery was not advisable and the nature of the problem required for its cure hysterectomy.

16. When the Deponent decided to perform hysterectomy, she told Dr Lata to intimate the mother of Ms. Samira Kohli of the fact that hysterectomy was going to be performed on her. No complications had arisen in the operation theater and the procedure being performed was in terms of the consent given by Ms. Samira Kohli herself."

In her affidavit dated 16.2.2002 filed by way of examination-in-chief, Dr Lata Rangan stated:

"14. I was in the operation theater along with Dr Prabha Manchanda. The laparoscopic examination revealed a frozen pelvis and considering the extent of the lesion it was decided that conservative surgery was not possible and that the nature of the problem required performance of hysterectomy.

15. When it was decided to perform hysterectomy the deponent was told by Dr Prabha Manchanda to intimate the mother of Ms. Samira Kohli of the fact that hysterectomy was now going to be performed on her. No complications had arisen in the operation theater and the procedure conducted therein was in terms of the consent given by Ms. Samira Kohli herself. I got the mother to sign the Form too so that the factum of intimation was duly documented."

Thus, the respondent's definite case is that on 9.5.1995, the respondent had provisionally diagnosed endometriosis and informed the appellant; that appellant had agreed that hysterectomy may be performed if the lesion was extensive; and that in pursuance of such consent, reiterated in writing by the appellant in the consent form on 10.5.1995, she performed the AH-BSO removing the uterus and ovaries on finding extensive endometriosis. In other words, according to respondent, the abdominal hysterectomy and bilateral salpingo-oophorectomy (AH-BSO) was not necessitated on account of any emergency or life-threatening situation developing or being discovered when laparoscopic test was conducted, but according to an agreed plan, consented by the appellant and her mother on 9.5.1995 itself, reiterated in writing on 10.5.1995. Therefore, the defense of respondent is one based on specific consent. Let us therefore examine whether there was consent.

38. The Admission and Discharge card maintained and produced by the respondent showed that the appellant was admitted "for diagnostic and (?) operative laparoscopy on 10.5.1995". The OPD card dated 9.5.1995 does not refer to endometriosis, which is also admitted by the respondent in her cross-examination. If fact, the respondent also admitted that the confirmation of diagnosis is possible only after laparoscopy test:

"On clinical and ultrasound examination, a diagnosis can be made to some extent. But precise diagnosis will have to be on laparoscopy."

The consent form dated 10.5.1995 signed by the appellant states that appellant has been informed that the treatment to be undertaken is "diagnostic and operative laparoscopy. Laparotomy may be needed." The case summary dictated by respondent and written by Dr Lata Rangan also clearly says "admitted for Hysteroscopy, diagnostic laparoscopy and operative laparoscopy on 10.5.1995". (Note: Hysteroscopy is inspection of uterus by special endoscope and laparoscopy is abdominal exploration by special endoscope.)

39. In this context, we may also refer to a notice dated 5.6.1995 issued by respondent to the appellant through counsel, demanding payment of ₹ 39,325/- towards the bill amount. Paras 1, 3 and 4 are relevant which are extracted below:

"1. You were admitted to our clinic Dr Manchanda, No. 7, Ring Road, Lajpat Nagar, New Delhi for diagnostic and operative laparoscopy and endometrial biopsy on 10.5.1995."

"3. The findings of laparoscopy were: a very extensive lesion of the endometriosis with pools of blood, extensive adherence involving the tubes of the uterus and ovaries, a chocolate cyst in the right ovary and areas of endometriosis on the surface of the left ovary but no cyst."

"4. The findings were duly conveyed to Ms. Somi Kohli who was also shown a video recording of the lesion. You and Mrs. Somi Kohli were informed that conservative surgery would be futile and removal of the uterus and more extensive surgery, considering your age and extensive lesion and destruction of the functions of the tubes, was preferable."

This also makes it clear that the appellant was not admitted for conducting hysterectomy or bilateral salpingo-oophorectomy, but only for diagnostic purposes. We may, however, refer to a wrong statement of fact made in the said notice. It states that on 10.5.1995 after conducting a laparoscopic examination, the video recording of the lesion was shown to appellant's mother, and the respondent informed the appellant and her mother that conservative surgery would be futile and removal of uterus and more extensive surgery was preferable having regard to the more extensive lesion and destruction of the function of the tubes. But this statement cannot be true. The extensive nature of lesion and destruction of the functions obviously became evident only after diagnostic laparoscopy. But after diagnostic laparoscopy and the video recording of the lesion, there was no occasion for respondent to inform anything to appellant. When the laparoscopy and video recording was made, the appellant was already unconscious. Before she regained consciousness, AH-BSO was performed removing her uterus and ovaries. Therefore, the appellant could not have been informed on 10.5.1995 that conservative surgery would be futile and removal of uterus and extensive surgery was preferable in view of the extensive lesion and destruction of the function of the tubes did not arise.

40. The admission card makes it clear that the appellant was admitted only for diagnostic and operative laparoscopy. It does not refer to laparotomy. The consent form shows that the appellant gave consent only for diagnostic operative laparoscopy, and laparotomy if needed. Laparotomy is a surgical procedure to open up the abdomen or an abdominal operation. It refers to the operation performed to examine the abdominal organs and aid diagnosis. Many a time, after the diagnosis is made and the problem is identified it may be fixed during the laparotomy itself. In other cases, a subsequent surgery may be required. Laparotomy can no doubt be either a diagnostic or therapeutic. In the former, more often referred to as the exploratory laparotomy, an exercise is undertaken to identify the nature of the disease. In the latter, a therapeutic laparotomy is conducted after the cause has been identified. When a specific operation say hysterectomy or salpingo-oophorectomy is planned, laparotomy is merely the first step of the procedure, followed by the actual specific operation, namely hysterectomy or salpingo-oophorectomy. Depending upon the incision placement, laparotomy gives access to any abdominal organ or space and is the first step in any major diagnostic or therapeutic surgical procedure involving (a) the lower port of the digestive tract, (b) liver, pancreas and spine, (c) bladder, (d) female reproductive organs and (e) retroperitoneum. On the other hand, hysterectomy and salpingo-oophorectomy follow laparotomy and are not themselves referred to as laparotomy. Therefore, when the consent form refers to diagnostic and operative laparoscopy and "laparotomy if needed", it refers to a consent for a definite laparoscopy with a contingent laparotomy if needed. It does not amount to consent for abdominal hysterectomy with bilateral salpingo-oophorectomy surgery removing the uterus and ovaries/fallopian tubes. If the appellant had consented for abdominal hysterectomy with bilateral salpingo-oophorectomy then the consent form would have given consent for "diagnostic and operative laparoscopy. Laparotomy, hysterectomy and bilateral salpingo-oophorectomy, if needed."

41. On the documentary evidence and the histopathology report, the appellant also raised an issue as to whether appellant was suffering from endometriosis at all. She points out that ultrasound did not disclose endometriosis and the histopathology report does not confirm endometriosis. The respective experts examined on either side have expressed divergent

views as to whether appellant was suffering from endometriosis. It may not be necessary to give a definite finding on this aspect, as the real question for consideration is whether appellant gave consent for hysterectomy and bilateral salpingo-oophorectomy and not whether appellant was suffering from endometriosis. Similarly, there is divergence of expert opinion as to whether removal of uterus and ovaries was the standard or recognized remedy even if there was endometriosis and whether conservative treatment was an alternative. Here again it is not necessary to record any finding as to which is the proper remedy. It is sufficient to note that there are different modes of treatment favored by different schools of thought among gynecologists.

42. Respondent contended that the term "laparotomy" is used in the consent form (by her assistant Dr Lata Rangan) is equal to or same as hysterectomy. The respondent's contention that "Laparotomy" refers to and includes hysterectomy and bilateral salpingo-oophorectomy cannot be accepted. The following clear evidence of appellant's expert witness—Dr Puneet Bedi (CW 1) is not challenged in cross-examination:
"Laparotomy is opening up of the abdomen which is quite different from hysterectomy. Hysterectomy is a procedure which involves surgical removal of uterus. The two procedures are totally different and consent for each procedure has to be obtained separately."
On the other hand, the evidence of respondent's expert witness (Dr Sudha Salhan) on this question is evasive and clearly implies laparotomy is not the same as hysterectomy. The relevant portion of her evidence is extracted below:
"**Q.** As per which medical authority, laparotomy is equal to hysterectomy.
Ans. Consent for laparotomy permits undertaking for such surgical procedure necessary to treat medical conditions including hysterectomy.
Q. I put it to you that the medical practice is to take specific consent for hysterectomy.
Ans. Whenever we do hysterectomy only, specific consent is obtained."

43. Medical texts and authorities clearly spell out that Laparotomy is at best the initial step that is necessary for performing hysterectomy or salpingo-oophorectomy. Laparotomy by itself is not hysterectomy or salpingo-oophorectomy. Nor does "hysterectomy" include salpingo-oophorectomy, in the case of woman who has not attained menopause. Laparotomy does not refer to surgical removal of any vital or reproductive organs. Laparotomy is usually exploratory and once

the internal organs are exposed and examined and the disease or ailment is diagnosed, the problem may be addressed and fixed during the course of such laparotomy (as for example, removal of cysts and fulguration of endometrial area as stated by respondent herself as a conservative form of treatment). But laparotomy is never understood as referring to removal of any organ. In medical circles, it is well recognized that a catch-all clause giving the surgeon permission to do anything necessary does not give roving authority to remove whatever he fancies may be for the good of the patient. For example, a surgeon cannot construe a consent to termination of pregnancy as a consent to sterilize the patient.

44. When the oral and documentary evidence is considered in the light of the legal position discussed above while answering questions (i) and (ii), it is clear that there was no consent by the appellant for conducting hysterectomy and bilateral salpingo-oophorectomy.

45. The Respondent next contended that the consent given by the appellant's mother for performing hysterectomy should be considered as valid consent for performing hysterectomy and salpingo-oophorectomy. The appellant was neither a minor, nor mentally challenged, nor incapacitated. When a patient is a competent adult, there is no question of someone else giving consent on her behalf. There was no medical emergency during surgery. The appellant was only temporarily unconscious, undergoing only a diagnostic procedure by way of laparoscopy. The respondent ought to have waited till the appellant regained consciousness, discussed the result of the laparoscopic examination and then taken her consent for the removal of her uterus and ovaries. In the absence of an emergency and as the matter was still at the stage of diagnosis, the question of taking her mother's consent for radical surgery did not arise. Therefore, such consent by mother cannot be treated as valid or real consent. Further, a consent for hysterectomy is not a consent for bilateral salpingo-oophorectomy.

46. There is another facet of the consent given by the appellant's mother which requires to be noticed. The respondent's specific case is that the appellant had agreed for the surgical removal of uterus and ovaries depending upon the extent of the lesion. It is also her specific case that the consent by signing the consent form on 10.5.1995 wherein the treatment is mentioned as "diagnostic and operative laparoscopy". Laparotomy may be needed includes the AH-BSO surgery for removal of uterus and ovaries. If the term "laparotomy" is to include hysterectomy and salpingo-oophorectomy

as contended by the respondent and there was a specific consent by the appellant in the consent form signed by her on 10.5.1995, there was absolutely no need for the respondent to send word through her assistant Dr Lata Rangan to get the consent of appellant's mother for performing hysterectomy under general anesthesia. The very fact that such consent was sought from appellant's mother for conducting hysterectomy is a clear indication that there was no prior consent for hysterectomy by the appellant.

47. We may, therefore, summarize the factual position thus:

    i. On 9.5.1995, there was no confirmed diagnosis of endometriosis. The OPD slip does not refer to a provisional diagnosis of endometriosis on the basis of personal examination. Though there is a detailed reference to the findings of ultrasound in the entry relating to 9.5.1995 in the OPD slip, there is no reference to endometriosis which shows that ultrasound report did not show endometriosis. In fact, ultrasound may disclose fibroids, chocolate cyst or other abnormality which may indicate endometriosis, but cannot by itself lead to a diagnosis of endometriosis. This is evident from the evidence of CW1, RW1 and RW2 and recognized textbooks. In fact, respondent's expert Dr Sudha Salhan admits in her cross-examination that endometriosis can only be suspected but not diagnosed by ultrasound and it can be confirmed only by laparoscopy. Even according to respondent, endometriosis was confirmed only by laparoscopy. [Books on "Gynaecology" clearly state: "The best means to diagnose endometriosis is by direct visualization at laparoscopy or laparotomy, with histological confirmation where uncertainty persists."] Therefore the claim of respondent that she had discussed in detail about endometriosis and the treatment on 9.5.1995 on the basis of her personal examination and ultrasound report appears to be doubtful.

    ii. The appellant was admitted only for diagnostic laparoscopy (and at best for limited surgical treatment that could be made by laparoscopy). She was not admitted for hysterectomy or bilateral salpingo-oophorectomy.

    iii. There was no consent by appellant for hysterectomy or bilateral salpingo-oophorectomy. The words "laparotomy may be needed" in the consent form dated 10.5.1995 can only refer to therapeutic procedures which are conservative in nature (as for example removal of chocolate cyst and fulguration of endometrial areas, as stated by respondent herself as a choice of treatment), and not radical surgery involving removal of important organs.

48. We find that the Commission has, without any legal basis, concluded that "the informed choice has to be left to the operating surgeon depending on his/her discretion, after assessing the damage to the internal organs, but subject to his/her exercising care and caution". It also erred in construing the words "such medical treatment as is considered necessary for me for" in the consent form as including surgical treatment by way of removal or uterus and ovaries. The Commission has also observed: "whether the uterus should have been removed or not or some other surgical procedure should have been followed are matters to be left to the discretion of the performing surgeon, as long as the surgeon does the work with adequate care and caution". This proceeds on the erroneous assumption that where the surgeon has shown adequate care and caution in performing the surgery, the consent of the patient for removal of an organ is unnecessary. The Commission failed to notice that the question was not about the correctness of the decision to remove the uterus and ovaries, but the failure to obtain the consent for removal of those important organs. There was also a faint attempt on the part of the respondent's counsel to contend that what were removed were not "vital" organs and having regard to the advanced age of the appellant, as procreation was not possible, uterus and ovaries were virtually redundant organs. The appellant's counsel seriously disputes the position and contends that procreation was possible even at the age of 44 years. Suffice it to say that for a woman who has not married and not yet reached menopause, the reproductive organs are certainly important organs. There is also no dispute that removal of ovaries leads to abrupt menopause causing hormonal imbalance and consequential adverse effects.

Re: Question Nos. (iv) and (v):

49. The case of the appellant is that she was not suffering from endometriosis and therefore, there was no need to remove the uterus and ovaries. In this behalf, she examined Dr Puneet Bedi (Obstetrician and Gynecologist) who gave hormone therapy to appellant for about 2 years prior to his examination in 2002. He stated that the best method to diagnose endometriosis is diagnostic laparoscopy; that the presence of

endometrial tissue anywhere outside the uterus is called endometriosis; that the histopathology report did not confirm endometriosis in the case of appellant; and that the mode of treatment for endometriosis would depend on the existing extent of the disease. He also stated that removal of uterus results in abrupt menopause. In natural menopause, which is a slow process, the body gets time to acclimatize to the low level of hormones gradually. On the other hand, when the ovaries are removed, there is an abrupt stoppage of natural hormones, and therefore, hormone replacement therapy is necessary to make up the loss of natural hormones. Hormone replacement therapy is also given even when there is a natural menopause. But hormone replacement therapy has side effects and complications. He also stated that on the basis of materials available on the file, he was of the view that hysterectomy was not called for immediately. But if endometriosis had been proven from history and following diagnostic laparoscopy, hysterectomy could be considered as a last resort if all other medical methods failed. What is relevant from the evidence of Dr Puneet Bedi, is that he does not say that hysterectomy is not the remedy for endometriosis, but only that it is a procedure that has to be considered as a last resort.

50. On the other hand, the respondent who is herself an experienced obstetrician and gynecologist has given detailed evidence, giving the reasons for diagnosing the problem of appellant as endometriosis and has referred to in detail, the need for the surgery. She stated that having regard to the medical condition of complainant, her decision to perform hysterectomy was medically correct. The complainant wanted a cure for her problem and the AH-BSO surgery provided her such cure, apart from protecting her against any future damage to intestines, bladder and ureter. She explained that if the uterus and ovaries had not been removed there was a likelihood of lesion extending to the intestines causing bleeding, fibrosis and narrowing of the gut; the lesion could also go to the surface of the bladder penetrating the wall and causing hematuria and the ureter could be damaged due to fibrosis leading to damage of the kidney; there was also a chance of development of cancer. She also pointed out that the complainant being 44 years of age, was in the premenopausal period and had menorrhagia which prevented regular ovulation which was necessary for pregnancy; that endometriosis also prevented fertilization and produced reaction in the pelvis which increased lymphocytes and macrophages which destroy the ova and sperm; and that the state of bodily health did not depend upon the existence of uterus and ovaries.

51. The respondent also examined Dr Sudha Salhan, Professor and Head of Department (Obstetrics and Gynecology) and President of the Association of Obstetricians and Gynaecologists of Delhi. Having seen the records relating to appellant including the record pertaining to clinical and ultrasound examinations, she was of the view that the treatment given to appellant was correct and appropriate to appellant's medical condition. She stated that the treatment is determined by severity of the disease and hysterectomy was not an unreasonable option as there was no scope left for fecundability in a woman aged 44 years suffering from endometriosis. She also stated that the histopathology report dated 15.5.1995 confirmed the diagnosis of endometriosis made by respondent. She also stated that she saw videotape of the laparoscopic examination and concurred that the opinion of respondent that the lesion being extensive conservation surgery was not possible and the problem could effectively be addressed only by more extensive surgery that is removal of the uterus and ovaries. She also stated that the presence of chocolate cyst was indicative of endometriosis. She also stated that medication merely suppresses endometriosis and the definitive treatment was surgical removal of the uterus and both the ovaries. She also stated that hysterectomy is done when uterus comes out from a prolapse and the woman is elderly, or when there is a cancer of the uterus, or when there are massive fibroids or when a severe grade of endometriosis along with ovaries or in cases of malignancy or the cancer of the ovaries.

52. The evidence therefore demonstrates that on laparoscopic examination, respondent was satisfied that appellant was suffering from endometriosis. The evidence also demonstrates that there is more than one way of treating endometriosis. While one view favors conservative treatment with hysterectomy as a last resort, the other favors hysterectomy as a complete and immediate cure. The age of the patient, the stage of endometriosis among others will be determining factors for choosing the method of treatment. The very suggestion made by appellant's counsel to the expert witness Dr Sudha Salhan that worldwide studies show that most hysterectomies are conducted unnecessarily by gynecologists demonstrate that it is considered as a favored treatment procedure among medical fraternity, offering a permanent cure. Therefore, respondent cannot be held to be negligent, merely because she chose to perform radical surgery in preference to conservative treatment. This finding, however, has

no bearing on the issue of consent which has been held against the respondent. The correctness or appropriateness of the treatment procedure does not make the treatment legal in the absence of consent for the treatment.

53. It is true that the appellant has disputed the respondent's finding that she was suffering from endometriosis. The histopathology report also does not diagnose any endometriosis. The expert witness examined on behalf of the appellant has also stated that there was no evidence that the appellant was suffering from endometriosis. On the other hand, the respondent has relied on some observations of the histopathology report and on her own observations which have been recorded in the case summary to conclude that the appellant was suffering from endometriosis. The evidence shows that the respondent having found evidence of endometriosis, proceeded on the basis that removal of uterus and ovaries was beneficial to the health of the appellant having regard to the age of the appellant and condition of the appellant to provide a permanent cure to her ailment, though not authorized to do so. On an overall consideration of the evidence, we are not prepared to accept the claim of appellant that the respondent falsely invented a case that the appellant was suffering from endometriosis to cover-up some negligence on her part in conducting the diagnostic/operative laparoscopy or to explain the unauthorized and unwarranted removal of uterus and ovaries.

Re: Question No. (vi):

54. In view of our finding that there was no consent by the appellant for performing hysterectomy and salpingo-oophorectomy, performance of such surgery was an unauthorized invasion and interference with appellant's body, which amounted to a tortious act of assault and battery and, therefore, a deficiency in service. But as noticed above, there are several mitigating circumstances. The respondent did it in the interest of the appellant. As the appellant was already 44 years old and was having serious menstrual problems, the respondent thought that by surgical removal of uterus and ovaries she was providing permanent relief. It is also possible that the respondent thought that the appellant may approve the additional surgical procedure when she regained consciousness and the consent by appellant's mother gave her authority. This is a case of respondent acting in excess of consent but in good faith and for the benefit of the appellant. Though the appellant has alleged that she

had to undergo hormone therapy, no other serious repercussions are made out as a result of the removal. The appellant was already fast approaching the age of menopause and in all probability required such hormone therapy. Even assuming that AH-BSO surgery was not immediately required, there was a reasonable certainty that she would have ultimately required the said treatment for a complete cure. On the facts and circumstances, we consider that interests of justice would be served if the respondent is denied the entire fee charged for the surgery and in addition, directed to pay ₹ 25,000/- as compensation for the unauthorized AH-BSO surgery to the appellant.

55. We accordingly allow this appeal and set aside the order of the commission and allow the appellant's claim in part. If the respondent has already received the bill amount or any part thereof from the appellant (either by executing the decree said to have been obtained by her or otherwise), the respondent shall refund the same to the appellant with interest at the rate of 10% per annum from the date of payment till the date of repayment. The Respondent shall pay to the appellant a sum of ₹ 25,000/- as compensation with interest thereon at the rate of 10% per annum from 19.11.2003 (the date of the order of commission) till date of payment. The appellant will also be entitled to cost of ₹ 5,000/- from the respondent.

CASE NO. 2

The second case deals with the problems we clinicians tend to face while dealing with insurance companies which manage the cashless services of our patients having mediclaim. Such cases can act as a deterrent for the insurance companies which try to refuse claims on flimsy grounds.

Apollo Munich Health Insurance Co. Ltd. & Another v/s Kirti & Another
Decided on 01-04-2014
National Consumer Redressal Commission
Hon Justice JM Malik and Hon Dr SM Kanitkar
Judgment
Dr SM Kanitkar, Member

1. The Petitioner filed the present Revision Petition under section 21(b) of the Consumer Protection Act 1986 against the order dated 28.11.2013 passed by the State Consumer Disputes Redressal Commission, (in short, "State Commission") in FA/427/2013 whereby the State Commission allowed the Appeal filed by the Respondent No. 1/Complainant.

2. Facts in brief relevant to dispose of this petition are: The complainant Mrs Kirti was advised diagnostic tests and surgery for symptoms of severe abdominal pain and menstrual problems. Accordingly, she underwent diagnostic laparoscopy and myomectomy at Ivy Hospital. As per policy conditions, prior to the admission a cashless request was sent to the Petitioner company—Apollo Munich Health Insurance Co. Ltd. (the OP-2). But, no avail came. Hence, the Complainant spent ₹ 73,510/- on her treatment and thereafter lodged a claim with the OPs for payment of the said amount. However, OP No. 1 and 2 repudiated the claim on the ground that said "hospitalization" is related to treatment of infertility (Primary infertility since 1½ years), which is excluded from policy under standard exclusion under section 6-e.

3. Therefore, alleging deficiency in service by OPs, who did not provide cashless facility, a complaint before the District Consumer Disputes Redressal Forum, (in short, "District Forum") was filed by the complainant. The District Forum dismissed the complaint.

4. Aggrieved by the order of District Forum, the complainant filed the first appeal before the State Commission.

5. The State Commission perused evidence, the medical records and concluded that, the OPs who repudiated the claim of Complainant are deficient in service, and held that, treatment for infertility, was not excluded from coverage of insurance policy issued to the complainant. The treatment taken by complainant was for fibroid uterus and not for primary sterility. Hence, the State Commission allowed the appeal and directed the Petitioners/OPs 1 and 2 to pay ₹ 73,510/- as compensation, plus ₹ 20,000/- towards mental agony, along with ₹ 10,000/- as costs to the complainant.

6. Against, the impugned order of State Commission, the OP-1 and 2 filed this revision.

7. We have heard the Counsel for the petitioner. He argued vehemently and denied of any deficiency in service by OPs and that the repudiation was correct, as per the terms and conditions of policy under exclusion clause. We have perused the hospital records, the policy and its terms and conditions.

8. The counsel for the OP/Petitioners stated that as per section 6(e)(ix) of the terms and conditions of the policy, the treatment for 'infertility', was permanently excluded. He further contended that, the preauthorization form for cashless facility was received on 28.02.2012 for the treatment of primary infertility, for 1½ years with Provisional/Different Diagnosis of Fibroid Uterus from Ivy Super Speciality Health Care, Mohali. The estimated cost was ₹ 85,000/-.

In the discharge summary, it mentions the diagnosis, as (a) Primary infertility (b) Fibroid uterus; hence, the cashless authorization was specifically denied by OPs, as the claim was not payable.

9. The evidence on record shows that the, complainant took a mediclaim policy, from the OPs, since 2009 and thereafter, it was being renewed, on yearly basis. The claim made by complainant was during subsistence of this policy period from 24.12.2011 to 23.12.2012. The discharge summary of Ivy Hospital clearly mentioned as follows:

Diagnosis:
(i). Primary infertility
(ii). Fibroid uterus

Procedure: A. Diagnostic laparoscopy myomectomy done under GA on 01/03/12.

Findings: Large posterior-superior fibroid uterus (9 × 10 cm) present in the post wall of uterus.

Clinical summary: A 35-years-old nondiabetic, normotensive female patient presented with H/O heavy bleeding during menses and lower abdominal pain, and inability to conceive after 1½ years of marriage.

10. No doubt the patient/complainant was diagnosed as a case of primary infertility, but she was also diagnosed as having fundal fibroid. The Ivy Hospital performed diagnostic laparoscopy and then myomectomy. This operation was necessary to control her symptoms of heavy menstrual bleeding and her abdominal pain. We are of the considered view that, removal of fibroid was an absolute necessity, for better health of patient. Fibroid is one of the causes of infertility, but many patients, may conceive, even in presence of fibroids. The analysis of the case reveals that the OP Company rejected the claim on the basis that the primary cause for the surgery was primary infertility. Hence, the repudiation of claim by the OPs, under exclusion clause section 6(e)(ix) is just an arbitrary act.

11. Yet, the insurance companies usually attribute a reason for an ailment which would make it convenient for them to reject the claim. If a reason is attributed, the onus would lie on the insurance company to medically prove the correctness of its contention. The medical records, ultrasound report and discharge card show that the insured was treated for fibroid, which was presented with heavy menstrual bleeding and lower abdominal pain. She got admitted to the hospital due to sickness or emergency health problems, not for primary infertility. Therefore, insurance companies cannot just assume a reason, for an ailment, according to its own convenience, and/or whims and fancies.

12. On the basis of forgoing discussion, we find no error or any illegality in the order passed by the State Commission. We dismiss this revision petition with a punitive costs of ₹ 25,000/- which the Petitioners, will pay to Mrs Kirti within 90 days, from the receipt of this order, otherwise it will carry 9% interest, till its realization.

■ CASE NO. 3

This case deals with ureteric injury following laparoscopic surgery for ovarian cyst in which the gynecologist tried to hide the complication from the relatives. This lack of transparency was not considered correct in the eyes of law.

Rizwana Shaikh v/s Loveleena Nadir (Dr) & Another
Decided on 05-08-2008
Delhi SCDRC
Hon Justice JC Kapoor and Hon Justice Rumnita Mittal

Judgment
JD Kapoor, President

1. On account of alleged gross and sheer negligence as well as professional misconduct apart from breach of trust on the part of the OP, the complainant has, through this complaint, sought the following reliefs:
   i. Direct the OPs to pay a sum of ₹ 1,500,000/- towards the compensation to the complainant along with interest at 24%.
   ii. Direct the OPs also to pay a sum of ₹ 25,000/- to the complainant towards the cost of litigation.

2. Allegations of the complainant, who is 42 years of age and a mother of three children, i.e. two sons and a daughter aged around 20, 19 and 12 years respectively, in brief, are that in the month of August/September 1999, she had pain in her abdomen and had a complete ultrasound of the whole abdomen on 1.9.1999. As per the report of the ultrasound, both her kidneys were absolutely normal in size, shape, position and echotexture and the conclusion of the report was large cystic, septated abdominopelvic mass ovarian.

3. That on 4.9.1999, the complainant consulted the OP No. 1 at Shyamlal Nursing Home, Daryaganj, New Delhi and she also confirmed that it is a case of ovarian cyst and advised the complainant for operation. The urine culture analysis was also done at the advice of the OP No. 1 which was also normal and pus cells were 0–2/HPF only. She again consulted the OP No. 1 on 8.9.1999 and the OP No. 1 again advised the complainant for operation by the method of laparoscopy/laparotomy under GA on 10.9.1999 at 8 am as the diagnosis was ovarian cyst. On 19.9.1999, laparoscopic operation was done by the OPs at Shyamlal Nursing Home, Daryaganj. OPs started the operation at around 8.30 am and continued it up to 3 pm, i.e. almost for 7 hours which got the complainants family members apprehended who were waiting outside the operation theater anxiously. It is pertinent to mention here that this type of operation generally takes 2 to 3 hours to complete. After the operation which was stated by the OPs to the complainant's family to be successful, the complainant was shifted to the ICU and it was observed at that stage by complainant's family that a catheter and one drain pipe in left side of the abdomen to the patient were attached. This fact coupled with the time taken by the OPs to complete the operation made the complainant's family assured that something wrong has been done to the patient. The complainant was in a very bad shape and her condition was deteriorating and due to this blood transfusion was done by the OPs on 11.9.1999.

4. That on 1.9.1999, the OPs removed the catheter and advised the complainant to take liquid/juice. In the afternoon, it was noticed by the complainant's family that the liquid was oozing out from drainage pipe abdomen hole and the complainant was in great pain and remained so the whole night. On 13.9.1999, both the OPs examined the complainant and immediately fixed the catheter once again. The complainant's family members kept asking the OPs reasons for not improving the condition of the patient and for the above mentioned problem but the OPs did not pay any heed to their queries and without the knowledge and permission of the complainant and her family members, very secretly got the complainant checked up by a urologist as suspicion of urinary bladder leakage was there. After the check-up, both the OPs insisted and compelled the complainant's family members to shift the complainant to their Pamposh Medicare Centre for IVP and further management and the complainant was shifted to the Pamposh Medicare Centre on 14.9.1999.

5. That concentration was given by the OPs and Dr GK Datar only on urinary bladder at the time of IVP and cystogram. Whereas actual leakage was due to urinary tract/left side ureter damage which was ignored by both the OPs. Laparoscopic operation of ovarian cyst was mainly in left side and damage to left ureter indicated that the operation was performed wrongly and negligently by the OPs.

6. That on 30.1.2001, the complainant consulted another Doctor namely Dr Rupam Arora (gynecologist) as the complainant was not satisfied by the treatment of the

OPs and got her ultrasound done once again and to the shock and surprise of the complainant and her family members, the report expressed doubt about the left kidney. On 16.3.2001, the complainant consulted Dr SN Rizvi (nephrologist) for kidney and on his advice got IVP (radiological examination of the urinary tract) at Diwan Chand Satyapal Aggarwal X-ray clinic. As per the report of the IVP, there was no contrast seen in the left kidney after 24 hours and the right kidney and ureter was normal.

7. That Dr Rizvi advised the complainant to consult a urologist in AIIMS and on 29.3.2001 the complainant consulted Dr Dogra at AIIMS who got completed DTPA renal scan with GFR evaluation for kidney which shows right kidney as normal in function and size whereas left kidney was poorly perfused, hydronephrotic, obstructed with extremely poor function and the renal function of the left kidney was only 4%. The ultrasound was also done which shows left kidney in shrink position with lesser size as compared to the right kidney. It was further revealed that the left side ureter is dilated and there is possibility of a stricture at the lower end.

8. That in view of the above stated facts, circumstances and in the light of various tests and examinations got conducted by the complainant from various medical experts, it became crystal clear and established that the OPs at the time of laparoscopic surgery conducted by them on 10.9.1999 have damaged the ureter/urinary tract in left side which is a case of gross and sheer negligence as well as professional misconduct apart from breach of trust on the part of the OPs. It was further clear and established that the urinary leakage was due to the damage in the urinary tract and this damage in the urinary tract slowly affected the functioning of the left kidney/ureter which ultimately became nonfunctional. This negligent act of the OPs has caused the complainant permanently physically weak and handicapped in many ways thus reduced the life expectancy of the complainant who is a mother of three young children. To recover completely, which is not guaranteed, she needs to have kidney transplant.

9. At the outset, the OP has denied the allegations of negligence in conducting the operation for removal of cyst and has averred that it was after more than a year of the operation that the tests showed that complainant's left kidney was not functioning properly. Ultrasound done at PD Gupta Mediscan Centre by the patient showed stone (calculi) in inferior calyx of left kidney. This development has nothing to do with the operation carried out by the OPs. It is quite possible that the patient ignored and neglected the stone in the kidney, which aggravated and caused pain to her.

10. All tests indicated that the left side kidney is not functioning and left side ureter is dilated. It is wrong and hence denied that it was a consequence of the operation. After the operation, all tests carried out on the basis of suspicion, proved normal. On the other hand, one ultrasound examination done in 2001, showed stones in left kidney which may have been neglected by the complainant, which caused her pain and predicament.

11. The OPs are not guilty of any act of negligence. Kidney transplant is done only when both kidneys are irretrievably damaged. It is absolutely possible to live a full life with only one functioning kidney. In any case, it has nothing to do with the operation carried out by the OPs.

12. So far as other allegations of removal of catheter from the urinary bladder the OP has come up with the following averments:

    i. That the complainant was alive to and aware of the risk involved in the operation and she would not hold the doctors guilty in case the operation was not successful. However, in the present case, the operation was successful.

    ii. That the investigation showed a large cystic swelling (fluid-filled) of the ovary. The OPs after examination recommended surgical removal of the ovarian swelling by laparoscopic surgery. Laparoscopic surgery is an established technique in which patient's recovery is faster and pain is much less. Surgery was undertaken after informing the complainant and her attendant and getting their consent. Thereafter, the cystic swelling was successfully taken out. After lengthy operation, the patients are shifted to Intensive Care Unit for observation. A catheter in the bladder is routinely introduced in all operation in the pelvic region and so was the case with the complainant. A drainage tube was left in place in the abdominal cavity of the patient so that it could drain any collection of fluid/blood near the site of the operation.

    iii. That the start of the operation is not the time that the patient is shelled into operation theater. Preparation and anesthesia takes time, thus it is wrong to presume that the operation took 7 hours. It is also wrong to mention that this type of operation takes 2 to 3 hours. The length of the operation depends on the actual finding at the operation site. After lengthy operation, the patients are shifted to Intensive Care Unit for observation and not because they are in a critical condition. A catheter in the bladder is routinely introduced in all operations in the pelvic region and so was the case with the complainant. A drainage tube was left in place in the abdominal cavity of the patient so that it could drain any collection of fluid/blood near the site of the operation. Obviously, some oozing was expected and that is why a drainage tube was left in place. No queries were avoided and it is a regular practice of the OPs to brief the persons attending the patients about the operation which was done in the present case.

iv. That for removal of catheter and allowing juice/ liquids to be taken by month is an indication of recovery of the patient as per expectations. Patient was shifted out from ICU, too since she had recovered satisfactorily. Though no mention is made of that liquid was oozing from the drainage pipe as expected. Pain after this kind of operation for a few days is also normal and expected.

v. That on 13.9.1999, the nature and smell of the liquid oozing from the drainage tube made OPs suspicious that may be dealing with a urinary leak and, therefore, the catheter was reintroduced to drain the bladder efficiently. This development was neither abnormal nor due to any negligence on the part of the OPs. The complainant's relatives were informed about the development and also about the proposal to seek the opinion of a urologist. There was nothing secretive about it as the relatives of the complainant were informed and the name and designation of the urologist Dr CM Goel was disclosed to them. Had there been anything secretive, a mention of suspected urinary leak in the case-sheet and discharge summary would not have been made and an announced official opinion would not have been sought from a qualified, renowned urologist. All these steps were taken in the best interest of the complainant. Complainant was shifted to Pamposh Medicare Centre because it was thought better care could be taken of the patient at the center as also proximity to a very renowned and qualified X-ray clinic.

vi. That cystogram was done to recheck for any urinary leak and was again found normal. Since the cystogram was found normal, catheter was removed from the urinary bladder. It may also be mentioned here that after operation of this

magnitude pain for few days in normal which subsides with time and medication.

vii. That IVP is meant to delineate the entire urinary tract, which was shown to be normal. Cystogram is meant to delineate the bladder. Left-sided ureter damage would have shown up as a leak on the IVP, which it did not. It is wrong and hence denied that operation was performed wrongly by the OPs.

viii. That the complainant did not seek any medical advice from the OPs in the whole year of 2000. If for 1 year after the operation, the complainant did not require any medical advice, it can be safely presumed that the operation was successful.

13. In support of her claim, the complainant has produced and proved the following documents:

    i. Copy of report of ultrasound dated 1.9.1999.
    ii. Copy of prescription dated 4.9.1999 given by the OP No. 1 giving details of the check-up of the complainant.
    iii. Copy of the report dated 6.9.1999 of urine culture.
    iv. Prescription dated 8.9.1999 written by the OP No. 1 advising and fixing the date of operation.
    v. Copy of the discharge file dated 14.9.1999.
    vi. Copy of report dated 15.9.1999 of IVP test.
    vii. Copy of prescription dated 22.9.1999 given by the OP No. 1.
    viii. Copy of the report of cystogram dated 2.10.1999.
    ix. Copy of prescription dated 2.10.1999.
    x. Copy of the bill raised by the OPs and paid by the complainant.
    xi. Copy of prescription dated 11.10.1999.
    xii. Copy of report dated 31.1.2001.
    xiii. Copies of reports/prescriptions of Dr Rizvi.
    xiv. Copy of report of IVP test dated 23.3.2001.
    xv. Copy of report dated 28.3.2001 by AIIMS.
    xvi. Copy of DTPA renal scan report dated 29.3.2001 and ultrasound.
    xvii. Copy of ultrasound report dated 21.5.2001.
    xviii. Copy of demand notice dated 14.8.2001.
    xix. Copies of postal receipts.

14. The complainant is also presuming the negligence on the premise of following queries:

    i. After such minor laparoscopic surgery of ovarian cyst, where was the need to shift the patient in ICU?
    ii. Where was the need for blood transfusion, if the condition of patient was good and laparoscopic operation was successful?
    iii. Why drainage tube was kept in abdomen for 21 days?

This clearly shows that something went wrong while performing surgery due to the gross and sheer negligence/professional misconduct of OPs.

15. While interlinking the damage to the left side ureter with the kidney, the complainant has come up with the following version:

"Due to damage to left side ureter, kidney was getting damaged slowly and when she consulted Dr Roopam Arora (gynecologist) and Dr PD Gupta, she came to know about damage to left side kidney. After consulting Dr SN Rizvi (nephrologist), detail check-ups/investigation at Diwan Chand Satyapal Aggarwal X-Ray Clinic (a fully equipped clinic with modern machines), she came to know the following facts:

    i. Left side kidney size reduced and not functioning.
    ii. Left side ureter was dilated and there was a possibility of stricture at the lower end.
    iii. There were no stones in kidneys.
    iv. Right side kidney and ureter were normal.

16. On the concept of medical negligence, we have culled out certain criteria from the ratio of large number of judgments starting from Bolam's case followed by various judgments of the Supreme Court, some of which are as under:

    i. Bolam's case reported in (1957) 2 All ER 118, 121 D-F.
    ii. Sidway vs. Bethlem Royal Hospital Governors and Others, (1985) 1 All ER 643.
    iii. Maynard vs West Midlands Regional Health Authority, (1985) 1 All ER 635.
    iv. Whitehouse vs Jordan and Another, (1980) 1 All ER 650.
    v. Indian Medical Association vs VP Shantha and Ors, III (1995) CPJ 1 (SC)=I (1996) CLT 81 (SC)=(1995) 6 SCC 651.
    vi. Jacob Mathew (Dr) vs State of Punjab and Anr., III (2005) CPJ 9 (SC)=III (2005) CCR 9 (SC)=VI (2005) SLT 1=122 (2005) DLT 83 (SC)=(2005) SCC (Cr.) 1369.

17. The conclusions are as under:

    i. Whether the treating doctor had the ordinary skill and not the skill of the highest degree that he professed and exercised, as everybody is not supposed to possess the highest or perfect level of expertise or skills in the branch he practices
    ii. Whether the guilty doctor had done something or failed to do something which in the given facts and circumstances no medical professional would do when in ordinary senses and prudence
    iii. Whether the risk involved in the procedure or line of treatment was such that injury or death was imminent or risk involved was up to the percentage of failures
    iv. Whether there was error of judgment in adopting a particular line of treatment. If so what was the level of error. Was it so overboard that result could have been fatal or near fatal or at lowest mortality rate?
    v. Whether the negligence was so manifest and demonstrative that no professional or skilled person in his ordinary senses and prudence could have indulged in
    vi. Everything being in place, what was the main cause of injury or death? Whether the cause was the direct result of the deficiency in the treatment and medication
    vii. Whether the injury or death was the result of administrative deficiency or postoperative or condition environment-oriented deficiency.

18. As is apparent from the aforesaid conspectus of facts, the allegations of medical negligence on the part of the OPs, the solitary point to be determined is whether there was any kind of possibility of damage to the ureter while performing the laparoscopic surgery of ovarian cyst and whether leakage was due to some damage done to the ureter or was due to the nondetection of the stone, i.e. calculus for a year or so, which aggravated and caused pain to the complainant.

19. The defense of the OP that the damage to the left ureter as well as left kidney got damaged due to nondetection of stones, i.e. calculus for a year or so is not tenable as the documents on record show that there was no stone/calculi in the left ureter/kidney of the complainant just prior to the performance of laparoscopic operation for removal of the ovarian cyst. In this regard, report of Dr Sucharita Jain's ultrasound dated 1.9.1999 is to the effect that both kidneys are normal in size, shape, position and echotexture and no calculus hydronephrosis or SOL seen. Furthermore, the diagram of the urinary tract placed on record by the complainant as well as OP points to the possibility that while removing the ovarian cyst by laparoscopic procedure, the left ureter was cut/damaged at the lower end and since a stitch was put there to close the cut, the same did not allow urine to pass out and started putting back pressure on the kidney, which resulted in damage to the left ureter as well as kidney.

20. Furthermore, ultrasound carried out at Diwan Chand Satyapal Aggarwal X-ray Clinic on 29.3.2001 (Ex. CW1/18) states as under:

"Lower abdominal ultrasound (hysterectomy with oophorectomy).

The right kidney measures 107 mm in length with a parenchymal thickness of 16 mm. No hydronephrosis/No calculus.

The left kidney measures 93 mm in length with a parenchymal thickness of 10 mm. There is marked dilation of the pelvicalyceal system and the dilated ureter is seen to have a tortuous course initially. Lower down it can be traced till the mid pelvis. No calculus can be identified. Possibility of a stricture at the lower end may be considered.

The urinary bladder is distended and is normal in appearance. No calculus is seen.

Right ovary is normal in size and appearance. Suggest clinical correction and further workings with CT/RGP."

21. Thus, it is apparent that even till 29.3.2001, there was no stone or calculus seen in the left kidney. Another ultrasound report of the urinary tract dated 21.5.2001 by Diwan Chand Satyapal Aggarwal Imaging Research Centre (Ex. CW1/19) showed that the left ureter is dilated in its entire course, no obvious ureteric calculus can be seen. It is only for the first time in the scan conducted by PD Gupta Mediscan Centre (P) Ltd. dated 31.1.2001, the existence of calculi was seen in the left kidney.

22. Besides the above evidence, the fact that laparoscopic operation of the ovarian cyst took about 7 hours instead of normal 2 to 3 hours and the OPs have not been able to give any satisfactory explanation for the said delay in conducting operation and has given a casual and generalized reply, which further raises the inference that something had gone wrong during the said surgery. Further the fact that when the complainant was brought after the surgery, there was a catheter which was kept on for 22 days, drain pipe for 12 days and a urologist had to be brought into check on the patient as there was suspicion of urinary bladder leakage also supports the theory projected by the complainant. It was explained by the patient that due to stricture at lower end of the left ureter, urine or fluid was not passing into urinary bladder and there was no way out for urine and, hence, it was putting pressure on the kidney.

23. The averment of the OP that it was after more than a year that the complainant had complained of the kidney damage and as such the same could not have any connection with the laparoscopic surgery carried out by the OPs also does not find favor with us as during the entire course various doctors were being consulted from time-to-time and it was only at a much later stage it was discovered that the ureter and the kidney had got damaged. Even otherwise the ultrasound report immediately before the laparoscopic operation on the complainant, both the kidneys were found to be normal and no stone or calculi were seen. It could only be during the surgery that a nick/cut was caused in the lower end of the left ureter which is in close proximity to the ovary and ovarian cyst and the likelihood of the ureter having been damaged cannot be ruled out.

24. Thus, because of nonpassing of urine to the bladder would have damaged the ureter as well as the kidney gradually. The OP has in no way proved that the existence of stone/calculi at a later stage could have caused such a damage to the ureter and kidney that as per report of Diwan Chand Satyapal Aggarwal X-Ray Clinic dated 2nd March, 2002, the left kidney could be barely visualized through the study and renal cortical function had worsened since the last scan.

25. Thus, in our view, OPs are guilty for negligence and deficiency in service in conducting the laparoscopic surgery/operation for removal of ovarian cyst on the complainant and causing immense physical pain and agony and unnecessary future medical expenses.

26. In our view, lumpsum compensation of ₹ 50,000/- besides ₹ 10,000/- as cost of litigation shall meet the ends of justice.

27. Payment shall be made within 1 month from the date of receipt of this order.

28. Complaint is allowed and disposed of in foresaid terms.

29. A copy of the order as per the statutory requirements be forwarded to the parties free of charge and thereafter the file be consigned to Record Room.

Complaint allowed.

▌CASE NO. 4

Deepak Kr Neogi and Another v/s Birendra Nath Das (Dr) and Another

Decided on 27-02-2006
West Bengal SCDRC
Hon SN Basu and Hon PK Chattopadhyay

This is a case of bowel injury during laparoscopic hysterectomy. The mishap was communicated to the relatives and well managed as per the routine norms.

Judgment
SN Basu, Member

1. This is an appeal directed against the orders and judgment passed by the learned Forum, South 24-Parganas in CDF Case No. 79 of 2003. The learned Forum in their Order dated 4.3.2004, directed the OP 1/Respondent No. 1 to pay compensation of ₹ 100,000/-

and also cost of ₹ 500/-. Being aggrieved by the above order, the present appeal has been preferred. The case was heard analogously with Case No. 152/A/2004 as the subject matter was the same and the parties to the other appeal case are also the same.

2. The facts of the case are that the complainant/appellant No. 1's wife Smt. Dipti Neogi was admitted in Ramkrishna Seva Pratisthan on 4.1.2003 under respondent No. 1 due to some gynecological problem. He was advised by the respondent No. 1 for removal of her uterus and accordingly laparoscopic surgery was done for removal of the uterus of the appellant No. 1's wife on 6.1.2003. The patient had reportedly felt severe pain in the abdomen besides having breathing trouble. But despite request made by the appellant No. 1/Complainant's wife and also her relatives, the respondent No. 1 allegedly did not attend to her to take necessary measures for alleviating pain. On 8.1.2003, the complainant/appellant No. 1 was told by the hospital authority that the patient was OK but subsequently in the afternoon the complainant/appellant No. 1 was requested over telephone to attend the hospital immediately. The complainant was also told to arrange blood for blood transfusion. On 8.1.2003, his consent was allegedly sought for surgical operation, but later on the complainant/appellant No. 1 came to know that the second operation had already taken place without his consent. The patient was taken to ICCU as her condition was critical. The respondent No. 1 informed appellant No. 1 that a perforation of intestine had been detected which happened in the course of the first operation. The appellant No. 1 alleged that all this happened due to sheer negligence on the part of the respondent No. 1. The patient expired on that date. She was found to have developed septicemia. The complainant/appellant No. 1 had, therefore, filed the complaint for proper compensation against the OPs.

3. The learned Forum had observed that the circumstances in which the patient had died left enough scope for doubt that something went wrong with the operation and also in its postoperative care. The learned Forum further observed that it was clear from the documents on record that the intestine of the patient had been perforated during the first operation which was not noticed or taken care of initially and as a result of which there was continuous bleeding resulting in falling of blood pressure and ultimately development of septicemia. Learned Forum, therefore, concluded that the attending doctors failed to give proper importance to the complaint of pain by the patient and her relatives and they only became active after it was detected that the blood pressure of the patient had come down alarmingly. The learned Forum further observed that transfusion of blood on the patient further proved that the patient was in need of blood due to drainage of her own blood on account of her perforated intestine. The respondent No. 1 in his written objection as well as in the Memo of Appeal had stated that the complaint was not based on personal knowledge of the complainant but on conjecture. The respondent No. 1 had further contended that it was not a fact that the respondent No. 1 had failed to notice the incidence of perforated intestine of the patient. He contends that it is not possible to identify or locate such a small perforation immediately after the operation and thus he had no scope to know that there had been an instance of perforation of the intestine. The patient was also found to be progressing on the following day though she had complained of pain in her abdomen. But such pains are very common after an operation of this nature. The respondent No. 1 had strongly denied that the attending doctors did not give any importance to the patient's complaint and had been aroused to action only after the blood pressure fell. He had further stated that after the blood pressure of the patient had fallen alarmingly, he had sent for the Medical Officer of the hospital for examining the patient and on receipt of the report he himself visited the patient and then found that something was wrong. He suspected a secondary abdominal bleeding or any abdominal injury, and accordingly he administered higher dose of antibiotic and the relatives of the deceased were informed over telephone. The respondent No. 1 added further that he had decided that the patient was in need of a laparoscopic operation under the given circumstances to find out the cause of her present clinical condition. Since the relatives of the patient did not turn up till 1.00 pm on 8.1.2003, he had decided to go in for the above operation with the help of another surgeon of the hospital. The respondent No. 1 had also stated in his written argument the actions taken by him regarding the operation. The bilious abdominal collection was sucked out and small perforation in small intestine was detected and locally repaired and abdomen was closed in single layer. He had further averred that such small perforation cannot be detected in an injury and clinical features do not develop before 36 to 48 hours after the primary surgery. He avers that this was more or less the time taken by him to detect that some internal bleeding was going on. The appellant has adduced excerpts from the book "Gynaecology (3rd edition) by RW Shaw, WP

Soutter and SL Stanton (page 149). [Publisher Churchill Livingstone] which says "Patients who have received more than minor laceration such as puncture with a Veress needle at the time of laparoscopy will normally present after 42 to 72 hours". The respondent No. 1/OP No. 1 had further stated in his WNA, which fact is also acknowledged by the learned Forum that after the second operation the blood pressure remained low and respiratory effort being unsatisfactory, the patient was put on a ventilator. Thereafter, she was sent to ICCU considering the respiratory problem faced by her. He states that in spite of his best efforts, he could not discuss the problems with the relatives of the patient till 6.30 pm on 8.1.2003, i.e. the date of second operation.

4. The appellant No. 1 in his written argument had stated that when the patient was taken to the hospital on 29.11.2002, the USG of lower abdomen and pelvis did not show any abnormality and the uterus was normal in shape and size. He has also made an allegation that the history sheet dated 4.1.2003 showed that Dr Das, the respondent No. 1 explained to his patient the modalities of management and the patient had opted for hysterectomy LAVH, but actual laparoscopy was done on 6.1.2003. The appellant had finally doubted the authenticity of the history sheet dated 4.1.2003. He further stated that ideal treatment should have been laparoscopy-guided ovariotomy, which is simple and less risky than laparoscopy and hysterectomy and so the respondent No. 1 should have opted for the safer option. But he did not do it. He also complained that no X-ray investigation of the lower abdomen was done on 7.1.2003 when the patient was complaining of severe pain and other troubles. The appellant No. 1 holds that by causing two perforations in the intestine of the patient, the respondent No. 1 is found guilty of murderous negligence. He further commented that the "surgeon was inefficient or negligent," which was ultimately responsible for developing septicemia causing death to the patient. He holds both the hospital and doctor responsible for being negligent.

5. We have perused the impugned orders passed by the learned Forum, Memo of Appeal and the written objection as well as the written notes of arguments filed by both sides. We have also heard the learned Advocates of both sides. In his complaint, the appellant No. 1/complainant had made allegations against the respondent No. 1 as well as respondent No. 2 for being negligent which caused death to his wife at the age of 42. After going through the facts and submissions made by both sides, we find that the complainant/appellant No. 1 had brought his wife to respondent No. 2 for a

hysterectomy operation, and was advised by the doctor after examining the various medical reports. But very unfortunately two perforations had been inflicted on the intestine of the patient by the attending surgeon Dr Das, who is the respondent No. 1. From the details noted in the case record of the hospital as well as submissions and written statements filed by both sides, we find that the patient had been complaining of severe pain after the operation. We also find that there had been routine visits by the attending surgeon after the operation and he prescribed some pain-killer medicines as he was of the view that the pain was due to the operation. The averment of the respondent No. 1 that the patient had shown some sign of improvement on the day following the operation is further corroborated by the fact that on the next day there was no sign of severe physical distress in the patient excepting the pain when the condition of the patient had suddenly deteriorated necessitating another operation. We also find that when the doctor had come to suspect that the pain coupled with falling blood pressure was not a normal one, he had immediately arranged second operation to give relief to the patient with the help of another surgeon. He also repaired the perforations caused during the first operation. However, when the patient's condition became critical she was put on ventilator to help her breathing problem and ultimately she was transferred to ICCU where she ultimately expired.

6. If the whole situation is analyzed, we find that it is a fact that the intestine was perforated while executing the first operation but when the same was suspected the attending surgeon as well as the hospital authority took all possible measures to combat the situation. It is a fact which has also been admitted by the respondent No. 1 that the detection of perforation was after some 36 hours, but there is nothing on record to show that it happened due to willful negligence on the part of the appellant. However, the authority adduced by the respondent No. 1 containing expert opinion in the matter of puncture of any internal organ at the time of operation is also supportive of the fact that it takes time to detect the damage. Under such circumstances, we do not think it proper to hold the attending surgeon and the hospital responsible for negligence in terms of section 2(1)(g) of the CP Act, 1986 though the untimely death of a young lady is certainly very unfortunate. In this context, it may be relevant to refer to the decision of the Hon'ble Apex Court in 2005 CTJ 1085 (SC) (CP), wherein it has been observed by the Hon'ble Court that "A simple lack of care, an error of judgment or of accident is not a proof of negligence on the part of

medical professional—so long as a doctor follows the practice acceptable to the medical profession of that day, he cannot be held liable for negligence merely because a better alternative course or measure of treatment was available or simply because a more skillful doctor would not have followed or resorted to that practice or procedure which the accused followed... whether he was negligent or not, the standard for judging him would be that of an ordinary competent person exercising ordinary skill in that profession". The above decision of the Apex Court clearly defines as to what should be called medical negligence and what should not. In the present case, we find that the hospital and the attending physician had taken all possible actions to save the situation after they came to know about the damage caused to the patient due to an accident on the part of the attending surgeon and the actions taken like the second operation, putting the patient on ventilator and sending her to the ICCU—all go to prove that there has not been any case of willful negligence, may be the doctor should have been more careful while undertaking the operation. In view of the facts and circumstances stated in the foregoing paragraphs, we are inclined to say that the learned Forum had misdirected itself to pass the above Order on 4.3.2004. It is, therefore, directed that the said Order of the learned Forum dated 4.3.2004 be set aside. The orders and judgment of this case will also govern Case No. 152/A/2004 as the subject matter and parties are the same.

7. The appeal is, therefore, dismissed on contest without any order as to cost in Case No. 158/A/2004 and allowed on context in Case No. 152/A/2004 without any order as to cost.

Appeal No. 158/2004 dismissed.

Appeal No. 152/2004 allowed.

■ CASE NO. 5

This is a case of laparoscopic surgery for endometrioma by a visiting surgeon from the USA. The charitable hospital did not have their own laparoscopic instruments. The instruments had to be hired from other hospital. During surgery, the instruments did not work properly. The condition of the OT was unhygienic. The assistant surgeons were not experienced in laparoscopy. Patient apparently had existing PID and colon got injured inadvertently (though denied by the surgeon). Patient died due to septicemia.

St. Antony Hospital Rep. by its Administrator v/s CL D'Silva

Decided by NCDRC on 12-04-2013
Hon Justice Ashok Bhan, Hon Vineeta Rai and Hon Dr SM Kanitkar

Judgment

Vineeta Rai, Member

1. This first appeal has been filed by St. Antony Hospital, Appellant herein and Opposite Party before the Tamil Nadu State Consumer Disputes Redressal Commission, Chennai (hereinafter referred to as the State Commission) being aggrieved by the order of that Commission, which had partly allowed the complaint of CL D'Silva, Respondent herein and Complainant before the State Commission alleging medical negligence against the Appellant.

2. FACTS:

In his complaint before the State Commission, Respondent-Complainant had stated that his wife Corrine D'Silva (hereinafter referred to as the Patient), who was gainfully employed in a foreign company in Chennai, complained of pain in the lower abdomen on the right side. Suspecting it to be a case of appendicitis, Respondent-Complainant took her to Pavithra Hospital, Erukkanchery, Chennai, wherein an ultrasound scan indicated that she had a small cyst on her right ovary and fibroid uterus was suspected. Respondent-Complainant took a second opinion from St. Thomas Hospital, where removal of ovaries was advised, which required surgery and 10 to 15 days' hospitalization. Since Respondent-Complainant and the patient were living in Madhavaram, they decided to go to the nearby Appellant in April, 2000 for fixing a date for admission and surgery. Appellant conducted preliminary tests like chest X-ray, ECG, etc., the results of which were normal. The Assistant Administrator of the Appellant advised the patient to postpone the surgery till 12.5.2000, as a reputed and experienced Doctor from the USA, one Dr Samuel Parra, was visiting their hospital to demonstrate his skills. Patient, therefore, applied for medical leave for 4 weeks from 12.5.2000 and was examined by Dr Samuel Parra on that date, who after diagnosis stated that he would remove the cyst by laparoscopy method and, if required, thereafter a surgery would also be done. Since the appellant did not have the laparoscopy instrument required by Dr Parra, it was arranged from a hospital in Tuticorin and the surgery was fixed for

24.5.2000. Patient got admitted on 23.5.2000 and was thereafter allotted a room which was very unhygienic as sewage water was stagnating nearby. At 8.30 a.m. on 24.5.2000, patient was taken to the operation theater for surgery and on its completion, she was brought back to the room at 12.45 pm. Same night, she developed high fever and also later complained of discomfort and severe pain in the abdomen. She was assured by Dr Parra that this was a routine pain after surgery. However, when her condition worsened, she was again examined on 26.5.2000 by Dr Parra who asked the Respondent–Complainant to arrange for 2 Pints of blood. Patient's condition continued to deteriorate and breathing became belabored and, therefore, she was put on oxygen. When Respondent–Complainant returned with the blood required for transfusion, he found that the patient had been taken to the operation theater for the second surgery. Thereafter at 11.20 pm Dr Parra informed the Respondent–Complainant that by mistake, colon of the patient was ruptured during the first surgery, as a result of which her body fluids and fecal matters had leaked into her system, but this was cleaned up and the mistake rectified during the second surgery. Respondent–Complainant was also informed that both ovaries had been removed and sent to the laboratory for tissue culture. Patient was breathing with great difficulty and the external incisions following her surgery were also not fully closed, which according to the Doctor was necessary in case another emergency surgery was required. Respondent–Complainant stated that he was fully confused with these sudden developments and on 27.5.2000 when he was permitted to see the patient, he found her in semiconscious state. He also reliably understood from discussions among Doctors that his wife's first surgery was an experimental one and the equipment used were not functioning properly. On 27.5.2000 at 7.00 pm Dr Parra and other Doctors from Appellant informed the Respondent–Complainant that they were not equipped to cope with patient's critical condition since there were no intensive care facilities and advised him to transfer her to Sri Ramachandra Medical College Hospital at Porur. When the patient was shifted late at night to Sri Ramachandra Medical College Hospital, she was taken to ICCU and put on ventilator there and doctors informed the Respondent–Complainant that his wife's recovery chances were only 5% as the internal organs were in septic condition due to presence of fecal matter, etc. causing severe internal damage. The Doctors at Sri Ramachandra Medical College Hospital also advised that the wounds may have to be reopened and

cleaned but this was very risky procedure, for which the Respondent–Complainant was required to sign a consent form. However, despite all efforts Patient passed away on 16.5.2000 at 2.20 am. As per the medical record, the cause of death was septicemia leading to multiorgan failure. Being aggrieved by the medical negligence and deficiency on the part of the Appellant and Doctors therein, including Dr Parra who used the patient as a guinea pig, in conducting a laparoscopy with ill-equipped equipment, which resulted in the rupturing of the colon of the patient, Respondent–Complainant issued a legal notice to the Appellant claiming ₹ 15 lakhs as compensation. However, since no reply was received from them, Respondent filed a complain before the State Commission on grounds of medical negligence and deficiency in service and requested that the Appellant be directed to pay him (i) ₹ 15 lakhs as compensation towards loss, hardships and mental agony suffered by him on account of gross deficiency in service and the medical negligence on the part of Appellant and its Doctors; (ii) ₹ 181,911/- being the refund in respect of medical treatment; and (iii) ₹ 10,000/- as litigation costs, as also any other relief as deemed appropriate in the interest of justice.

3. Appellant on being served filed a written rejoinder denying that there was any medical negligence on their part. It was stated that the Appellant is a charitable hospital which was rendering service to deserving and poor patients. Respondent–Complainant's wife had been admitted in the Appellant hospital where after examination she was diagnosed with endometrial cyst and fibromas of the uterus. Patient had agreed to the laparoscopy after she was clearly informed about the pros and cons of the same, including the possible complications, which could require converting it into an open procedure. On 24.5.2000, after conducting all the preoperative tests, the laparoscopy was conducted, which confirmed that patient had extensive endometriosis, inflammatory changes and also pelvic inflammatory disease. There were extensive adhesions and some fibrinous fluid. All these were attended to through a time consuming procedure. At 8.00 pm on the same day, patient's hemoglobin dropped to 9.3 and she complained of shoulder pain which was common after laparoscopy. However, there were no other problems. She was given IV fluids and antibiotics. The next day when she was not responding to conservative management and was showing systemic sepsis and peritonitis, Respondent–Complainant was advised about the need for exploratory surgery. It was denied that Dr Parra had informed the patient or the

respondent that her colon had ruptured during the first surgery and fecal matter and other body fluids had leaked into the system which needed to be immediately rectified. The second surgery was conducted by Dr Parra assisted by other qualified doctors and it was found that she had severe sepsis with peritonitis endometriosis associated with pelvic inflammatory disease, from which she had been suffering prior to the surgery. Because patient required prolonged ventilator support and other intensive care facilities, which were not available in the Appellant hospital, she was in her own interest advised admission in an advanced medical center for which necessary arrangements were made by the Appellant and she was transferred to Sri Ramachandra Medical College Hospital at about 9.00 p.m. accompanied by Dr Parra, an anesthetist and a nurse. It was reiterated that there was no medical negligence or deficiency in the treatment of the patient and the entire medical expenses came to only ₹ 25,330/- which was borne by the Appellant.

4. The State Commission after hearing the parties and on the basis of evidence filed before it, particularly the statement of Dr Parra, who admitted that there were some technical problems and defects with the laparoscopy equipment which he had faced while conducting the laparoscopy, concluded that medical negligence and deficiency in service was clearly established. In this connection, the State Commission, inter alia, observed as follows:

"So far as the present case is concerned, there is concrete unimpeachable evidence in the shape of the report of Dr Parra. The equipment was not in good shape; the persons who were assisting him were novices and had no previous experience with the use of laparoscope; during the surgery, there was some malfunctioning of the equipment; there was a tear in the colon and as to how it happened Dr Parra could not explain; the opposite party hospital was unhygienic. There is least doubt that the opposite party had been negligent and there was deficiency in service."

The State Commission while recording that it would be difficult to quantify the amount of compensation in the case of death of one's spouse, after taking into account all the facts of the case, held that a compensation of ₹ 500,000/- would be just and reasonable and accordingly directed the Appellant to pay the Respondent–Complainant the said amount together with ₹ 5,000/- as litigation costs within a period of 2 months.

5. Aggrieved by the order of the State Commission, the present first appeal has been filed.

6. Learned Counsel for the Appellant made oral submissions. Learned Counsel for the Respondent-complainant was not present but written submissions were taken on record.

7. Counsel for the appellant stated that the medical records filed in evidence clearly indicated that there was no deficiency or negligence on the part of the appellant in the treatment of the patient, including the laparoscopy as also the surgery. It was stated that the patient had been brought to the appellant with endometrial cysts and fibromas of the uterus, for which a diagnostic laparoscopy was necessary, and the procedure was conducted after all the preoperative tests. It was found during the laparoscopy that the patient also had pelvic inflammatory disease which caused complications leading to sepsis and peritonitis. This was not the result of any negligence as alleged, including accidental perforation of the colon, and despite the best medical care and treatment, including a second surgery, these complications persisted. No payment was taken from the patient by appellant which was a charitable institution and which also paid for her entire treatment at Sri Ramachandra Medical College Hospital, where she expired. All the Doctors, including Dr Parra, were well-qualified and professional Doctors and, therefore, the findings of the State Commission were not based on correct appreciation of the facts as also the evidence on record.

8. Counsel for the Respondent–Complainant in the written arguments contended that from the statement of Dr Samuel Parra before the State Commission, it was clear that the laparoscopy procedure conducted by him was totally botched up. There was malfunctioning of the equipment and during the procedure, colon of the patient got ruptured resulting in the fecal matters entering into her system, because of which another emergency surgery had to be conducted on 27.5.2000, which was also not conducted properly and even the surgical wounds were not properly incised and closed. These facts were confirmed by the Doctors in Sri Ramachandra Medical College Hospital, who despite their best efforts could not save the patient because by then the whole system of the patient had collapsed. The State Commission had, therefore, rightly concluded in its well-reasoned order that during the surgery there was a mistake which resulted in the tearing of the colon and subsequent complications which could not be managed and rectified by the appellant and its Doctors.

9. During the pendency of the present first appeal before this Commission, Respondent–Complainant died and his legal representatives were brought on record.

10. We have considered the oral and written submissions made by learned counsels for the appellant and the Respondent–Complainant respectively. Patient's admission in the Appellant hospital with a diagnosis of ovarian cyst and her examination by a Doctor from USA, Dr Samuel Parra, who confirmed the diagnosis and offered to remove the cyst by laparoscopic method, is not in dispute. It is further a fact that following this procedure, complications developed, because of which a second surgery became necessary, during which it was found that body fluids and fecal matters had leaked into the system and also that both ovaries had to be removed and sent to a laboratory for tissue culture. It is further a fact that on the appellant's own advice, patient was shifted to a higher health facility, i.e. Sri Ramachandra Medical College Hospital, where despite her being in the ICCU, she could not be saved. Dr Parra while denying that there was any medical negligence and deficiency in service on appellant's part in conducting the laparoscopy as also the subsequent surgery had also admitted on oath before the State Commission that the laparoscopy equipment was not available in the appellant hospital and had to be obtained from another hospital just 2 days prior to the surgery. It was further admitted by Dr Parra that right from the beginning, there were technical difficulties while conducting the procedure since the insulator needle was not working properly so the umbilical trocar was placed by open technique. Further, there were problems with the suction irrigation system as the "rubber tubing of the suction were collapsing when applying the suction" which was time consuming. Dr Parra has also admitted that on 26.5.2000, there were intra-abdominal infections and there was also possibility of peritonitis, which was not responding to conservative management. Therefore, a second exploratory surgery was conducted, wherein Dr Parra stated that the patient was explored with the finding of a small tear of the sigmoid colon and there was also a residual fluid from the irrigation during the laparoscopy. However, despite stating all these facts, Dr Parra concluded that patient's death was not because of any complications that can arise in such surgeries and was because of pelvic inflammatory disease. We are not able to accept this contention of Dr Parra in view of the fact that he has clearly stated that there were serious technical difficulties while conducting the laparoscopy which confirmed the Respondent–Complainant's contention that the patient was used as a guinea pig. Further, the appellant and Dr Parra were not able to satisfactorily explain the tear in the colon which led to the sepsis and peritonitis, except to say that "a non-fault irreparable damage had occurred". From the evidence of Dr Parra, it is also clear that soon after the surgery, the patient continued to face a number of medical problems and blood was also transfused to her. These facts are confirmed from the medical records of both appellant hospital and Sri Ramachandra Medical College Hospital filed in evidence by the Appellant. The State Commission after considering the evidence on record had, therefore, concluded that there was medical negligence and had specifically stated in Para-9 of its order as follows:

"It is thus clear that during the surgery, there was a mistake done which resulted in the tearing of the colon. We have also noticed that the equipment was also defective. When even according to Dr Parra, the equipment was defective it is a moot question whether Dr Parra and his associate doctors and assistants should have proceeded further and done the operation. Even, according to Dr Parra, there was a concealed non-noticeable injury of the colon that manifested itself in the postoperative course. He had also realized that a non-fault irreparable damage had occurred. In such a situation, the one and only conclusion that could be reached is that there was negligence which resulted in serious complications. The patient had to be shifted to the tertiary for management and of course, things had become unmanageable and ultimately the patient collapsed and died."

11. We are in agreement with the finding of the State Commission that appellant was guilty of medical negligence and deficiency in service right from the beginning in not checking whether the laparoscopy equipment were working, because of which admittedly several problems arose during the laparoscopic procedure, including a tear in the colon. If indeed, the laparoscopy had gone smoothly as contended by appellant, then there would not have been need for a second surgery, which was done to redress the deficiency of the first surgery. Further, doctors in the appellant hospital themselves admitted that they were unable to treat the patient in their hospital, which clearly indicates that by the time she was referred to higher medical facility, her condition was very critical and could not be reversed. Sri Ramachandra Medical College Hospital where she was transferred has also confirmed that the patient's condition at the time of admission was very critical.

12. The principles of what constitutes medical negligence is now well established by a number of judgments of this Commission as also the Hon'ble Supreme Court of

India, including in Indian Medical Association vs. VP Shantha [(1995) 6 SCC 651]. One of the principles is that a medical practitioner is expected to bring a reasonable degree of skill and knowledge and must also exercise a reasonable degree of care and caution in treating a patient (emphasis provided). In the instant case, it is very clear from the facts stated in the foregoing paragraphs that a reasonable degree of care was not taken in the treatment of the patient. This is apparent, as stated earlier, from the fact that even the laparoscopy equipment were not checked before they were used because of which several problems arose with its functioning during the procedure as admitted by the doctor who conducted the procedure. Apart from this, the doctors from the appellant hospital have not been able to explain how the colon tear occurred and why a third surgery may have been necessary because of which even the surgical wounds were not properly sutured. The instant case is a case of res ipsa loquitur where medical negligence is clearly established.

13. We, therefore, agree with the order of the State Commission and uphold the same in toto. The present first appeal is dismissed. Appellant is directed to pay to the Respondent–Complainant a sum of ₹ 500,000/- as compensation together with litigation costs of ₹ 10,000/- within a period of 2 months. No costs.

CASE NO. 6

Another case of bowel injury during laparoscopic surgery.

Smt C Rekha v/s M/s R C P M Hospital & Others

Decided on 16-04-2011 by Kerala SCDRC
Hon Justice KR Udayabhanu and Hon S Chandramohan Nair

Judgment
Shri KR Udayabhanu, President

The complainant has claimed a sum of ₹ 4,824,000/- towards compensation on the ground that the surgery, etc. conducted by the opposite parties 2 to 5, at first opposite Party hospital was vitiated by negligence and lack of adequate care. As per the averments in the complaint, she consulted the 3rd opposite party gynecologist of the hospital in January 2006 on account of continuous back pain. After undergoing ultrasonogram, she was informed the 2nd and 3rd opposite parties/doctors that she is having an ovarian cyst and the same has to be removed by laparoscopic surgery. She was told that it is a minor procedure. The complainant was admitted at the hospital on 28.02.2006. She was taken to the operation theater 01.03.2006 at about 8 am. It is alleged that the procedure was done in a careless and negligent manner. Instead of removing the ovarian cyst, they caused a serious full thickness injury to the rectum, the ascending, mid-transverse and descending colon of the large intestine. On realizing the serious error, they summoned the 5th opposite party/surgeon working in a nearby hospital without the knowledge of complainant's relations and continued the operation. At about the 12.30 pm, the 2nd opposite party summoned the husband of the complainant and informed as to the error occurred and got him sign certain papers. By the evening, it was informed that colostomy was done to the complainant by the 5th opposite party. In the next morning, itself the complainant was removed to the Medical College Hospital (MCH), Trivandrum in an ambulance of the opposite parties and accompanied by the junior doctor of the hospital. It is alleged that the colostomy done was also in a careless manner and resulted in further injury to the internal organs. The doctors of MCH conducted a major operation and removed the injured and infected organs. The distal racial stump was closed and colostomy was refixed. She was discharged on 15.6.2006. On 26.6.2006 she was again admitted and underwent a major operation on 5.7.2006 to remove colostomy. The same was not successful. Another major operation was done on 8.7.2006 and the colostomy was retained. She was told that she will have to continue with the colostomy during the entire life. The complainant was aged 32 years and has passed MSc (Zoology) and BEd She was working as a teacher of +2 course in Sri Narayana Central School, Kayamkulam from 1998 onwards. She has also passed the State Eligibility Test (SET). She was drawing a monthly salary of ₹ 9,000/-. She is married and is having two minor children. On account of the present physical condition, she is unable to lead a normal family life. The complainant has lost her employment and would not be able to do any work with a permanent colostomy bag. She needed treatment forever and assistance even for her daily needs. She has claimed the compensation under various heads ₹ 300,000/- for treatment expenses, loss of income including future income, i.e. ₹ 3,024,000/-, and ₹ 500,000/- for loss of amenities, etc.

2. The opposite parties have failed a joint version. It is stated that the complainant consulted the 3rd opposite party on 3.11.2005 with a request for laparoscopic sterilization. She gave a history of having at her 2nd delivery in 2000 in the hospital. She wanted the procedure to be done in April. On 6.2.2006, she again came to the same doctor with complaints of feeling heaviness in the lower abdomen, frequency of micturition and backache. After taking a detailed history and examination, the 3rd opposite party felt

a cystic mass, on the right side. She was advised an ultrasound scan. It was found as per the ultrasound scan report that the uterus is anteverted, measuring 97 × 51 × 65 mm. Submucosal seedling fibroid was seen in the fundus. Copper-T was seen in the cervical canal. Multiloculated cystic lesion 150 × 90 × 123 mm, possibly arising from left ovary (sic.) was seen. Diagnosis of ovarian cyst was made and she was advised surgery for the same. Her blood sugar test was done the same day, which turned out to be high and she was referred for medical opinion for control of her hyperglycemic state. The patient reported again to 3rd opposite party on 25.2.2006, with a fitness certificate from a physician, for undergoing surgery. Preanesthetic check-up was done by the 4th opposite party and she was posted for surgery on 1.3.2006. The 3rd opposite party discussed in detail the merits and demerits of laparotomy and laparoscopic approach in dealing with her ailment. The patient opted for laparoscopy procedure. She was thus admitted on 28.2.2005 for cystectomy and interval tubal sterilization. Bowel wash and preanesthetic medication were given. She underwent surgery on 1.3.2006 by the 2nd and 3rd opposite party with the 4th opposite party as the anesthetist after taking an informed consent.

3. Since the cyst was large in size, the cystic fluid had to be aspirated out, after which the cyst is to be removed. Hence, while the cyst was being removed, the cyst got ruptured exuding the cystic material into the peritoneal cavity. Since the patient had requested and given consent for sterilization, right salpingo-oophorectomy was done. The sterilization procedure was completed on the left side by application of Fallope rings and cauterization of the left tube. The copper-T was removed from the uterus through the vaginal route. A seedling fibroid was removed from the uterus. After this, the specimen was removed through a colpotomy incision and it was sent for histopathological examination. At that time, rectal injury was suspected. The 5th opposite party an expert surgeon was called in. After examining the patient, he opined laparotomy as the only way to deal with the situation. The condition of the patient was discussed with her husband and some other relatives by the 2nd and 5th opposite parties and consent was obtained for colostomy, if required. On opening the abdomen, it was found that there was a rectal tear, descending colon appeared hemorrhagic with a longitudinal tear, along the tinia. Mucosa of the descending colon and transverse colon were found separated from the seromuscular layer.

4. The patient was shifted to the MCH, Trivandrum on the next day. During shifting two doctors accompanied the patient along with a detailed medical summary. The allegations of the complainant are denied. The 4th opposite party is anesthetist and is in no way associated with the complications that developed. It is contended that the surgery was done with almost care and caution. During colpotomy, a partial injury to the anterior rectal wall occurred. This injury, did not enter into the rectal lumen, but stopped short of the mucosal layer. As there was carbon dioxide in the peritoneal cavity, for pneumoperitoneum the gas could have entered into this layer and effected a pneumatic dissection. Also, with the pulling of the specimen, the dissection of the mucosa, extended to a higher level. As regards tear of the serosal surface of the colon; while the patient was under pneumoperitoneum, there was no tear visible. Once colpotomy was done and the intra-abdominal pressure decreased, the pressure inside the seromuscular tube of the colon, could have resulted in rupture of the tube.

5. It is contended that every care was taken during the surgery. Complications are always unexpected. In the instant case even though all precautions were taken, a known but rare complication, of injury to the neighboring viscera has occurred. It is contended that the claims made are exorbitant and exaggerated. A person who uses a permanent colpotomy bag can lead an otherwise normal life. The opposite parties have sought for dismissal of the complaint with compensatory costs.

6. The evidence adduced consisted of the testimony of PWs 1 & 2, DWs 1 to 4 and exts.A1 to A10, B1, X1(a) and X2.

7. PW1 is the complainant herself and PW2 is the head of the Surgical Gastroenterology Department at Medical College Hospital who conducted the surgeries on the complainant subsequent to her admission at the Medical College Hospital on reference from on the first opposite party hospital. DW1 is the second opposite party gynecologist who is also the proprietor of the first opposite party hospital. It was he who conducted the laparoscopic surgery on the complainant that ended in complications. DW2 is the third opposite party gynecologist who assisted the second opposite party in the laparoscopic surgery. DW3 is the 4th opposite party anesthetist at the first opposite party hospital who induced anesthesia on the complainant. DW4 is the 5th opposite party surgeon working in another hospital who was called in to conduct colostomy on the complainant. DW5 is the Professor and Head of Department of Obstetrics and Gynecology at the Medical College Hospital, Thiruvananthapuram. Ext.

P10 is the discharge card of the complainant from the Medical College Hospital. Ext.X1 is the case sheet of the complainant at Medical College Hospital. Ext.X1 (a) is the referral letter from the first opposite party hospital attached with Ext.X1. Ext.X2 is the case sheet of the complainant from the Medical College Hospital wherein she was again admitted and underwent another surgical procedure. Ext.B1 is the case sheet of the complainant at the first opposite party hospital.

8. It is an admitted case that the complainant was admitted at the first opposite party hospital for cystectomy and internal tubal sterilization through laparoscopic surgery. It is the admitted case of the opposite parties that during the procedure cystectomy was done as well as the salpingo-oophorectomy. The sterilization procedure was completed on the left side by application of Fallope rings and cauterization of the left tube. It is also their case that Copper-T was removed from the uterus through the vaginal route. A seedling fibroid was removed by the uterus. According to the opposite party at that time rectal injury was suspected. The details as mentioned in Ext.X1 (a), the reference letter is as follows:

Ultrasound done multiparous - cyst - small fibroid - displaced copper-T - multiloculated hemorrhagic cyst laparoscopy was done on 1.3.2006/10 mm main port and 3 accessory ports pneumoperitoneum with carbon dioxide—uterus normal in size - left tube and ovary normal - right ovary cystic ruptured while dissection spilling hemorrhage - chocolate material - right salpingo-oophorectomy done - colpotomy done to retrieve the dissected matter on pulling tubular structure coming out. Rectal injury noted— surgeon called in emergency laparotomy done on examination; ascending, mid and descending colon found hemorrhagic—longitudinal tear of the tinea— whole mucosal tube, separated from the muscular layer - rest of the viscera found normal - pneumodissection of the mucosa through the tear - linear tear repaired after putting the mucosal tube inside - colostomy done. The procedure was done at 4.58 pm. According to the complainant at 8 am, she was taken to the operation theater for laparoscopy. Subsequent to the complications, the 5th opposite party surgeon was called in and he performed laparotomy and colostomy. What has been stressed by the counsel for the complainant is that in Ext.B1 case sheet of the first opposite party/hospital, an important factor that has been mentioned in Ext.X1 (a) reference letter has been suppressed. The same is the fact mentioned in Ext. X1 (a) on pulling tubular structure coming out. What

has been stressed is that after putting the colpotomy incision, opposite parties 1 and 2 caused on injury to the large intestine and that what has been pulled out is the mucosal tube which is the inside part of the large intestine instead of the burst remains of the cyst and the right ovary. On resulting the mistake, the 5th opposite party/surgeon was urgently called in and laparotomy was done and the dissected matter from the large intestine was put inside and colostomy was done. The same has caused infection which has further complicated the matters. The very suppression of the words that tubular structure came out on pulling is sufficient to establish negligence on the part of the opposite parties 1 and 2, it is submitted. On the other hand, it is the contention of the counsel for the opposite parties that what is happened is a freak accident, the like of which is not recorded in medical journals. According to the opposite parties, a tear in the rectum was occasioned during the procedure and the same resulted in a tear in the large intestine, and the gas used for the procedure infiltrated into the tear in the large intestine and the pressure resulted in separating the mucosa of the intestine from the rest of the large intestine. As is evident, the above explanation would not explain the words in Ext.X1 (a) reference letter that on pulling tubular structure came out. PW2, the surgeon who attended the complainant at the Medical College Hospital has also explained the relevant notes in Ext.X1 (a). He has stated that it is mentioned in the referral letter that while doing the procedure, the cyst was burst, and when incision was put in the vagina for removing the ovary, a tubular structure came out. PW2/Surgeon of Medical College Hospital removed the damaged portions of the large intestine and did a colostomy. Subsequently, the complainant was again admitted for connecting the large intestine with the remaining portion of the rectum in order to avoid the colostomy. As the rectal portion was very short, the operation was not successful, and hence the colostomy was retained. The fluid collection was also aspirated. Both the above operations were done under general anesthesia. He has also stated that at the time of laparoscopy at the first opposite party hospital, it was on account of the pressure of the gas that the injury of the large intestine happened during the procedure, and the mucosa inside the large intestine separated from the muscular layer. He has specifically stated that during the procedure the large intestine ought not to have been injured. He has also stated that on account of a minor mistake such an injury can take place. He has also stated that the portion of the ovary that has been cut for removing and the portion of the large intestine can be separately identified through the laparoscopic. He has also stated that the complainant will have to live with the colostomy throughout her life. He has also stated in the cross-examination that a rectal injury during such procedure takes place very rarely. On a pointed the question, he has stated that such percentage of mistakes can be 1% and even if experts do the surgery the same can take place. He has denied the suggestion that it would not be possible to detect such an injuries immediately. He has also stated that the injury taken place in the laparoscopic procedure is such that can be detected immediately. He has also stated that after detecting the injury the further treatment carried out was as per the standard procedure. He has also stated that the mucosal tube removed by him could be around 90 cm as suggested. Usually, on account of illness if the mucosal layer is to be removed the maximum length removed, would be 10 cm. He has also stated that in certain persons the vagina and rectum will be adjoining and in such cases when the vagina is opened there is likelihood of rectal injury.

9. DW5, the Head of Department of Gynecology of the Medical College Hospital who was examined at the instance of the opposite parties as an expert. He has stated that while doing colpotomy rarely rectal injuries can take place. He has also stated that even if colpotomy is done correctly while pulling out the tissues sometimes the colpotomy incisions may tear and affect the other organs, especially in the case of ladies who have given birth to more than one child.

10. DWs 1 & 2 are the surgeons who conducted the laparoscopy and the gynecologist who assisted respectively has deposed in support of the averments in the version. According to him, he used to conduct the laparoscopy procedure since 1998. He had worked in the Medical College Hospital earlier. The 5th opposite party/Surgeon is attached to another hospital was summoned in the light of the emergency and he conducted laparotomy as well as colostomy. He has stated that he did the colostomy and the affected portion, i.e. the transverse colon and descending colon were retained for the purpose of joining it later. He has submitted that the tubular structure was put inside and switched. There is no suggestion to DW4 that what he did has resulted in infection as contented by the counsel for the complainant.

11. Another point that has come out the explanation of colpotomy by DW5, the Professor for the Medical College Hospital he has stated that colpotomy is done at posterior fornix which is above the posterior valve of vagina. Incision is put above the posterior valve of the vagina for entry into the peritoneal cavity. Evidently, in the instant case the injury that has taken place is the portion of the vagina which is not at the spot mentioned by PW5. If the incision was put at the posterior fornix of the vagina there is no possibility of a rectal injury. Further, the injury noted in Ext.X1 case sheet of the Medical College Hospital is at sigmoid colon. It is also mentioned that it is a full thickness tear. The serosal tear (longitudinal) of the proximal colon up to mid transverse colon has taken place. The case of the opposite parties is that the right dissected ovary, fallopian tube and the cyst was taken out through the incision also has to be suspected. What has come out while pulling is a tubular structure. It is possible that while pulling the large intestine got further dissected inside. Opposite parties 2 & 3, gynecologists being experts ought not to have committed such a mistake. The complainant has reposed trust in them under the impression that they are experts. Very serious consequences have been ensued on account of the mistake committed by the opposite parties 1 & 2. The above conduct on the part of the opposite parties 1 & 2 cannot be treated as a possible eventuality of such a surgery. Even PW2, the surgeon of the Medical College Hospital who has otherwise deposed as to the possibility of such injuries has stated that such injuries should not have been taken place while performing laparoscopic surgery at the above portion. We find that the above conduct of the opposite parties 2 & 3 amounts to actionable negligence.

12. There is no evidence to show that the 4th opposite party/anesthetist was negligent. Hence, we find that the 4th opposite party is not liable. In the case of the 5th opposite party/surgeon, it is alleged that he conducted the procedure of colostomy in a careless manner and that it is his act of putting back the mucosal tube back inside the large intestine that caused the infection. There is no proper evidence in this regard to substantiate the allegation although the 5th opposite party has admitted that he has placed the mucosa layer inside the intestine. We find that there is no sufficient evidence to indict the 5th opposite party/surgeon as well.

13. So far as the compensation is concerned, the complainant has produced the certificate of date of birth, the copies of the BEd certificate, and the postgraduate degree certificate which would show that she has passed the examinations in first class. She has also produced the certificate of State Eligibility Test.

As per Ext.A9, the certificate of the Principal of the Sri Narayana Central School she is working therein as a teacher of the +2 classes from June 98 to February 2006. The salary is not mentioned therein. According to the complainant, she was getting ₹ 9,000/- per month. There is nothing to discredit the version of PW1, the complainant that she has stopped working and is unable to work as a teacher on account of the fact she has to carry a permanent colostomy bag. She was aged only 32 at the time of undergoing the surgery at the first opposite party hospital. According to her, she is unable to have a proper marital life. We find that in the circumstances there is nothing to disbelieve the evidence to PW1 in this regard.

14. In the circumstances, we find that it would be reasonable to award a sum of ₹ 25,000/- towards the pain and suffering undergone on account of the multiple surgeries and ₹ 50,000/- towards loss of amenities during the treatment as well as in future. A sum of ₹ 30,000/- is awarded towards loss of earning during the period of treatment. A sum of ₹ 20,000/- is awarded towards loss of expectation of life. A sum of ₹ 5 lakhs would be reasonable towards her future loss of earning taking into account the unpredictables as well. A sum of ₹ 50,000/- is awarded towards the treatment expenses including the amount required for future treatment. The complainant will be entitled for 6.75 lakhs altogether. The complainant will also be entitled for interest at 7% per annum from the date of complaint, i.e. 27.12.2006. The complainant will be entitled to cost of ₹ 7,000/-. The opposite parties 1 to 3 would be jointly and severally liable to pay the amount. The amounts are to be paid within 4 months from the date of receipt of this order failing which the complainant will be entitled for interest at 12% on the amount of 6.75 lakhs from 16.4.2011, the date of this order.

■ CASE NO. 7

This is a case done by a laparoscopic surgeon against a vendor supplying laparoscopic instruments for negligence due to supply of faulty set of equipment.

Picker India Ltd. v/s Dr Jamal Ara

Decided on 22-03-2007 by NCDRC
Hon Justice SN Kapoor and Hon BK Tamini

Judgment
BK Tamini, Member

1. Appellant was the opposite party before the State Consumer Disputes Redressal Commission, Orissa (hereinafter referred to as State Commission), where the respondent/complainant had filed a complaint alleging deficiency in service on the part of the appellant.

2. The basic facts leading to filing the complaint, as alleged in complaint, were that the respondent/complainant who is a doctor by profession, decided to purchase a Laparoscopy Set, Type-III, Model 3, from the appellant/opposite party for use in her operation theater to give better service to the patient. Invoice was provided by the Regional Sales Manager Mr Ghosh. The equipment was supplied. But it was the case of the complainant that certain parts such as Silicon Tube, Carbon Dioxide Cylinder and Spatula were never supplied despite having received full payment by the appellant. The complainant approached their Kolkata office but when the complainant's representative reached Kolkata office to find out about the details of supply of these parts, he came empty handed as the appellant's office had shifted its known address to some other place without giving out the new address. In such circumstances, the matter was taken up with the appellant's head office at Delhi requesting for resale the machine and refund the complainant's money with interest as the equipment was not demonstrated within 2 months from the installations and Kolkata office has been closed. It is only on 22.2.1997 that the Regional Kolkata office informed them about the new address in which they also informed that on 10.2.1997 they have sent silicon tube through one Dr Samal of Bhubaneswar. According to the complainant an assurance was given that the appellant's engineer Mr Arijit Ghosh will meet the complainant on 26.2.1997 and give the demonstration of the machine. No one turned up on that date. As per the complainant Mr Ghosh informed her on phone to arrange a patient on whom he will demonstrate. The demonstration was given on 4.4.1997. During the demonstration of the machine CO_2 "insufflator" did not work, causing a great damage and loss of credibility. This CO_2 "insufflator", as advised by Mr. Ghosh, engineer of the appellant company, was sent for replacement on 5.4.1997 which was received by the appellant on 7.4.1997. Till the date of filing the complaint this CO_2 "insufflator" was not replaced. It is in these circumstances, that a complaint was filed praying for taking back the machine and refund the money with interest at 18% per annum along with cost of CO_2 cylinder, color TV and loss of credibility and litigation cost. The matter was contested by the appellant before the State Commission on several grounds. The State Commission, after considering all the grounds and perusal of material on record, allowed the complaint in the following terms:

"In the result, the OP is directed to refund a sum of ₹ 600,000/- along with interest from the date of payment to the O.P. till realization. Besides the OP do pay an amount of ₹ 133,452/- as calculated above. The entire amount be paid within 8 weeks from the date of communication of this order."

3. Later on an application made by the complainant, the State Commission by order dated 6.9.2001 passed the following order:

"Heard Mr Jena, the learned Counsel for the complainant and Mr Paikraythe, the learned Counsel for the OPs. in the matter of correction of the judgment. So far rate of interest is concerned, this has been already mentioned in the original judgment.

The portion, i.e., quotation in page 5 of the judgment be substituted as follows:

"If any antisituation arises in between and you are not able to start by 12 months, we also assured you to resale the equipment at a good price."

Judgment be corrected accordingly. Corrected judgment be supplied to the parties at our cost."

4. Aggrieved by this order this appeal has been filed before us.

5. We heard the learned Counsel for both the parties at considerable length and perused the material on record. It is important to note that this is a second round of litigation. Earlier aggrieved by order on dated 13.11.1997 passed by the State Commission, the appellant had filed an appeal before this Commission and after hearing the parties the matter was remanded back to the State Commission after imposing a cost of ₹ 15,000/- on the appellant. On being remanded and after hearing the parties the impugned order was passed by the State Commission.

6. The learned Counsel for the appellant took four pleas. Firstly, no expert inspection report is on record despite request from the appellant; secondly, after having passed the order, the State Commission could not pass a subsequent order by way of clarification; thirdly that the complainant has shown complete "rigidity" by not allowing inspection of the equipment despite directions of this Commission resulting in the Commission not getting a first-hand report of the status of the machine in order to appreciate the status of the machine and fourthly, there is no allegation on the point of machine being defective.

7. As far as the first plea is concerned, we see on record an application by the appellant made before the State Commission for production of the machine for examination which was opposed and objected to by the respondent/complainant, hence the State Commission by two different, orders decided to pass orders on merit and deal with this point at the time of passing final order. We appreciate that it would have helped the State Commission to arrive at the more realistic conclusion, had the machine been got inspected through an "expert". This is a fact that the State Commission has not passed any order on this point.

8. As far as the second plea is concerned, we see that as per settled law the State Commission could not have entertained the application for clarification and subsequently passed the order but as we see that no damage seemed to have been caused to the appellant which affecting the right of the appellant hence we see no merit in this plea as well.

9. Dealing with the third and fourth pleas together, we find that the complainant's case in the complaint was that certain parts had not been supplied and subsequently when the "insufflator" was supplied, it did not work in view of which the machine was not demonstrated, hence by a letter dated 20.2.1997, the complainant asked for refund of money. But before that, we see that when the equipment was delivered to the respondent/complainant, a certificate dated 18.12.1996, was signed by the complainant as well as by the engineer of the appellant, which reads as under:

"Laparoscopy set delivered, installed and tested found OK."

10. We have no manner of doubt that once this letter of satisfaction and installation has been given/signed on 18.12.1996 by the complainant and further payment of ₹ 550,000/- made on 9.12.1996, we are in no doubt that the total equipment with the parts were delivered and the signature on the installation report as also the payment of the balance amount of ₹ 550,000/- is testimony to this effect. We have seen the affidavits of Mr Arijit Ghosh as also affidavits filed by the complainant as also by Dr Samal as well as their cross-examination. In the worst case scenario, even if we accept that these parts, namely "insufflator", silicon tube, CO_2 cylinder were not supplied with the machine, but when we see the affidavit of the said Mr Ghosh—who has since changed his job and working with a competitor company—even he states in his affidavit that "insufflator" was supplied albeit with some delay. There is no dispute that as per affidavit filed by Dr Samal, silicon tube was brought by him in February, 1997 and given over to the complainant. In the affidavit filed by Jai Singh George, GM (Tech) of the appellant, he clearly states that the "insufflator" supplied to the complainant was found to be having some problem. In early April 1997, it was called back

for replacement after it was found that the "insufflator" is not helping pass the CO_2 for which a replacement was sent only in May, 1997, i.e. after a delay of a month or more thus depriving the complainant the use of the equipment, which again as per the affidavit of the appellant developed some problem in June 1997, upon which the respondent/complainant insisted on returning the entire set. There is no material on record that any replacement or any engineer was sent to remove these defects. There is only a statement on oath by the appellant that they were ready to replace the "insufflator" and asked the respondent to return the same in terms of warranty. No positive action appears to have been taken by the appellant to make the equipment functional by way of repairing or replacing the "insufflator" and demonstrate its functioning at the site, i.e. the premises of the complainant.

11. We also see that admittedly the equipment was having warranty of 1 year. As per the material on record, we also see that an inspection report from the appellant's side dated 17.6.1997, about "insufflator", reads as under:

"insufflator" (LMS 930) is not working since the beginning.

"insufflator" taken back to office and repaired it, tested without gas. But, here with CO_2 gas, it tested and found no gas flow from "insufflator". The total set is not used. No surgeons are ready to operate by this set. So, customer is in trouble.

....

Re-service status—not working.........

Customer is not willing to use this set. She wants to return it back."

12. Chronologically, if we see even according to the appellant the first time "insufflator" went "bad" in early April 1997, which was sent to the appellant and they took almost one and a half months to replace it with a new one. There is no dispute that without the "insufflator" the equipment cannot be put to any gainful use, thus, depriving the user/buyer of the benefit of the costly equipment. This is also not in dispute that as per the affidavit of GM (Tech) of the appellant, the "insufflator" again developed defects in June 1997, which is borne by the report of 17.6.1997 reproduced earlier. This is a costly equipment and perhaps could be damaged in transit. In our view, it was the responsibility of the appellant to have sent service engineer to collect the equipment and then send it back after repairs or supply a new one by way of replacement, and test/demonstrate the equipment on the site. This is the least which can be expected

from a seller of sensitive and sophisticated equipment. On our record, there is nothing to show that any effort was made by the appellant to repair or replace the "insufflator" and make it work on the site. What was expected was that the complainant will send the defective equipment to the appellant, which we are unable to accept. Chronology and history of working of "insufflator" leaves much to be deserved on the part of the appellant. When a person buys costly equipment he or she does not buy a headache. Undisputedly the complainant is in Orissa and the appellant is in Kolkata. It is also not in dispute that the appellant has Service Engineers. Frequent breakdown of insufflator within 6 to 7 months of the purchase of the equipment and non-replacing it or demonstrating its functioning properly at the premises of the complainant is a clear case of deficiency in service on the part of the appellant. The plea of the appellant that the complainant was not qualified or adept at handling the equipment, does not wash with us. We have seen the affidavit and cross-examination of the complainant. In our view, the appellant has failed to prove the allegation with the help of any material on record. There is no dispute that all these activities were within the warranty period. Delayed supply, in the first instance, delayed replacement, in May/June 1997 and again non-replacement of "insufflator" after June 1997 has resulted in depriving the respondent/complainant use of the equipment worth ₹ 6 lakhs.

13. On the other hand, we also see there are mitigating circumstances, in favor of the appellant. Firstly, there is his written application filed before the State Commission for production of machine so that the truth could come out but it was opposed by the complainant on account of reasons best known to her. We are constrained to derive adverse inference from this fact.

14. Vide our order dated 20.4.2004, we passed the following order:

"Learned Counsel for the appellant states that appellant would send expert from Delhi to examine whether the machine, which was purchased by the complainant, can be made workable. He further states that the expert would report the defects, if there are any, in the said machine and report the same to this Court. Learned Counsel for the respondent states that respondent would fully cooperate in inspection of the said machine or making the same in workable condition. Learned Counsel for the appellant states that expert would visit the premises of the complainant where the machine is lying either on 7th or 8th May

2004. For this purpose prior telephonic information would be given to respondent."

To which the follow-up action is summarized vide our order dated 21.5.2004, which reads as under: "Learned Counsel for the appellant submitted that the expert who was sent by them to inspect the machine was not permitted to inspect the machine except allowing him to see it from a distance. Learned Counsel for the appellant has submitted an application for direction. Learned Counsel for the respondent seeks time to file the reply.

List for disposal of the application and for arguments on 7.10.2004 before the Bench presided over by the Hon'ble President of this Commission."

15. The above series of actions on the part of the complainant lead us to conclude that they were not ready to cooperate. In the aforementioned circumstances, while equipment supplied had developed defect within the warranty period and taking almost a month and a half for replacement and that too, not found working within a short span, reflects upon the quality of the material supplied, which in our view, was not up to the mark because we cannot accept that any good equipment can develop defects within a short time. This happened not once but twice within a period of 6 months of its installation and then lack of effort on the part of the appellant to send their own engineer to repair or to transport for replacement, is a clear case of deficiency in service on the part of the appellant as far as the question of "insufflator" is concerned.

16. We see that the order passed by the State Commission is entirely based on non-supply of the three parts mentioned earlier, which in our view, is belied by the "certificate" given by the complainant on the point of delivery installation and test, and the equipment was found to be OK and secondly at best it could be said that "insufflator" was supplied albeit with some delay and when it was found to be not working in April 1997, replacement was also sent, with which the equipment started functioning but it again developed some defects in June 1997. As already mentioned silicon tube was carried in the month of February 1997 by Dr Samal and delivered to the complainant. The entire order of the State Commission which is based on non-supply of these items, does not stand the scrutiny as per material on record, in view of which, it cannot be sustained.

17. As discussed in earlier part of the order, while holding the appellant deficient in rendering service limited to non-repair/non-supply of workable "insufflator" to the complainant, depriving her of the use of the equipment and in view of the mitigating circumstances enumerated earlier, we are not inclined to order refund of whole amount at which machine was purchased. As per the quotation on record, the digital "insufflator" is priced at ₹ 188,843/-, to which, in our view, the complainant is entitled. Hence, the appellant is directed to pay ₹ 188,843/- being the cost of the "insufflator" along with interest at 10% per annum from the date of filing of the complaint till the date of payment and the respondent/complainant shall return the "insufflator" lying with her after receiving the awarded amount. The respondent/complainant is also entitled to compensation which we fix at ₹ 50,000/- in view of the fact that the complainant was deprived of use of equipment for a long period.

18. All the above payments be made by the appellant to the respondent/complainant within 6 weeks from the date of passing of this order failing which the complainant shall be at liberty to proceed against the appellant under sections 25/27 of the Consumer Protection Act, 1986.

Appeal dismissed.

Section 6

HYSTEROSCOPY

- Instrumentation in Hysteroscopy
- Hysteroscopic Septum Resection
- Office Hysteroscopy
- Hysteroscopic Cannulation of Proximal Tubal Block
- Hysteroscopic Myomectomy
- Complications in Hysteroscopic Surgery—Prevention and Management

"I did then what I knew how to do. Now that I know better, I do better."

Maya Angelou

CHAPTER 20

Instrumentation in Hysteroscopy

Meenu Agarwal

"Hysteroscope is no more an exclusive toy in the hands of few endoscopic surgeons."

INTRODUCTION

Hysteroscopy was one of the very first endoscopic procedures performed to look into the uterine cavity with a candle as the light source. Hence, it is rather strange that hysteroscopy had to wait for the innovations in other endoscopic procedures before its present status of an important armamentarium of a gynecological setup.

The major hindrance was the difficulty faced for the distention of the uterine cavity and the friable nature of endometrium causing bloody field and difficulty in vision.

Modern hysteroscopy represents 200 years of innovative ideas that put into practice in the form of instrumentation, techniques and clinical applications. We need to pay our deepest gratitude to the scientists who have made safe hysteroscopy possible by their continuous work on illumination, uterine distention and instrumentation.

Philip Bozzini (1773–1809) was a German doctor who designed an instrument which could reflect external light for visualization of body cavities. He called this device a "Lichtleiter, or Light Conductor". It was a constructed of a hollow tube divided by a partition septum and had various attachments. This hollow tube was fitted with a concave mirror and a candle light was used as the light source. He is rightfully considered today as the father of endoscopy.

The Bozzini Lichleiter is displayed at American College of Surgeons in Chicago (Table 1).

As seen from this table ever since the beginning of 1980, hysteroscopy has taken a quantum leap and has revealed the limitation of the blind dilatation and curettage. Now we have understood the superiority of a diagnostic hysteroscopy over cervical dilatation and curettage and that of a visual biopsy over fractional curettage.

The improvement in the optics, particularly in fused fiber bundle systems, mini hysteroscopes with 2–3 mm diameter, have changed the marketing strategies from focusing to endoscopic surgeons to a routine use by general gynecologists.

ROOM SETUP

As with all endoscopic procedures, surgical dexterity plays a major role. It is important to have the screen in front of the surgeon while doing the hysteroscopy, be it diagnostic or operative (Fig. 1).

For a right handed surgeon, the screen should be between the left shoulder and the left leg of the patient. Make sure that the surgeon's head is always between his two hands while looking at the screen; this will ease the procedure and also avoid neck muscle strain for the surgeon.

Table 1: The milestones in the development of hysteroscopy

Year	Contributor	Findings
1807	Bozzini	First endoscope (the "light conductor")
1869	Pantaleoni	First hysteroscopic examination in a living patient
1914	Heineberg	System for irrigating the uterine cavity
1925	Rubin	CO_2 for uterine distention
1926	Seymour	Hysteroscope with in-flow and out-flow channels
1928	Gauss	Intrauterine photography
1934	Schroeder	Measurement of intrauterine pressures
1934–43	Segond	Irrigation systems and biopsies
1942–70	Norment	Rubber balloon: practical irrigation system
1957	Englund et al.	Evaluation of abnormal uterine bleeding
1968	Menken	Tubal cannulation
1974	Parent et al.	Contact hysteroscopy
1978	Neuwirth	Use of resectoscope
1980	Hamou	Microhysteroscope
1996	Stephano Bettochi	Office operative hysteroscope

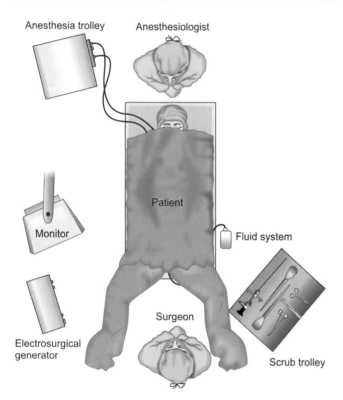

Fig. 1: Room setup

SYSTEMS USED FOR THE FLOW RATE AND IRRIGATION PRESSURE

Although hysteroscopy was described by Lindeman as early as in 1880, when he used a candle light to look into the uterine cavity in a postmenopausal woman and diagnosed a uterine polyp, it remained a challenge as the uterine potential space and its distention were difficult to attain and sustain. The endometrial cavity is a virtual space that is only distended in pathological situations. Under normal circumstances, the uterine walls are in close opposition to one another. To achieve panoramic view of the uterus, the walls must be forcibly separated. The thick muscle of uterine walls requires a minimum pressure of 40 mm Hg to distend the cavity sufficiently to see with a hysteroscope.

Various systems commonly used to control flow rate and irrigation pressure are:

A. Gravity fall of liquid: The bag is suspended at a suitable height on an IV stand about 100 cm above from the patient which would give a pressure of about 70 mm Hg. The outlet tubing is left in a bucket.

B. Pressure cuff: This device is based on BP sphygmomanometer. The normal saline bottle is placed in the cuff. The cuff has a measurement meter exactly like the BP sphygmomanometer. The pressure is obtained by inflating the pressure cuff and must be kept around 30 mm Hg. It must be understood that the progressive emptying of the bottle will give an inner effective pressure. A transurethral resection (TUR) cannula and two bottles of normal saline, preferably with two pressure cuffs should be used, so that as soon as one is getting over, the irrigation can be shifted to the second bottle, without compromising on the vision and speed of the procedure (Fig. 2).

C. Air insufflations: It probably is an indigenous system developed by individual surgeons (Fig. 3).

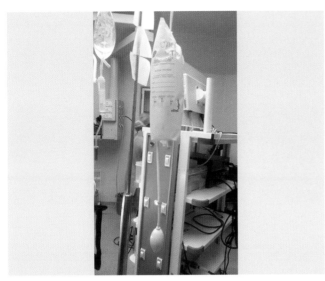

Fig. 2: Pressure cuff to control flow rate and irrigation pressure

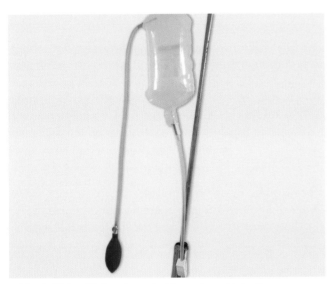

Fig. 3: Air insufflations to control flow rate and irrigation pressure

Herein air pressure is created about the fluid level which pushes the fluid with force into the uterine cavity.

Drawback: There is no monitoring of the effective IV pressure and if used for resection of myoma, it can suddenly push a lot of fluid within seconds and put the patient in fluid and electrolytic imbalance suddenly before the surgeon realizes. Also if the venous channels are open and the fluid gets over with only air getting pushed inside, there is a risk of life threatening air embolism.

D. Electronic suction and irrigation pump: This is the most important equipment for a hysteroscopy setup for optimal visualization and reducing the complications. There is an automatic control of irrigation and suction pressure to give a constant distention of the uterine

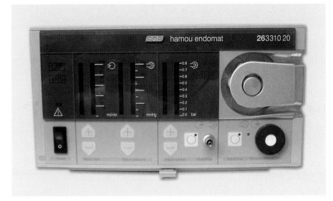

Fig. 4: Electronic suction and irrigation pump (Endomat; Karl Storz GmbH & Co.)

cavity and a clear vision throughout the surgical procedure. We use Storz Hysteromat which is an intelligent pump to maintain intrauterine pressure. It has a pressure controlled double roller pump which along with maintaining a constant preset intrauterine pressure also ensures good dilatation of the uterine cavity with a clear view during hysteroscopic procedures at any time.

The uterine cavity distension pressure should be the lowest pressure necessary to distend the uterine cavity and ideally should be maintained below the mean arterial pressure (MAP). Normally the settings are kept at 75 mm Hg inflow and 0.25 bar suction and a flow rate of 200 mL/min, but for myoma resection the intrauterine pressures are kept lower as the myoma pops out in lower intrauterine pressures (Fig. 4).

■ COLD LIGHT SOURCE

As in any other endoscopic surgery, the technical specifications of cold light source have a major impact on the image quality. A good quality light source with a xenon lamp will give good illumination. Light is transmitted though fiberoptic or a fluid light cables with a diameter of 3.5–5 mm and a length of 180–350 cm for standard hysteroscopy procedure. Cold light cables with a diameter of 5 mm and a length of 180 cm are most commonly used. A 175 watt source is sufficient for routine procedures whereas 300 watt source is recommended for office hysteroscopy.

■ IMAGING SYSTEM

Different types of video cameras are available. The image quality depends on:
1. Resolution (number of lines or pixels)
2. Sensitivity (Lux)

A high signal to noise ratio indicates that the vision will not be impaired if there is bleeding in the uterine cavity. Modern high definition (HD) camera offers very high resolution and almost natural color inside the uterine cavity. HD camera has proved to be really superior to the earlier innovations in the camera systems and has improved the vision greatly.

Complete systems with video-recorders are also available but they are expensive, so separate recorder software on a computer can be used which can act as a second screen in budgeted settings.

TELESCOPES

The hysteroscopes are available in various diameters 1 mm, 2 mm, 2.9 mm (Bettochi) and 4 mm (standard). There are different viewing angles 0°, 12° and 30°. A 30° forward oblique telescope is ideal for diagnostic purpose, and a 12° telescope probably would be ideal for resectoscope which requires the loop electrode in the field of vision all the time. For all practical purposes, a 2.9 mm (Bettochi) (Fig. 5)and a 4 mm (standard and resectoscope) telescope with 30° forward oblique angle would suffice for a complete hysteroscopic setup, although many other combinations are possible depending upon personal preference.

OFFICE HYSTEROSCOPY

❑ Bettochi hysteroscope (2.9 mm) (Stephano Bettochi)
❑ Trophyscope (2 mm) (the CAMPO compact hysteroscope)
❑ Bettochi integrated office hysteroscope (BIOH)

Bettochi hysteroscope (2.9 mm) can be used with a single flow operating sheath (4.3 mm) in combination with an outer sheath (5 mm) as a continuous flow operating system. It has an oval shaped design which perfectly fits the anatomy of the cervical canal of 4 mm opening diameter. Now Bettochi integrated office hysteroscope is also available which is a more compact system fitted with a fiberoptic light connection and inflow and outflow connectors.

Trophyscope (2 mm) has a diameter of 2.9 mm and can be loaded with an operating sheath of 4.4 mm. The trophyscope designed by Rudy Campo has an outer diameter of only 2.9 mm. As a rule no cervical dilatation is required. Light transmission is also enhanced by adding more optical fibers to get good image quality even with a smaller diameter. An innovative feature of this system is additional outer sheath in active and passive position. Two

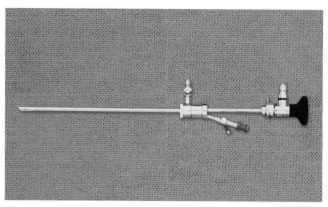

Fig. 5: Bettochi hysteroscope

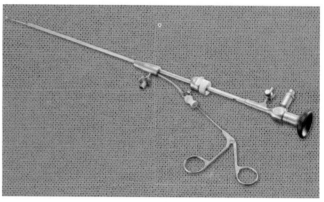

Fig. 6: Trophyscope

types of outer sheaths are available: one for continuous flow and second with a 5-french operative working channel. For the diagnostic procedure, the outer sheath is in passive position but can be advanced distally into active position. With a simple push of the button and distal movement, the cervix is gently dilated with the help of the outer sheath. The sliding mechanism makes it possible to use the sheath without having to remove the hysteroscope.

The trophyscope is particularly useful in infertility patients, nulliparous women as well as evaluation of postmenopausal patients (Fig. 6).

Bettochi integrated office hysteroscope: BIOH is fitted with a handle compatible for use with the Bettochi system and consists of operating sheath, fiberoptic light connector and connectors for irrigation and suction all fitted into the handle directly making it an easy assembly and it allows the surgeon a faster approach to the procedure especially in an outpatient setting. It has a small diameter of 4 mm and has an oval sheath. The telescope is integrated into the inner sheath. Both single and continuous flow applications are available (Fig. 7).

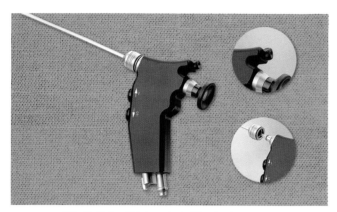

Fig. 7: Bettochi integrated office hysteroscope

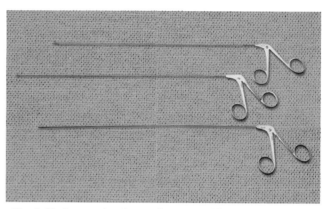

Fig. 9: Hysteroscopic scissors, Grasper and Punch biopsy forceps

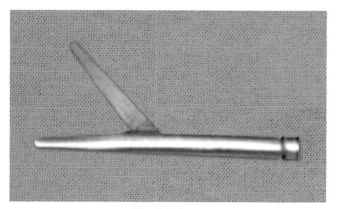

Fig. 8: Scissor

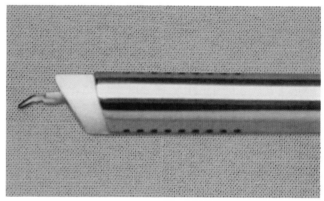

Fig. 10: Resectoscope loop assembled with the hysteroscope

MECHANICAL INSTRUMENTS

Most of the operative hysteroscopic instruments have a semi-rigid design and a diameter of 1.67 mm (5 french).

☐ **Scissors:** These scissors have one fixed and the other movable jaw. It is a good idea to rest the immovable scissor jaw on the tissue and cut the tissue in-between with the movable jaw. The scissors' jaws tend to go out of alignment after a few cases due to their fine delicate design and are generally not repairable and have to be replaced with a new pair of scissors (Fig. 8).

☐ **Alligator grasping forceps:** These forceps are helpful for remaining small polyps, foreign body, intrauterine contraceptive device (IUCD) and endometrial biopsies.

☐ **Spoon biopsy forceps:** Excellent for remaining small polyps and can be used for taking endometrial biopsy and can get a substantial tissue for biopsy.

☐ **Punch biopsy forceps**: For resistant tissue biopsies like from atrophic endometrium for myometrial biopsy (Fig. 9).

☐ A pediatric sponge holder can come handy to remove small polyps or fibroids which have been cut at the base with scissors and are too big to be taken out with the help of hysteroscopic graspers. The pediatric sponge holder is used like ovum forceps to hold the specimen blindly and take it out.

ELECTRICAL INSTRUMENTS

☐ Monopolar needle electrode
☐ Bipolar needle electrode
☐ Monopolar retracting loop for polypectomy
☐ Resectoscope.

The resectoscope consists of a classic endoscope, with diameters ranging between 2.9 mm and 4 mm—preferably with a 12-degree viewing angle to keep the electrode within the field of view—combined with a cutting loop operated by a passive spring mechanism, and two sheaths for continuous irrigation and suction of the distension medium. Apart from the cutting loop, other instruments, such as Collin's knife and a variety of vaporizing or coagulating electrodes, can be used with the working element of the resectoscope. All these instruments are available for both the 22-Fr and the 26-Fr resectoscope (Fig. 10).

☐ Hysteroscope with diameter ranging from 2.9 mm to 4.0 mm with a 30° angular view (although 12° is preferable for resectoscope to keep the cutting loop within the field of view all times, though it is not feasible to have too may telescopes).

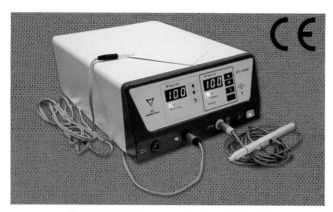

Fig. 11: High frequency electrosurgical unit

❑ Cutting loop operated by passive spring mechanism.
❑ Two sheaths of continuous irrigation and suction of the distention media.

Resectoscope can be used with bipolar and monopolar current. It is important to note that you can use the same resectoscope for monopolar or bipolar technique by changing the working element and the electrode with the respective media which will be normal saline for bipolar and glycine for monopolar current. It is a good idea to have the staff/self check and assemble the resectoscope before starting the case.

HIGH FREQUENCY ELECTROSURGICAL UNITS

Modern high frequency (HF) electrosurgical units can be operated both in monopolar and bipolar mode (Fig. 11). In monopolar mode, the electrodes from the HF electrosurgical units pass through the cutting loop of the resectoscope before passing through the body tissues to the neutral electrode and then returning to the electrosurgical unit. So the body tissue between the neutral electrode (body plate) and the resectoscope becomes a path for the current causing a theoretical risk for electrical burns.

In the bipolar system, the electrical arc is formed the loop itself and is passed through the tissues only between the two ends of the loop and hence it is safer.

ADVANTAGES OF BIPOLAR ENERGIES OVER MONOPOLAR

Electrolytic solutions include normal saline and Ringer lactate.

Current recommendation is to use the electrolytic fluids in diagnostic cases, and in operative cases in which mechanical, laser or bipolar energy is used. Since they conduct electricity, these fluids should not be used with monopolar electrosurgical devices.

Non-electrolytic fluids eliminate problems with electrical conductivity, but can increase the risk of hyponatremia. These solutions include glycine, glucose, dextran, mannitol, sorbitol and a mannitol/sorbitol mixture. Each of these distention fluids is associated with unique physiological changes that should be considered when selecting a distension fluid.

Glucose is contraindicated in patients with glucose intolerance.

High-viscous dextran also has potential complications which can be physiological and mechanical. It may crystallize on instruments and obstruct the valves and channels. Coagulation abnormalities and adult respiratory distress syndrome (ARDS) have been reported.

Glycine metabolizes into ammonia and can cross the blood brain barrier, causing agitation, vomiting and coma. Although it is most commonly used, all the safety precautions need to be exercised while using this distension media.

When fluids are used to distend the cavity, care should be taken to record its use (inflow and outflow) to prevent fluid overload and intoxication of the patient. Normal saline should be used wherever possible for operative hysteroscopic surgery to reduce the risk of hyponatremia and hypoosmolarity. Normal saline should be used for distention during operative hysteroscopic procedures not requiring the use of monopolar electrosurgical instruments.

The surgical team should be prepared to accurately monitor distending fluid medium input and output, including all three potential sources: (1) return from the hysteroscope, (2) spill from the vagina and (3) loss to the floor.

MAINTENANCE AND STERILIZATION OF INSTRUMENTS

The hysteroscope can carry vaginal infection to the uterine cavity. Hysteroscopy should be preceded by proper disinfection of the vagina. Along with the cleaning of the vagina, proper sterilization of equipment is equally important.

In case of office hysteroscopy, the vaginoscopy performed with normal saline at the beginning of the procedure gives a normal saline wash to the vagina and cervix so an intense vaginal cleaning can be avoided.

After the completion of procedure, the hysteroscopic set should be disassembled and each part should be washed with water and detergent. Soft brushes and syringes should be used to flush the lumen and the narrow parts. An orthodontic brush can be used to clean stubborn stains.

If tap water is used, the rinse should be followed by 70% alcohol washing as the tap water may inoculate the inside lumen of channels with water borne microorganisms. After this the instruments should be kept on a clean and dry surface.

Glutaraldehyde (2%): For sterilization, 2% glutaraldehyde is approved as an effective agent against all vegetative bacteria, fungi and microorganisms. Before use, the clean and dried instrument should be soaked for 20 minutes in the solution. It is removed and washed with distilled water before use.

Saline is not recommended with metallic pieces as it has got ionizing properties that can cause rusting and pitting of equipment.

Ethylene oxide sterilization (ETO): This takes approximately 8–12 hours. The instrument should be completely dried before this treatment.

Autoclave sterilization is the cheapest system, and owing to the diffusion of steam, it cleans even the smallest gaps and openings. Only the instruments which are specifically certified for the autoclave may be sterilized with a 20-minute cycle at 121°C or 7 minutes at 134°C (Fig. 12).

Autoclave sterilization of the telescope can be hazardous, so should be done by self or by trained staff. The endoscopes require certain special steps—they must be placed in a perforated metal container, wrapped in suitable gauze. It is better to allow natural cooling in order to prevent damage to the shafts. Special care must be taken while cleaning the lenses and scopes. They can be cleaned with warm water or 90% alcohol and then dried with cotton balls. Look through the scope to look for any spots or blurred vision. This can

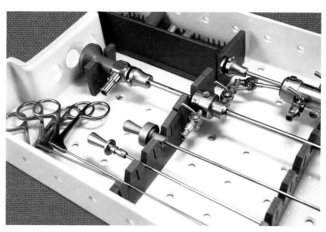

Fig. 12: Autoclave sterilization

be removed by cleaning the lens with 90% alcohol. If the problem persists after repeated cleaning, please check for any damage to the lens.

At the end of the surgery, the fiberoptic cables should always be arranged in large loops to avoid twisting the bundles of fibers. The cables can be cleaned with alcohol or spirit before the procedure.

FUTURE OF HYSTEROSCOPIC INSTRUMENTATION

What we see today must have been the future dream of hysteroscopic surgeons 200 years ago. The future probably would be simplification of instrumentation, better distension equipment, safer and easier delivery of electrocautery, bipolar energy will become the order of the day and perhaps, if the morcellation controversy gets us there, we would be using hysteroscopic morcellators routinely.

CHAPTER 21

Hysteroscopic Septum Resection

Madhuri Kashyap

INTRODUCTION

Uterine septum is the most common Müllerian anomaly and one which is easily correctable. Hysteroscopic septum resection or metroplasty is a common and rewarding surgery in terms of achieving a full term pregnancy.

EMBRYOLOGICAL ANTECEDENTS OF THE SEPTUM

The uterus develops by the midline fusion of the two paramesonephric ducts (Müllerian ducts), which is completed by 12 weeks of intrauterine life. The medial walls of both ducts fuse to form the intrauterine septum. This septum gets absorbed in a caudal to cranial fashion and results in a single cavity at the end of 20 weeks. Partial or complete failure of resorption leads to persistence of a partial or complete septum (Fig. 1).

American Fertility Society Classification of Müllerian Duct Anomalies[1] [American Society of Reproductive Medicine (ASRM)] (Fig. 2).

The prevalence of uterine malformation is about 6.7% in the general population, slightly higher at 7.3% in infertile women and significantly higher in women with a history of recurrent miscarriages at 16%.[2]

SPECTRUM OF REABSORPTION FAILURE

❑ Arcuate/subseptate uterus 7%: Class VI. Refers to a slight midline septum

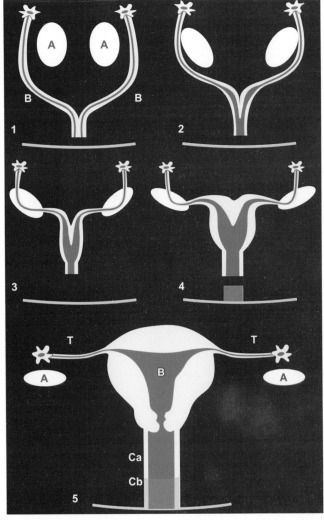

Fig.1: Scheme showing the embryological development and sequence (1–4) of Müllerian ducts fusion (B), (A) indicates the ovaries. Number 4 demonstrates the formation of the uterine body after fusion

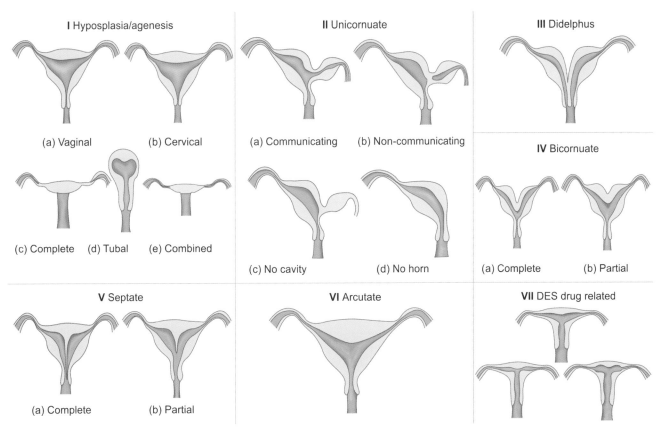

Fig. 2: Classification of uterine malformations according to the American Fertility Society

❑ Septate uterus 35–55%: Class V (Fig. 3). Most common Müllerian anomaly. It is of two types:
1. Complete: Any septum reaching up to the internal os.
2. Partial: Any septum short of the internal os.

The septum may extend further down into the cervix and vagina.

Because of the close embryologic relationship of the Müllerian structures to the mesonephric ducts, when Müllerian anomalies occur, renal anomalies should be ruled out.

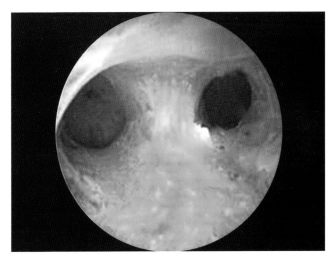

Fig. 3: Septate uterus

ROLE OF THE SEPTUM IN INFERTILITY AND REPEATED PREGNANCY LOSSES AND INDICATIONS FOR TREATMENT

The relationship between the septate uterus and infertility remains controversial. However the recent consensus is to treat the septum prophylactically in cases of primary infertility, especially if it is long standing or if the patient is to undergo sophisticated assisted reproductive technology (ART) procedures.

On the other hand there is a uniform consensus that the septum increases pregnancy wastage with abortion rates varying from 26% to as high as 94%. In patients with recurrent pregnancy losses, the septate uterus was the most common anatomical problem.

Pregnancy losses are attributed to two reasons:
1. Implantation on the septum which is relatively avascular and fibrotic, deprives the blastocyst of sufficient nutrients due to poor placentation and it is eventually aborted.

2. Space restriction for the growing fetus due to the septum.

CLINICAL PRESENTATION

❑ May go unnoticed since full term pregnancies are known
❑ Infertility
❑ Spontaneous abortion
❑ Preterm labor
❑ Malpositions
❑ Intrauterine growth restriction (IUGR).

CLINICAL EXAMINATION

It is important to differentiate a cervical septum from a double or dicollis cervix. On speculum examination, the double cervix has an hourglass appearance, whereas a septate cervix shows a normal contour with a septum. Sometimes, there may also be a vaginal septum where again duplication anomalies must be ruled out.

DIAGNOSTIC MODALITIES

The uterine septum has to be differentiated from a bicornuate uterus which has two uterine horns, i.e. two cavities while a septate uterus has a single uterine body with a single but divided cavity. Most diagnostic modalities aim to differentiate between these two conditions since the management of both differs greatly.

Hysterosalpingography

Before the advent of newer imaging modalities, hysterosalpingography (HSG) was used to detect uterine anomalies. It cannot however differentiate between a uterine septum and a bicornuate uterus. Also it may miss small septa. Hence newer imaging techniques are now preferred. However, it still has a place in infertility evaluation when an unsuspected uterine anomaly may be detected and tubal patency assessed simultaneously. Also it is a comparatively cheaper and simple test (Figs 4 to 6).

2D Ultrasound

The uterine morphology is best evaluated in the luteal phase because the thick, echoic secretory endometrium has a better contrast with the adjoining myometrium. 2D ultrasound or ultrasonography (USG) is a simple and minimally invasive test which can detect many uterine

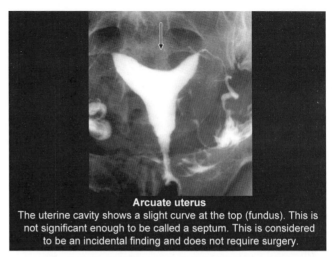
Arcuate uterus
The uterine cavity shows a slight curve at the top (fundus). This is not significant enough to be called a septum. This is considered to be an incidental finding and does not require surgery.

Fig. 4: Hysterosalpingograhy image of arcuate uterus

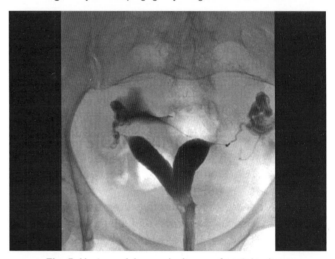
Fig. 5: Hysterosalpingograhy image of septate uterus

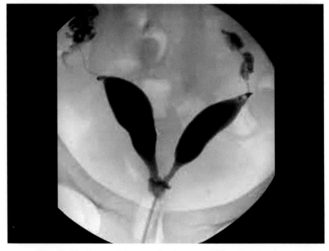
Fig. 6: Hysterosalpingograhy image of bicornuate uterus

anomalies. A better evaluation with 2D USG can be achieved by combining the abdominal and transvaginal approaches which better assess the fundus and cervical regions respectively. However, unicornuate uterus can be missed and it is difficult to distinguish between septate and bicornuate uterus. The coronal view is the best one for diagnosing the type of anomaly, a view that is difficult to obtain with 2D USG. Hence, a suspicion of a uterine anomaly on 2D USG can be accurately differentiated on 3D USG which gives excellent coronal plane images. Recently saline infusion sonohysterography has also been used to diagnose Müllerian anomalies with a high sensitivity of 98% and specificity of 100%.

3D Ultrasound

This is an excellent tool to diagnose and differentiate a septate uterus from a bicornuate or didelphic uterus and is better than 2D USG, HSG and hysteroscopy and equivalent to magnetic resonance imaging (MRI) in diagnostic accuracy for Müllerian anomalies.[3]

To distinguish bicornuate from septate uteri using 3D imaging, a line is traced joining both horns of the uterine cavity at the level of the ostia. If this line crosses the fundus (Fig. 7A) or is 5 mm or less from it (Fig. 7B), the uterus is considered bicornuate; if it is more than 5 mm from the fundus (Fig. 7C) it is considered septate, regardless of whether the fundus is dome-shaped, smooth or discretely notched.[3,4] The fundus also appears broader in the septate uterus and indented in bicornuate and didelphic uterus.

3D ultrasound can also differentiate between a septate and a bicornuate uterus when the fundal contour is normal.

Comparison between the ESHRE-ESGE and the ASRM criteria for diagnosis of a septate uterus on 3D USG.

The European Society of Human Reproduction and Embryology-The European Society for Gynaecological Endoscopy (ESHRE-ESGE) and ASRM have suggested guidelines for differentiating between the septate and bicornuate uterus, based on the internal fundal indentation.

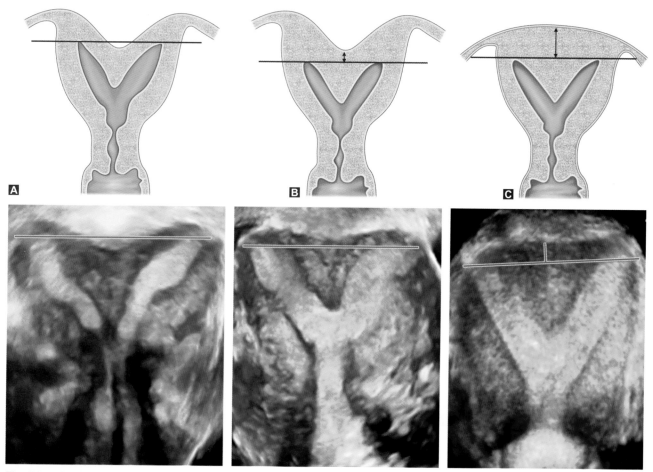

Figs 7A to C: To distinguish bicornuate uteri from septate uteri with three-dimensional ultrasound we can use the formula proposed by Troiano and McCarthy[5]—(A and B) A line is traced joining both horns of the uterine cavity. If this line crosses the fundus or is ≤5 mm from it, the uterus is considered bicornuate; (C) If it is >5 mm from the fundus it is considered septate, regardless of whether the fundus is dome-shaped, smooth or discretely notched

The ASRM diagnosis of septate uterus was confirmed if the depth of the external fundal indentation was less than 1 cm and the internal fundal indentation was more than 1.5 cm. The indentations were measured after obtaining a coronal view with visible intramural parts of both fallopian tubes. Internal fundal indentations more than 50% of the uterine wall thickness were diagnosed as septate uterus by ESHRE-ESGE criteria.

Though the diagnosis of septate uterus by both classifications showed moderate agreement, septate uterus was diagnosed with a significantly higher frequency (almost three times) by the ESHRE-ESGE classification. The morphology of septa differed between the ESHRE-ESGE and ASRM criteria. The use of uterine wall thickness to define uterine deformity is a serious shortcoming of the ESHRE-ESGE classification. Most diagnosis of septa by the ESHRE-ESGE corresponded to an arcuate or normal uterus diagnosed by the ASRM.

Thus, there is a serious risk of overdiagnosis and over-treatment of septate uterus associated with the ESHRE-ESGE criteria. Therefore, the ESHRE-ESGE criteria should not be used to diagnose septate uterus and deem the patient eligible for hysteroscopic resection if the uterus is classified as normal by ASRM.[6]

In arcuate uterus, the fundal indentation appears as an obtuse angle at the central point less than 1.5 cm deep (Fig. 8A), while a septate uterus has an acute angle fundal indentation with a depth of 1.5 cm or more (Fig. 8B).[4]

3D ultrasound can measure the dimensions of the septum and assess its vascularity thus allowing prediction of the degree of difficulty that will be met during hysteroscopic metroplasty. It has a high accuracy of 99–100% in diagnosing and differentiating uterine septum from other types of Müllerian anomalies with corresponding high sensitivity and specificity. A study in Egypt in 2014 done to assess whether 3D USG can replace traditional hysteroscopy and laparoscopy and MRI in the accurate diagnosis of a septate uterus reveals that 3D ultrasound can differentiate between a septate, arcuate and bicornuate uterus with great accuracy with a 100% sensitivity and specificity and absolute concordance between 3D USG and the gold standard laparoscopic and hysteroscopic evaluation. The study further recommends that hysteroscopic septum resection may be done safely without the need for invasive laparoscopic confirmation of a septum, depending solely on 3D USG.[4]

Figures 9 to 11 show superior 3D images of the septate uterus with digital subtraction techniques.[7]

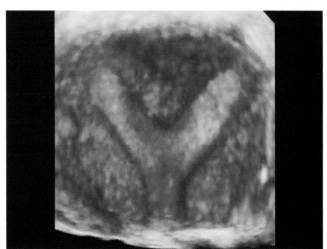

Fig. 9: Coronal view of a septate uterus on 3D volumetric ultrasound. Observe the secretory pattern of the endometrium

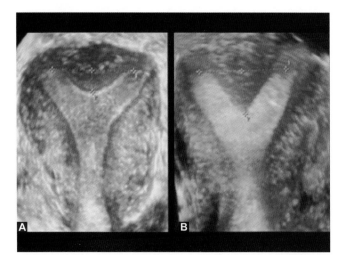

Figs 8A and B: (A) Three-dimensional surface rendered ultrasound image (coronal view) showing the normal outer uterine contour of a uterus that was identified as arcuate (rather than partial septate) because the fundal indentation appeared as an obtuse angle at the central point, <1.5 cm deep; (B) A partial septate uterus characterized by a normal outer uterine contour, which could be differentiated from arcuate uterus because the fundal indentation was an acute angle at the central point, >1.5 cm deep

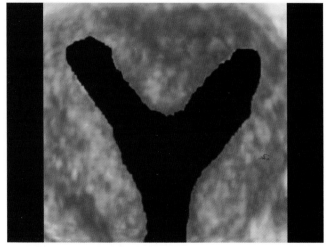

Fig. 10: Coronal view of a septate uterus on 3D volumetric ultrasound with digital subtraction of the endometrium

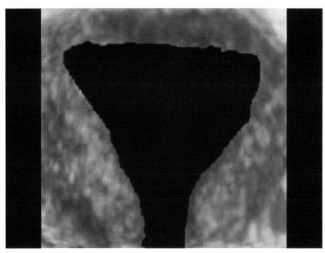

Fig. 11: Coronal view of a septate uterus on 3D volumetric ultrasound with digital subtraction of the septum

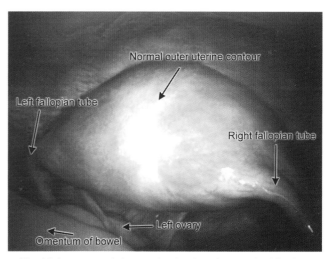

Fig. 12: Laparoscopic image showing broad, unnotched fundus, typical of the septate uterus

MRI

This is an excellent diagnostic technique for uterine anomalies with a high accuracy rate for the diagnosis of the septate uterus. However, it is not usually considered as the first line diagnostic test due to its cost and more cumbersome nature. MRI and 3D ultrasound show a high degree of concurrence in the diagnosis of Müllerian anomalies and may be employed together in difficult cases.

Diagnostic Hysteroscopy with Laparoscopy

Hysteroscopy is a practical way to evaluate the uterine cavity as the problem can be treated at the same time. However since it cannot evaluate the external fundal contour, a concomitant laparoscopy is mandatory to differentiate between a septate and a bicornuate uterus which is also useful to diagnose and treat any other factors which may contribute towards infertility.

On hysteroscopy if a blind wall is seen opposite a tubal ostial opening, then a differential diagnosis of a unicornuate, bicornuate, septate and didelphic uterus must be considered. As the scope is withdrawn from the fundus to the cervix, if another cavity is seen then the diagnosis narrows down to either a septate or bicornuate uterus. But if a separate cavity is not seen then a complete septum and didelphic uterus must be ruled out before diagnosing a unicornuate uterus (Figs 12 and 13).

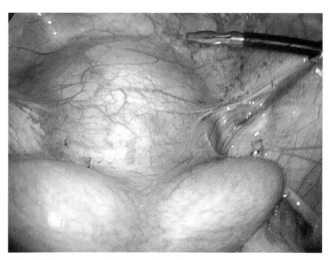

Fig. 13: Laparoscopic image of two clearly separated uterine horns with fundal indentation is a definite indication of the bicornuate uterus

PREOPERATIVE EVALUATION

It is important to rule out other factors such as endocrine and autoimmune conditions and karyotyping, that may lead to pregnancy wastage before deciding on surgical treatment of septum.

HYSTEROSCOPIC RESECTION OR METROPLASTY

The advent of hysteroscopy has revolutionized the treatment of uterine septum. It offers minimal discomfort and morbidity to the patient and can even be performed as an outpatient procedure. The surgery should be performed in the early proliferative phase when endometrial thickness is least. There are various ways in which the resection can be done.

Resection Methods Employing Electrolyte Distending Media

Any electrolyte containing distending media can be used such as normal saline. This minimizes all the complications associated with nonelectrolyte media like electrolyte imbalance and glycine toxicity.

Hysteroscopic Scissors

Septal resection using scissors is the method of choice in small and thin septa. The septum is divided in its middle from its lowermost end to its base, using systematic, delicate and shallow cuts while observing the symmetry of the cavity at all times. The fibrotic nature of the septum permits this division without bleeding. The scissors can be used both with the office hysteroscope as well as the regular hysteroscope. The office hysteroscopy can be done as an outpatient procedure since it does not require cervical dilatation.

Since the use of scissors entails only a mechanical cut, there is minimal damage to the endometrium unlike the resectoscope which uses thermal energy. Hence, intrauterine scarring and fibrosis is definitely much less when scissors are used. Studies have demonstrated that pregnancy rates are much higher when scissors are used for septal resection rather than the resectoscope. A perforation

with the scissors if it occurs is less likely to bleed since the scissors has a very small diameter. The learning curve for septum resection using scissors is very short and the technique can easily be reproduced and mastered (Fig. 14).

Versapoint™

This uses bipolar energy and can hence be used with saline and causes less endometrial damage as compared to the use of monopolar energy. Its only drawback is that it is costly and hence not used widely.

Bipolar Needle Electrode and Laser

Both these give good results and can be used with normal saline. The fiberoptic lasers like the neodynium:yitrium aluminum garnet (Nd:YAG), potassium titanyl phosphate (KTP) or Argon can all be used since they do not use conductive energy. The Nd:YAG laser is the preferred laser for hysteroscopic surgery. Light energy from lasers is transformed to thermal energy by electron flow. Fears of lateral thermal damage with the laser are unfounded because the endometrium has an inherent ability to heal itself.

Bipolar Resectoscope

The bipolar resectoscope has an advantage over the monopolar resectoscope in that saline can be used as the distending medium thus avoiding the complications associated with glycine. It requires an underwater bipolar generator. It is a safer procedure as compared to monopolar resection.

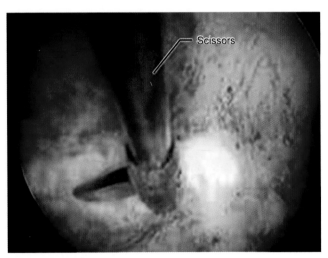

Fig. 14: Septal resection using scissors

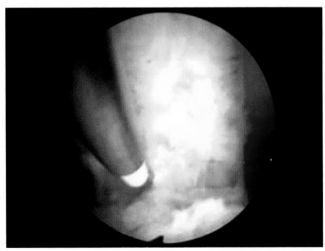

Fig. 15: Septal resection using Versapoint™

Resection Methods Employing Nonelectrolyte Distending Media

Nonelectrolyte distending media are used when monopolar energy is to be used to avoid conduction of current. Glycine 1.5% is the medium of choice. Monopolar underwater cutting current of 80–120 watt is used for the resection. Glycine input and output is monitored and recorded. Since the distending medium does not contain electrolytes, the fluid deficit that may have been absorbed by the patient should be strictly noted. A limit of 800–1,000 mL is paramount. A vigilant watch must be kept for hyponatremia and the signs of glycine toxicity especially with fluid deficits around 1,000 mL.

In expert hands the procedure does not take more than 20–30 minutes, so hyponatremia is rare especially if the hysteromat is used for distension.

Monopolar Needle Electrode

This has an advantage over the resectoscope in that it can be introduced through the operating channel of the conventional hysteroscope and hence requires less cervical dilatation than if the resectoscope were to be used. It is a very cost-effective method but the endometrial damage is more compared to the scissors or Versapoint™.

Resectoscope

Resection is usually done using a right angled knife called Collins knife inserted through the resectoscope (Fig. 16). It is the preferred method for broad thick septa that may be difficult to tackle with the scissors. A loop electrode may also be used (Fig. 17).

Cervical dilatation up to number 10 Hegar is required. Care must be taken to resect the septum equidistant from the anterior and posterior walls in order to have better healing and a uniform cavity. Resection using energy does cause more scarring and fibrosis due to thermal energy spread compared to hysteroscopic scissors. This can be minimized using bipolar current.

Assessment of the endpoint of resection: Septum resection begins carefully in the midline. It is crucial to stay in the same linear plane. As the resection progresses cephalad, it is important to continuously back away from the septum and reassess the progress. The septum is cut till the level of the fundus, so that both tubal ostia are in one line and can be seen together in a panoramic view. Care must be taken to remain at a safe distance from the ostia to avoid damage to the thin endometrium in this area. Resection should be stopped the moment pinkish myometrial fibers are seen. Another way to determine the endpoint of resection is by partially deflating the cavity. If the resected area shows bleeding points, then the resection should be stopped. It is preferable to leave a small portion of septum rather than damage the myometrium or perforate the uterus. Many studies demonstrate that septal remnants of less than 1 cm may not worsen the reproductive outcome. The cut ends of the septa merge easily into the anterior and posterior walls thus obviating the need for removal. Laparoscopic guidance does not add to the safety of the procedure and does not prevent a perforation but just helps to identify one. It only helps to differentiate between a septate and bicornuate uterus and its routine use is not recommended. However concomitant laparoscopy is still used by some gynecologists, wherein the transillumination from the hysteroscopy light is visible through the laparoscope which has dimmed or no light. The procedure should be stopped

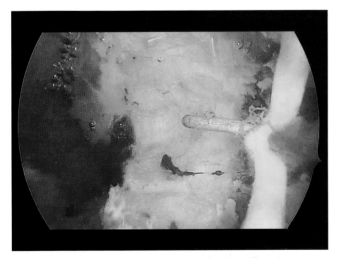

Fig. 16: Resectoscope with Collins knife

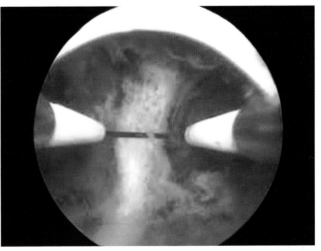

Fig. 17. Septal resection using a loop electrode

as soon as a faint light appears, otherwise the resection will have already damaged the myometrium. The best guide if so desired is simultaneous abdominal USG, but it becomes cumbersome to maintain the uterus and the sonographic transducer in the same plane while the surgeon is operating and moving the uterus.

CERVICAL SEPTUM

This can be cut with the help of long scissors by inserting each half into either half of the cervical canal. Since these septa are avascular, they do not bleed much. There is no need for cervical encerclage in any future pregnancy.

VAGINAL SEPTUM

These are vascular compared to uterine septa and hence require monopolar open cautery for their resection. It is imperative that the resection is done in the midline to avoid injury to bowel and bladder.

POSTOPERATIVE MANAGEMENT

❑ Antibiotics
❑ The healing process with re-epithelialization of the uterine cavity takes only 4–5 weeks. The use of postoperative hormonal therapy is controversial but it may be considered after resection of a large septum especially when unipolar energy has been used. Estradiol valerate 2 mg TDS for 21 days with oral progesterone 10 mg from day 16 for 10 days helps rapid re-epithelialization of the large raw surface to prevent adhesions
❑ Postoperative insertion of a balloon or an intrauterine contraceptive device (IUCD) is not recommended since it poses the risk of infection and adhesion formation
❑ The septate uterus is likely associated with cervical incompetence like all Müllerian anomalies and would benefit by a cervical encerclage during pregnancy
❑ Due to rapid healing of the resected area, pregnancy may be allowed after three cycles and delivery need not be by cesarean section.

COMPLICATIONS

These are rare though perforation can occur with all methods of resection. Perforation was reported in 1% of women in the National Institute for Health and Care Excellence (NICE) review of 2,528 women. Perforation with scissors does not require any treatment, but perforation

with the resectoscope mandates careful observation for bowel injury. If any doubt exists laparoscopy should be done to identify the extent of the perforation and assess the bowels for any injury. Secondary hemorrhage is very rare and can be managed by an intrauterine balloon. Uterine rupture during subsequent pregnancy or delivery is known. There is usually a history of a uterine perforation at the time of the septum resection which in most cases is due to the resectoscope. The NICE review of 2,528 women identified 18 reports of uterine rupture during pregnancy or delivery. In 10 out of the 18 cases, uterine perforation had occurred at the time of the resection. [8]

SURGICAL RESULTS AND GUIDELINES

❑ A Cochrane review[9] on metroplasty compared with expectant management for women with a history of recurrent miscarriage and a septate uterus was published in 2011. It states that since the effectiveness of hysteroscopic metroplasty has never been considered in a randomized controlled trial, there is insufficient evidence to support this treatment in these women. Nevertheless, in women with a history of repeated miscarriages, the viable pregnancy rate after septal resection varies from 60% to 90% in different studies. A review and meta-analysis by Valle and Ekpo in 2013 differs from the Cochrane review. It states that hysteroscopic metroplasty gives good results in pregnancy and live birth rates, despite the lack of prospective randomized controlled studies. A careful review of the published results supports this type of treatment. Their meta-analysis using strict exclusion criteria reports a 63.5% pregnancy rate.[10]
A case series of 170 women in the NICE review with recurrent pregnancy losses reported that 92% pregnancies ended in miscarriage before hysteroscopic metroplasty compared with 13% after hysteroscopic metroplasty.
A meta-analysis of 2,074 women in the NICE study in 2013, reported a live birth rate of 50% after hysteroscopic metroplasty. Similarly, Valle and Ekpo reported a 50.2% live birth rate.
❑ Septal resection in patients with primary or unexplained infertility is controversial, since no study has been published that randomizes infertile women to treatment versus no treatment, yet it remains in use. However, studies have shown that such surgery has resulted in increased number of viable pregnancies and live birth rates in women with unexplained infertility.[11,12] Recent NICE guidelines of 2013 indicated the uncertainty of performing metroplasty.

■ CONCLUSION

The advent of hysteroscopic septum resection has radically changed the management of repeated pregnancy losses due to the uterine septum, from traditional abdominal metroplasties to minimally invasive and safe day care or outpatient procedures with superior results and far less morbidity.

Septal resection may be considered before expensive ART procedures and in patients with long standing infertility. Such patients should undergo resection with small diameter hysteroscopes and with the hysteroscopic scissors wherever possible.

The learning curve for hysteroscopic septum resection using the scissors is very short and the requisite skill can be easily acquired. The electrosurgery technique however should only be attempted after sufficient training with the scissors and familiarity with the anatomical landmarks of the procedure. Moreover a thorough understanding of the principles of electrosurgery and knowledge of the sophisticated instruments to be used is vital especially if monopolar current is to be used.

■ REFERENCES

1. The American Fertility Society classification of Müllerian anomalies. Fertil Steril. 1988;49:944-55.
2. Saravelos SH, Cocksedge KA, Li TC. Prevalence and diagnosis of congenital uterine anomalies in women with reproductive failure: a critical appraisal. Hum Reprod Update. 2008;14(5):415-29.
3. Bermejo C, Martínez Ten P, Cantarero R, Diaz D, Pérez Pedregosa J, Barrón E, et al. Three dimensional ultrasound in the diagnosis of Mullerian duct anomalies and concordance with magnetic resonance imaging. Ultrasound Obstet Gynecol. 2010;35:593-601.
4. Role of 3D USG in the diagnosis of double uterine anomalies and concordance with laparoscopic and hysteroscopic diagnosis. The Egyptian Journal of Radiology and Nuclear Medicine. 2014;45(2):555-60.
5. Troiano R, McCarthy S. Mullerian duct anomalies: imaging and clinical issues. Radiology. 2004;233:19-34.
6. Ludwin A, Ludwin I. Comparison of the ESHRE-ESGE and ASRM classification of Müllerian duct anomalies in everyday practice. Hum Reprod. 2014:deu344.
7. Ferreira A, Filho FM, Nicolau LG, Pancich Gallarreta FM, de Paula WM, Gomes DC. Three-dimensional ultrasound in gynecology: uterine malformations. Radiologia Brasileira. 2007;40(2).
8. The National Institute for Health and Care Excellence (NICE). Interventional procedures overview by the RCOG and British Fertility Society, April 2014.
9. Kowalik CR, Goddijn M, Emanuel MH, Bongers MY, Spinder T, de Kruif JH, et al. Metroplasty versus expectant management for women with recurrent miscarriage and a septate uterus. Cochrane Database Syst Rev. 2011;(6):CD008576.
10. Valle RF, Ekpo GE. Hysteroscopic metroplasty for the septate uterus: review and meta-analysis. J Minim Invasive Gynecol. 2013;20:22-42.
11. Mollo A, de Franciscis P, Colacurci N, Cobellis L, Perino A, Venezia R, et al. Hysteroscopic resection of the septum improves the pregnancy rate of women with unexplained infertility: a prospective controlled trial. Fertil Steril. 2009;91(6):2628-31.
12. Bakas P, Gregoriou O, Hassiakos D, Liapis A, Creatsas M, Konidaris S. Hysteroscopic resection of uterine septum and reproductive outcome in women with unexplained infertility. Gynecol Obstet Invest. 2012;73(4):321-5.

CHAPTER 22

Office Hysteroscopy

Meenu Agarwal

"What we have to learn to do , we learn by doing."

Aristotle

■ INTRODUCTION

Office procedures do not necessarily mean that they need to be done in the doctor's office but to be done as an outpatient procedure.

Pantaleoni first performed hysteroscopy in 1869 but it took almost a century for it to become an essential part of gynecologist's armamentarium. The main obstacle to the progress in hysteroscopy was distension. The uterine cavity being a potential space needed distension and the presence of blood in the cavity due to fragility of endometrium would blur the quality of the image, hence making the visualization difficult. There was also resorption (vascular) and loss (cervix) of the distention media making the distension more difficult and messy.

Once the good insufflators were designed, the era of diagnostic hysteroscopy was heralded in 1980s with the conventional hysteroscopes under anesthesia.

With the modified slimmer oval designs of the telescopes and sheaths, the technique of diagnostic hysteroscopy became an ambulatory, well-tolerated office procedure.

The approach to the cervix through vaginoscopy without the use of speculum and tenaculum made it a more outpatient-friendly procedure with minimal discomfort.

■ DEFINITION

Diagnostic hysteroscopy and some hysteroscopic procedures can be conducted outside of the conventional formal operation theater without anesthesia in an appropriately equipped and staffed ambulatory situations yet taking utmost care of patient's safety and privacy.

■ INDICATIONS

- ❑ Unmarried/adolescent/sexually inactive females
- ❑ Infertility
- ❑ Uterine malformations
- ❑ Uterine synechiae
- ❑ Evaluation of abnormal uterine bleeding:
  - ❖ Heavy menstruation
  - ❖ Postmenopausal
- ❑ Postpartum menorrhagia
- ❑ Abnormal ultrasound findings:
  - ❖ Thick endometrial echoes
  - ❖ Suspected pathologies in the uterine cavity
- ❑ Endometrial biopsy
- ❑ Lost IUCD or foreign bodies in uterine cavity
- ❑ Correction of placement of mirena/IUCD
- ❑ Embryoscopy.

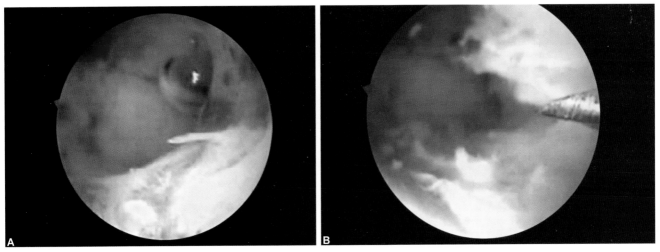

Figs 1A and B: Uterine synechiae cut as an office procedure

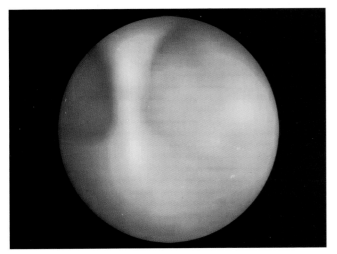

Fig 2: Uterine synechiae on office hysteroscopy

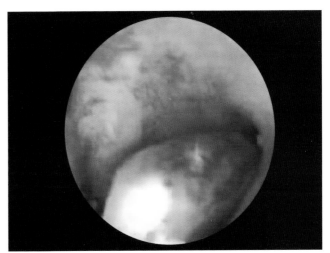

Fig 3: Endometrial polyp on office hysteroscopy

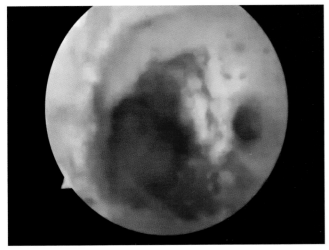

Fig 4: Anteroposterior adhesion band on office hysteroscopy

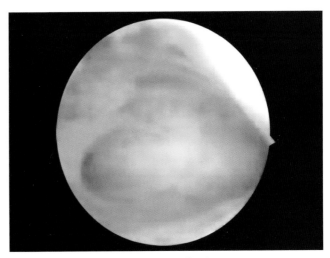

Fig. 5: Normal cavity on office hysteroscopy

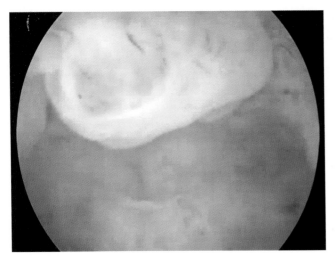

Fig. 6: Endometrial polyp

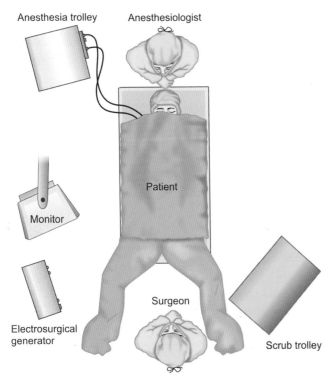

Fig. 7: Procedure in a lithotomy position

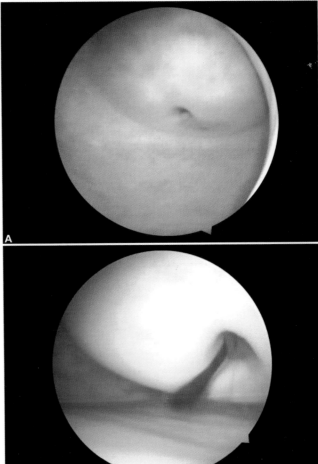

Figs 8A and B: Vaginoscopy (The trick is to keep the labia closed with a gauze to prevent any leakage of fluid)

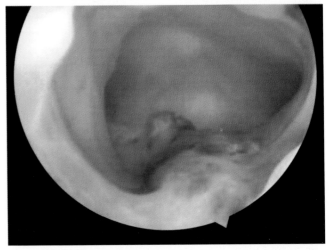

Fig. 9: Thickened posterior endometrium

▌TECHNIQUE

The procedure is performed in a lithotomy position. The patient is in supine position with legs supported on leg rests, buttocks at the edge of the table slightly beyond the table end. Extreme flexion, abduction and lateral rotation of hip should be avoided to prevent femoral nerve compression.

The surgeon should be positioned between the legs of the patient with the screen between his hands. This eases

the procedure and also prevents the strain to the neck muscles of the surgeon (Fig. 7).

While assembling the instruments, always put the light cable from below (sun shines from below) and the inflow

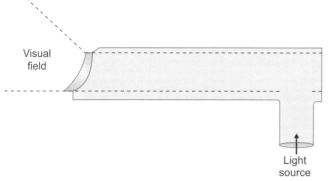

Fig. 10: 30° Hysteroscope showing the visual field

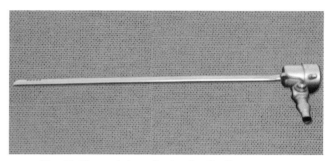

Fig. 12: The oval-shaped outer sheath of hysteroscope

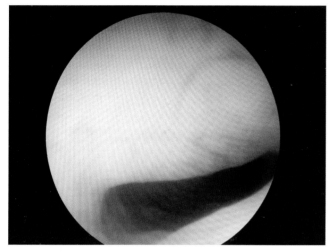

Fig. 11: The internal os is anteroposteriorly flattened

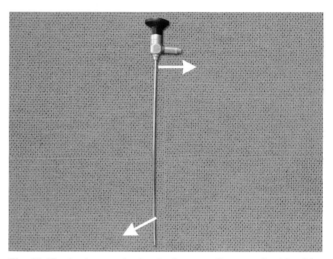

Fig. 13: The hysteroscopic view is always on the opposite side of the direction of light cord

cable from above (waterfalls from above) as that would prevent the entanglement of the cables. White balancing and focusing remains the mainstay before starting any endoscopic procedure.

Vaginoscopy

It is an essential part of office hysteroscopy. For beginners, they should always start with vaginoscopy for patients under anesthesia. The scope is placed in the vagina with the inflow on. Both lips of the labia are gently closed with the help of gauze.

As the vagina gets filled up with saline you can clearly visualize the vaginal walls, cervix and external os. Any lesions on the vagina/cervix can be clearly seen as a magnified view. The patient perceives no pain at the time of vaginoscopy. The inexperienced surgeon may find it difficult to find the cervix. It must be remembered that the cervical tissue and the vaginal tissue are different (Figs 8A and B).

Once the external os is seen, the scope is placed very gently into the external os and slowly maneuvered with the cervical canal and then through the internal os into the uterine cavity.

Care should be taken that the scope does not touch the walls of the cervix to minimize discomfort. The maneuver should resemble a train passing through a tunnel.

As a 30° telescope is being used, the visual hole should always be kept eccentric at 6 o'clock position with the light cable from below.

This would ensure that the entry is straight into the visual hole. For the beginners, a few office hysteroscopy procedures without the use of speculum and tenaculum with vaginoscopic approach can be performed under anesthesia. Once the internal os is reached, the pressure of the fluid helps in the opening of the internal os. The internal os is oval-shaped, i.e. it is flattened anteroposteriorly, so if the light cable is moved on the right or left side, it will make the telescope horizontal and this will ease the entry into the uterine cavity without causing any pain to the patient.

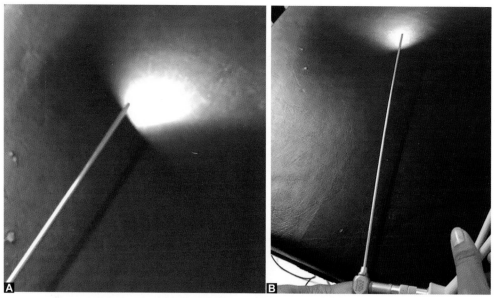

Figs 14A and B: The direction of throw of light is opposite to the position of light cable

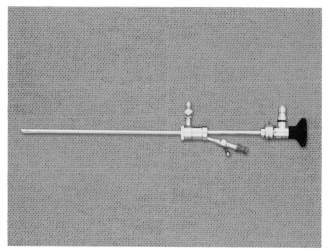

Fig. 15: Office hysteroscope (Bettochi)

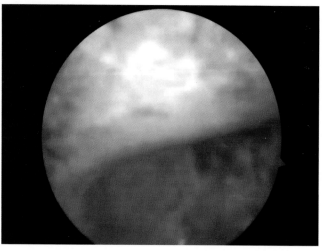

Fig. 16: Early pregnancy sac seen on office hysteroscopy

At all times, the ergonomics should be kept in mind while performing office hysteroscopy.

As a 30° scope is used, only the cable movement outside the body will show the entire uterine cavity so the entire contraption remains steady with only the light cable movement in all directions—right up to and around in 180° in each direction.

Operative Procedures

Office hysteroscope has a side operative channel through which 5 French instruments can pass through such as scissors, grasper, monopolar/bipolar needle, etc.

As endometrium has no sensory nerve fibers, small procedure in the uterine cavity does not cause any pain, e.g. procedures like synechiolysis, polypectomy, endometrial biopsy, removal of IUCD can be routinely done as an outpatient office procedure. It must be kept in mind that the polyp size is not bigger than the internal os as in that case patient would experience pain at the time of extraction of the polyp from the uterine cavity.

We have now given up using preoperative intravaginal misoprostol; however, the intrauterine pressures are kept at around 50 mm Hg to minimize the discomfort during the procedure.

■ CONTRAINDICATIONS

❑ Active pelvic infection
❑ Pregnancy
❑ Heavy per vaginal bleeding.

■ SUCCESS RATES

In our series of 2,600 diagnostic office hysteroscopy since 2004 with Bettochi 2.9 mm hysteroscope, it could be completed in almost all cases. In nine cases where we had to abandon the procedure were due to:
❑ Patients anxiety (4)
❑ Cervical stenosis (3)
❑ Pain (2).

■ ADVANTAGES

❑ No anesthesia/analgesics
❑ No speculum/tenaculum
❑ Outpatient procedure
❑ See and treat
❑ Small learning curve
❑ Low complication rate
❑ Minor operative procedures are possible using scissors and bipolar diathermy
❑ The technique can be used in virgins under anesthesia and is minimally invasive in the true sense.

CHAPTER 23

Hysteroscopic Cannulation of Proximal Tubal Block

Nalini Bagul

▌ INTRODUCTION

Tubal factor accounts for 25–35% of female infertility. 10–25% of them are due to proximal tubal occlusion (PTO). 40% of women have tubal spasm (Fertility and Sterility, 1999). Fallopian tubes can be blocked at the proximal (the portion near the uterus) or at distal (fimbrial) end. Mid piece obstruction can be present but is relatively uncommon. Distal tubal occlusion may lead to hydrosalpinx.

▌ ANATOMY OF PROXIMAL TUBE

❑ Normal intramural part of the tube ranges from 1.5 cm to 2.5 cm in length and it takes straight to slightly curved course at uterotubal junction.
❑ Diameter: 0.8–1.2 mm can accommodate the cannula of 1–1.2 mm diameter without epithelial damage.

▌ PATHOLOGY

In 1985, Fortier and Haney described the pathologic spectrum of disease in woman with proximal tubal occlusion.

The most frequent lesion was obstructive fibrosis in 35%, followed by salpingitis isthmica nodosa in 24%, intramucosal endometriosis in 14% and chronic tubal obstruction in 12% (Figs 1A and B).

Salak et al. resected tubal segments and found that 11 out of 18 patients with no demonstrable tubal occlusion. But six of them had amorphous material of unknown etiology within tubal lumen.

"Tubal spasm" can be a cause for PTO when hysterosalpingography (HSG) dye is forcefully injected.

▌ CLASSIFICATION OF PROXIMAL TUBAL OCCLUSION

❑ Nodular: Salpingitis isthmica nodosa
❑ Non-nodular: True fibrotic occlusion
❑ Pseudo-debris, polyp or hypoplastic tubes.

▌ MECHANISM OF RESTORING FERTILITY

❑ Separation of mild agglutination of mucosal fold
❑ Dislodgement of debris or mucosal plugs.

▌ SURGICAL METHODS OF REMOVAL OF PROXIMAL TUBAL OCCLUSION

❑ Macrosurgical cornual reimplantation
❑ Microsurgical tubocornual anastomosis
❑ Radiographic treatment: Selective salpingography and tubal catheterization
❑ Hysteroscopic transcervical tubal cannulation.

Hysteroscopic cannulation has much higher pregnancy rate than other procedures (Fertility and Sterility 1999, 2007). Pregnancy rates reported 9–57%.

Advantages of Hysteroscopic and Laparoscopic-guided Tubal Cannulation

❑ Prevent surgery
❑ Proper assessment of distal tubes and ovaries done at the same time

HSG with blocked tubes

HSG with dilated tubes (hydrosalpinx)

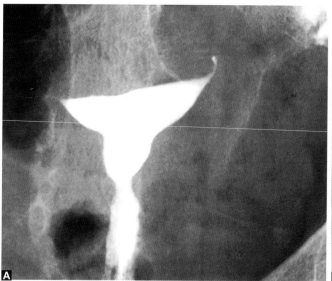 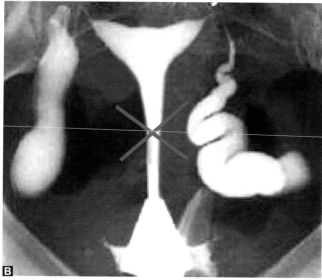

Figs 1A and B: (A) Proximal tubal occlusion can be treated with TC; (B) Distal tubal occlusion (hydrosalpinx) cannot be treated with TC

❑ Eliminate spasm as tubal factor
❑ Therapeutic confirmation of tubal patency.

Conditions associated with proximal tubal occlusion and their potential to respond to catheterization technique.

Response to Catheterization
Conditions: Frequently
Muscular spasm, stromal edema, amorphous debris, mucosal agglutination, viscous secretion
Conditions: Occasionally
Cornual polyps, chronic salpingitis endometriosis, salpingitis isthmica nodosa, intrauterine synechiae, parasite infection
Conditions: Never seen
Luminal fibrosis, failed tubal reanastomosis, leiomyomata, congenital atresia, tuberculosis

(*Source:* Das S, Nardo LG, Seif MW. Proximal tubal disease: the place for tubal cannulation. RBM Online. 2007;15:383-8.)

Instruments

❑ Hysteroscope
❑ Tubal catheterization/cannulation set contains
 ❖ Tubal cannula 30 cm long with guard (steel)–0.018 mm
 ❖ Inner Teflon catheter (special coating makes it slippery and easy to manipulate into tubal lumen).

Procedure

❑ To be performed in follicular phase of menstrual cycle
❑ Done under general anesthesia or local anesthesia
❑ Distension media: Normal saline
❑ Under all aseptic precautions, office operative hysteroscope is introduced through the cervix
❑ Right ostium located
❑ Tubal cannulation set with guard is introduced through operating sheath and passed into right ostium
❑ Guard withdrawn
❑ Chromopertubation done through outer cannula to rule out spasm of tube
❑ Concomitant laparoscopy done to confirm patency or block
❑ If block present, inner Teflon catheter is introduced through outer sheath and passed beyond the point of occlusion into distal tubal lumen and is moved in a to and fro manner to further open up the tube. This is similar to what a plumber does to open up a blocked pipe!
❑ Laparoscopically, see the entry of catheter. Sometimes tube can be stretched to negotiate the catheter.
❑ Withdraw guidewire
❑ Selective chromopertubation done through outer cannula to confirm the patency of tube
❑ Same procedure is repeated on the other side
❑ Patient can be discharged after 8 hours

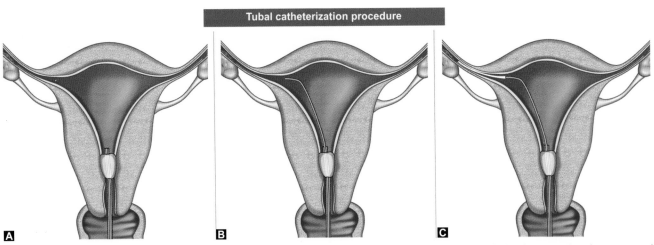

Figs 2A to C: (A) Cervical cannula in place for HSG. The balloon prevents dye from leaking. If tubal occlusion is encountered, we proceed with tubal catheterization; (B) A selective salpingography (SS) catheter is inserted through the cervical cannula and manipulated into the tubal opening. Dye is injected directly into the tubal opening in an effort to open the tube; (C) If the tube remains blocked, a wire-guide is next inserted through the SS catheter into the tubal opening to further by and open up the tube

❑ Follow-up HSG should be done after 1 month if required (Figs 2A to C).

Complications

❑ Perforation of guidewire through proximal potion of fallopian tube 1–10%
❑ Ectopic pregnancy in 8% of cases
❑ Bleeding—Rare
❑ Infection—Rare.

Contraindications

❑ Age more than 35 years
❑ Active *pelvic inflammatory disease* (PID)
❑ Genital TB
❑ Obliterative fibrosis causing extensive scarring in fallopian tubes
❑ Previous Fallopian tube surgery
❑ Severe tubal damage
❑ Male subfertility
❑ Distal blockage (hydrosalpinx).

▮ CONCLUSION

Hysteroscopic tubal cannulation is the first treatment option in cases of proximal tubal occlusion (National Institute for Health and Care Excellence (NICE) guidelines 2004]—in women less than 35 years of age, in absence of other causes of subfertility, and if surgical skills are available.

Case selection for hyteroscopic tubal cannulation is based upon the nature of problem:
❑ Debris
❑ Cornual polyps
❑ Pericornual synechiae
❑ Mucus agglutination (Woolcott, 1996).

CHAPTER 24

Hysteroscopic Myomectomy

Nagendra Sardeshpande

"Science is cumulative. The apprentice of the next generation can outdo the master of the last."

■ INTRODUCTION

Hysteroscopy involves viewing and operating in the endometrial cavity via a transcervical approach using a long, narrow telescope connected to a light source and a camera which is further linked to a monitor to provide illumination and magnified vision.

Although the concept of hysteroscopy has existed since 140 years since Pantaleoni first attempted the procedure in 1869, the technique has become extremely popular in the last few decades because of rapid advances in optics and instrumentation. Hysteroscopy has become the gold standard for diagnosis and treatment of intrauterine and endocervical pathology such as uterine septae, submucous fibroids and intrauterine adhesions and for procedures such as tubal cannulation and hysteroscopic tubal sterilization.

Uterine leiomyomas also called fibroids, fibromyomas, myomas or myofibromas are one of the most common benign tumors in women seen on ultrasound in 20-25% of women. Interestingly, histological evaluation has shown a much higher incidence of up to 70% suggesting that the vast majority of fibroids are asymptomatic with only 20-50% of women with fibroids experience symptoms directly related to the fibroids.[1] It should also be remembered that fibroids often coexist with other benign pelvic conditions such as adenomyosis, endometriosis, functional ovarian cysts or pelvic adhesions and symptoms of these conditions may overlap, mimic or mask symptoms of each other.

■ SUBMUCOUS FIBROIDS

The symptoms attributable to uterine fibroids depend upon the size of the fibroids, number and location. These factors determine the incidence and severity of symptoms. Around 20-30% of all myomas are submucous myomas.[2] Submucous fibroids are more likely to arise from the junctional zone myometrium, a zone of myometrium adjacent to endometrium, and myocyte shows cyclical changes during the menstrual cycle. These myomas have higher estrogen and progesterone receptors and fewer karyotype abnormalities.[3,4] Submucous myomas are associated with reduced HOXA-10 & 11 gene expression in adjacent endometrium and endometrial sloughing over it possibly contributing to subfertility.[5]

Abnormal menstrual bleeding is the most common symptom reported by women with fibroids. Menorrhagia is common with submucous leiomyomas (21% vs 1% with a range of 7.5-23%). Submucous fibroids as a cause of abnormal uterine bleeding is more common in premenopausal than menopausal women (23.4% vs 4.55%). Menometrorrhagia is more commonly seen with prolapsed pedunculated fibroids undergoing necrosis. These fibroids may also be responsible for postmenopausal bleeding. Submucous fibroids may also cause dysmenorrhea of variable severity.[2,6-8]

Submucous fibroids may be associated with subfertility, pregnancy wastage and preterm labor. However, this association is not always clear and many theories have proposed for these complications such as mechanical obstruction and vascular or endocrine dysfunction.[9] The incidence of myomas in women without another obvious etiology for infertility is small, estimated to be 1–2.4%.[10] Submucous fibroids causing distortion of the endometrial cavity may adversely influence fertility.[5] Hysteroscopic myomectomy has been reported to yield pregnancy rates of 16.7–76.9%.[11,12] However, no randomized controlled trials have been conducted to evaluate the effect of hysteroscopic myomectomy on fertility. Hysteroscopic myomectomy reduces abnormal uterine bleeding successfully in 62–90.3% of women.[13,14] For patients with recurrent miscarriage and intracavitary fibroids, surgery increases rates of viable pregnancy outcomes (RR 1.68, 95% CI: 1.37–2.05).[15,16]

DIAGNOSIS OF LEIOMYOMAS

Most submucous fibroids require an ultrasound to confirm the clinical diagnosis and to study the location and size of other coexistent fibroids. A uterus embedded with uterine fibroids will appear clinically enlarged, firm and bosselated. A solitary large submucous fibroid may cause uniform globular enlargement of the uterus. A cervical fibroid or a pedunculated submucous fibroid displaced into the cervical canal can cause enlargement of the cervix with a relatively normal uterus sitting on top. The cervical canal may appear patulous in such cases. Occasionally a prolapsed fibroid polyp may fill up the whole vagina. A prolapsed submucous fibroid may have to be differentiated from a uterine inversion.

Additionally, it is necessary to rule out additional pelvic pathology coexisting with uterine fibroids. Before deciding therapy, it is also necessary to know the number, size and location of leiomyomas and their relation to adjacent structures such as the bladder, bowel and ureters. Hence, more often than not, there is a need of performing a radiological evaluation to supplement the clinical diagnosis of uterine fibroids.

INVESTIGATIONS FOR UTERINE FIBROIDS

The various investigations done to diagnose and evaluate submucous uterine fibroids can be classified as follows:

I. **Radiological procedures:**
   1. Hysterosalpingography
II. **Ultrasonography:**
   1. Routine transabdominal and transvaginal ultrasound with or without a color Doppler
   2. Hysterosonography
   3. Three dimensional ultrasonography
III. **CT scan**
IV. **MRI**
V. **Surgical procedures:**
   1. Hysteroscopy with or without concomitant laparoscopy.

Hysterosalpingography

Hysterosalpingography (HSG) is one of the most common radiological procedures performed during investigation for infertility and occasionally, recurrent pregnancy wastage.

Submucous myomas create a crescent shape configuration as the contrast material passes around it during an HSG (Fig. 1). Submucous myomas in the lower segment of the uterus cause ballooning of this area and, on HSG, the lower uterine cavity appears distended. In addition, since the endometrium overlying the leiomyoma is often thinned out, marked extravasation may be noted. An intramural myoma encroaching on the endometrial cavity may cause distortion and broadening of the uterine cavity (Fig. 2). An HSG also allows one to evaluate the patency of the Fallopian tubes.[17]

Hysterosalpingography has its drawbacks. The amount of contrast fluid required to delineate leiomyomas varies from 1–20 cc depending upon the degree of distention of the uterine cavity caused by the fibroid. Too little fluid, especially with admixed air may cast false shadows and too much of contrast medium may obscure a small leiomyoma. A fundal myoma will cause widening of the fundal shadow and increase the distance between the cornua. This finding may also be noted in an arcuate or a bicornuate uterus. Uterine spasm or hypercontractility can cause intrauterine

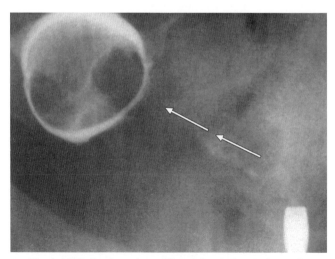

Fig. 1: HSG showing a large filling defect in the uterine cavity

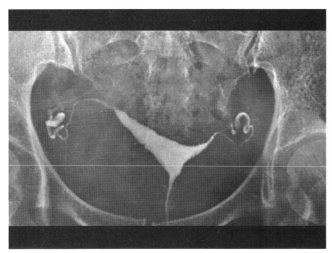

Fig. 2: Splayed out fundus due to a fundal fibroid

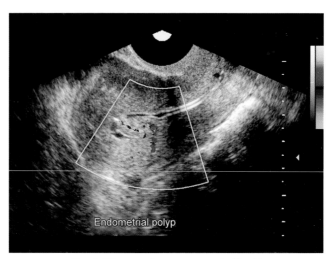

Fig. 3: Ultrasound appearance of a fibroid

filling defects and distorted shadows. Very rarely, an incidental intrauterine pregnancy at the time of an HSG can be mistaken for a leiomyoma.

An HSG can be a very valuable tool for diagnosis of intrauterine and tubal pathology. However, factors such as skilled performance of the procedure and interpretation of the findings decide its utility.

Ultrasonography

Today, ultrasound has become the commonest modality used to diagnose uterine fibroids.

Any pelvic pathology is best evaluated by a combination of transabdominal and transvaginal sonography for better image resolution except when an extremely large uterus lies beyond the range of the transvaginal probe and a satisfactory image can be obtained by abdominal ultrasound alone.

Myomas typically appear as hypoechoic or heterogeneous masses of varying size with a well-defined margin (Fig. 3). A border of hyperechoic tissue may be seen surrounding the myomas possibly representing the compressed surrounding connective tissue (pseudocapsule). The central area of especially large myomas may appear hypoechoic or heterogeneous (necrosis) or hyperechoic (calcification).

Distortion of the endometrial lining, especially if scanned in midcycle, may be noted in cases of submucous and large intramural fibroids encroaching on the cavity.

Cystic degeneration may occur in a fibroid. A degenerated submucous myoma may appear as a honeycomb pattern of multiple cystic areas surrounded by hyperechoic tissue. This may, occasionally, be difficult to differentiate from endometrial hyperplasia, molar degeneration or a missed abortion.

Transperineal ultrasound, although having limited use in gynecology, can be utilized to study uterine fibroids in a prolapsed uterus especially with an associated cystocele where the bladder can be used as an acoustic window.[18]

Transvaginal sonography has a sensitivity of 90%, specificity of 98% and a positive predictive value of 90% in diagnosing uterine fibroids.[19]

Contrast Hysterosonography

With conventional TVS, submucous fibroids may be difficult to locate as they transmit sound poorly, attenuate the beam and have ill-defined borders. Also, they may obscure endometrial measurements due to the irregular interface between the endometrium and myometrium.[20]

Contrast hysterosonography or saline infusion sonography (SIS) allows clear visualization of submucous fibroids as well as large intramural fibroids and their classification according to location, size and degree of intramural extension (Fig. 4). SIS offers the most accurate measurement of uterine fibroids with a variation of not more than 5–10%.[19]

A classification of intracavitary fibroids by SIS has been proposed:[21]

❑ SIS class I: Completely intracavitary fibroids, no myometrial component, base or stalk seen by SIS, amenable to hysteroscopic resection.
❑ SIS class 2: Fibroids with a submucosal component, involve less than 50% of the myometrium, amenable to hysteroscopic resection.
❑ SIS class 3: Intramural component of fibroid more than 50%, less amenable to hysteroscopic resection with greater likelihood of surgical complications.

Despite its benefits, SIS may not offer satisfactory visualization in very large uteri (more than 12–14 weeks), submucosal fibroids larger than 4–5 cm and large intramural fibroids.[14] Acutely retroverted uteri, intrauterine synechiae, septae and cervical stenosis may pose additional problems. Endometrial pseudopolyps and air bubbles in the endometrial cavity may pose a diagnostic dilemma. Imaging may also be difficult in acutely anteverted, retroverted or retroflexed uteri.

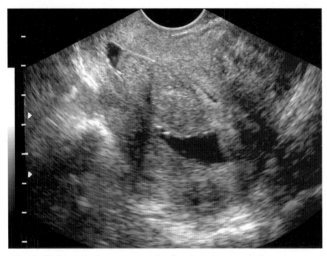

Fig. 4: Saline infusion sonography (hysterosonography) appearance of a submucous fibroid

Three-Dimensional Ultrasound

Three-dimensional ultrasound (3D USG) is an extension of 2D ultrasound. The target organ is scanned in three planes, the images fed into a computer which provides a composite 3D volumetric image of the target organ. In addition to diagnosing the location and number of fibroids, volume measurements of the fibroid are possible.

Similarly, 3D hysterosonography is useful in diagnosing submucous and submucous component of intramural fibroids. Using surface rendering and light, it is possible to demonstrate the round, the smooth surface of the myoma and obtain the feeding of depth inside the uterine cavity.[22]

This technology is as yet expensive. Any additional details and benefits of 3D USG over conventional 2D ultrasound in evaluating uterine fibroids are yet to be seen. Another new technology FlyThru 4D scanning can produce realistic 3D images of intrauterine pathology from all angles including through uterine myometrium (Fig. 5).

CT Scan

CT scan, while offering excellent visualization of extrauterine lesions, is of very little value in evaluating intramyometrial or intrauterine lesions. CT scan provides only transverse

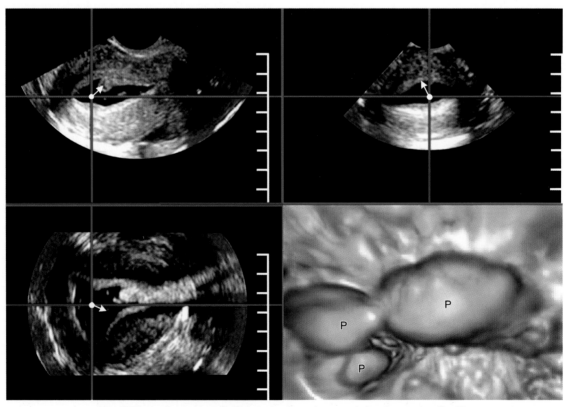

Fig. 5: Three-dimensional FlyThru technology ultrasound showing uterine fibroids

axial images. The CT scan also cannot readily differentiate the cervix from the body of the uterus. Hence, the CT scan has no genuine advantage over ultrasound for evaluation of uterine fibroids.

Magnetic Resonance Imaging

If not for the cost factor, magnetic resonance imaging (MRI) would today be the prime modality and gold standard for diagnosis and evaluation of uterine fibroids.

On T2 weighted images, leiomyomas appear as sharply marginated homogeneous areas with decreased signal intensity and margins distinct from the surrounding myometrium (Fig. 6). The signal intensity is less than the surrounding myometrium and similar to that of the junctional zone. Degenerated leiomyomas, containing calcified or cystic areas, hyaline material and occasionally blood, fat or mucin, have a heterogeneous appearance.[21]

Hysteroscopy

Hysteroscopy can diagnose submucosal myomas and intramural myomas distorting the uterine cavity.

The first sign of an intrauterine pathology such as a fibroid is the difficulty in achieving distention and separation of the anterior and posterior uterine walls producing a characteristic pillow shaped image. However, a small intramural myoma may become flattened on distention of the cavity and remain unnoticed. Reducing the fluid pressure and distention during a panoramic view will reveal this pathology.

Submucosal fibroids appear yellow-white, firm and smooth in consistency. The overlying endometrium is usually normally developed and sometimes thickened. The myoma appears brighter in contrast to the surrounding tissue since it reflects light. The surface often shows dense, arborescent vascularization.

A pedunculated myoma is easy to diagnose due to its characteristic color (yellow-white) and firm, smooth consistency. The overlying endometrium is usually thin, highly vascular and may be ulcerated. The opposing uterine wall is concave shaped. Myomas usually, due to their firm consistency, indent the uterine wall, whereas endometrial polyps, because of their softness, conform to the shape of the uterus.

Intramural myomas encroaching on the cavity produce characteristic asymmetry and distortion of the endometrial cavity. The tumor usually appears as an indentation or bump protruding into the cavity especially when observed under low fluid pressure.

Endocervical fibroids have similar characteristics as other myomas. However, their demarcation from the surrounding cervical tissue may not be distinct.[23]

Adenomyomas can be mistaken for uterine fibroids. However, during resection, there is a lack of characteristic pseudocapsule. Also, during resection, adenomyotic crypts may be noted.

Cervical ectopic pregnancy, especially an old, degenerated ectopic, may be difficult to differentiate from a degenerated cervical fibroid (Fig. 7). Although these pregnancies bleed more than a fibroid and have a freshly appearance, histopathological evaluation may be needed to settle the diagnosis.

Hysteroscopically, submucous myomas are classified as Figs 8 to 10:

Type 0: No intramural extension.

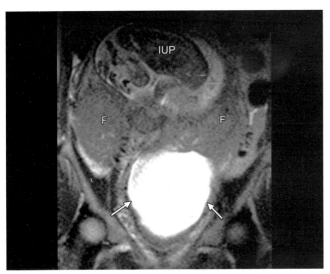

Fig. 6: MRI view of fibroids with pregnancy

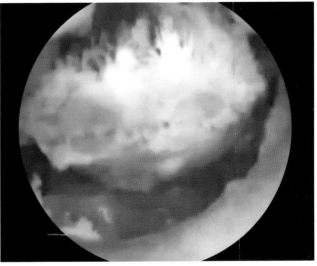

Fig. 7: Cervical ectopic pregnancy appearing as an intracervical mass

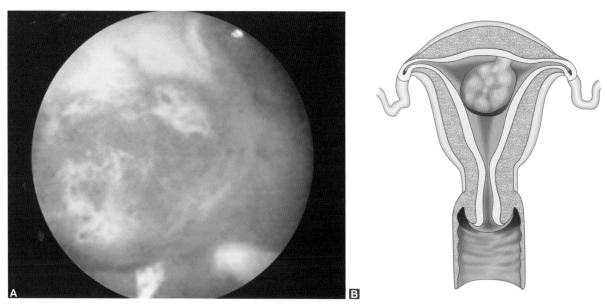

Figs 8A and B: (A) Type 0 fibroid; (B) Type 0 fibroid

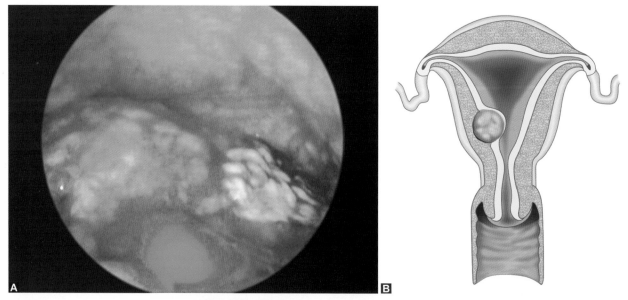

Figs 9A and B: (A) Type I fibroid; (B) Type I fibroid

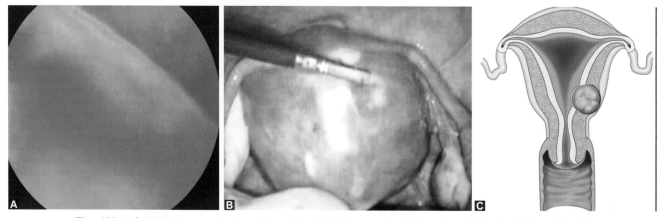

Figs 10A to C: (A) Hysteroscopic view of type II fibroid; (B) Laparoscopic view of type II fibroid; (C) Type II fibroid

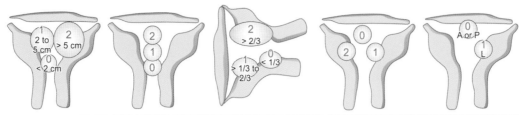

	Size (cm)	Topography	Extension of the base	Penetration	Lateral wall	Total
0	<2	Low	<1/3	0		
1	>2–5	Middle	>1/3–2/3	<50%	+1	
2	>5	Upper	>2/3	>50%		
Score	+	+	+	+	+	

Score	Group	Complexity and therapeutic options
0 to 4	I	Low complexity hysteroscopic myomectomy
5 to 6	II	High complexity hysteroscopic myomectomy Consider GnRH use? Consider two-step hysteroscopic myomectomy
7 to 9	III	Consider alternatives to the hysteroscopic technique

Fig. 11: STEPW classification of submucous fibroids

Type I: Intramural extension less than 50%.

Type II: Intramural extension more than 50%.

Type 0 and I are amenable to hysteroscopic removal. Type II fibroids are usually managed by abdominal approach. Hysteroscopic management requires great skill and, often, is done as a two-stage procedure.[13]

Another more detailed system of evaluation of submucous fibroids (STEPW classification) is the one proposed by Lasmar in 2005 (Fig. 11). This system includes the depth of penetration of the myoma, largest myoma diameter, extension of myoma to endometrial cavity surface and location along the uterine wall.[24] This is important since the volume of tissue to be resected increases exponentially with increase in diameter of the myoma from 0.52 cc for a 1 cm myoma to 65 cc for a 5 cm myoma (Fig. 12). This, in addition to factors such as increased myometrial penetration, increases the time of surgery and fluid absorption along with risk of complication such as fluid overload, electrolyte disturbances and uterine perforation.

CONTRAINDICATIONS TO HYSTEROSCOPIC MYOMECTOMY

❏ Active cervical or uterine infection
❏ Suspected pregnancy (missed periods)
❏ Suspected cervical malignancy.

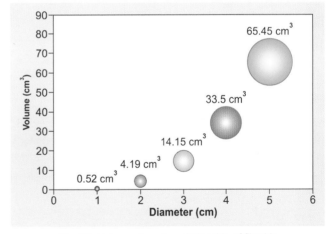

Fig. 12: Volume-diameter relationship of fibroids

PREOPERATIVE INVESTIGATIONS

Hematological and Cytological Investigations

❏ CBC, blood sugar, and a urine routine and microscopy.
❏ Blood typing and screening: especially prior to hysteroscopic myomectomy.
❏ Electrolyte determinations: In patients with medical disorders that predispose them to metabolic abnormalities (e.g. diuretic use).

❑ Determination of human chorionic gonadotropin (hCG) levels (urine or serum), if pregnancy is suspected.

❑ Investigations for infertility including TSH and partner's semen analysis.

❑ Hysterosalpingogram or sonohysterogram/pelvic ultrasound.

■ PREOPERATIVE PREPARATION

Preoperative Clinical Evaluation

Appropriate preoperative management includes accurate history taking and physical examination.

Antibiotic Prophylaxis

A diagnostic hysteroscopy does not warrant prophylactic antibiotics except in the presence of valvular heart disease, immunosuppression or suspected PID. A combination of antibiotics covering aerobic (doxycycline) and anaerobic (metronidazole) bacteria is appropriate during operative hysteroscopic procedures.

Difficult Cervical Dilatation or Cervical Stenosis

In patients with known cervical stenosis or tortuous cervical canals, preoperative vaginal or oral misoprostol (400 mg orally or vaginally 6 hours prior to procedure), or intraoperative vasopressin 1% administered paracervically may be used to assist in cervical dilation. Paracervical block with xylocaine 2% administered 6–7 ml each at 4 and 8 o'clock position may facilitate cervical dilatation and reduce postoperative discomfort.

Endometrial Preparation

For large submucosal fibroids, the use of a GnRH agonist decreases uterine volume by approximately 30%. Preoperative administration of a GnRH agonist helps resolve preoperative anemia, thins out the endometrium reducing vascularity and helps in elective scheduling of surgery. It may decrease blood loss and allow for an easier and more complete resection. For some large submucous fibroids requiring a two-stage procedure, a repeat GnRH analogue may be administered immediately following the primary procedure (1–2 doses at monthly intervals) and the subsequent procedure performed 6–8 weeks later.[12]

The most popular and relatively inexpensive GnRH analogue is Leuprolide 3.75 intramuscular 10–14 days prior to the procedure.

Aromatase inhibitors and GnRH antagonists have been used prior to hysteroscopy but have not become popular because of repeated dosing, expense and a dose-dependent effect.

Diagnostic Hysteroscopy

A 30° 4 mm hysteroscope used with isotonic sodium chloride as a distention medium has remained the standard practice for decades. A 30° hysteroscope allows visualization of the tubal ostia and the lateral uterine walls especially in a cavity with convergent lateral walls, recessed tubal ostia and distorted cavities because of septae, adhesions or fibroids. Diagnostic hysteroscopy can also be performed with 1.9 or 2.9 mm flexible or rigid hysteroscopes. An outflow sheath, although marginally increasing the diameter of the system, allows rapid clearing of blood and debris and better visualization.

Operative Office Hysteroscopy

Small, more sophisticated instruments and improved flow systems now allow an operative therapy to be performed at the same time as initial diagnosis. These procedures can be performed with paracervical block and sedation.

The 5-mm Office Continuous Flow Operative Bettocchi Hysteroscope includes a 2.9-mm rod lens system with an outer diameter of 5-mm which includes an inflow and outflow sheath and a channel for introducing operating instruments.

The Versapoint system includes a 1.9-mm hysteroscope with a flexible sheath through which operating instruments can be passed.

■ SURGICAL PROCEDURES

General Principles

The route of myomectomy is determined by the number of fibroids, location and relation of myoma with the serosal aspect of the uterus. A large type I fibroid, fibroid larger than 5 cm or a fibroid score of 5–6 by Lasmar's classification entails the increased possibility of a two-step procedure with intervening GnRH analogue therapy. A type II fibroid or a Lasmar classification score of 7 or more usually requires an abdominal myomectomy. However, this may vary depending on the size of the fibroid and surgeon's expertise.

While resecting a lateral wall fibroid, it has to be kept in mind that the relatively thinner lateral wall does not form a hollow cavity cradling the myoma but tends to bulge in with removal of the fibroid (Figs 13A to D). Hence the surgeon

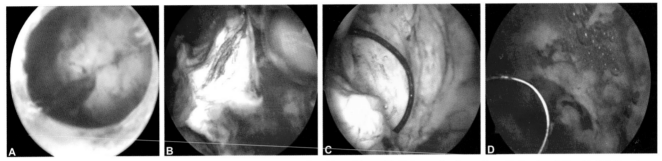

Figs 13A to D: (A) Lateral wall type 0 fibroid; (B) Lateral wall fibroid excision; (C) Retrograde dissection of lateral wall fibroid; (D) Basal myometrium after lateral wall fibroid myomectomy

must keep in mind the pink striated appearance of normal myometrium as opposed to the whorled white appearance of myomas especially while dealing with a lateral wall fibroid. The proximity of the uterine vessels and their main branches to the lateral uterine wall also may cause slightly more bleeding during the procedure.

While dealing with multiple submucous fibroids, two factors are kept in mind:

1. Resect the largest fibroid first since this can take more surgical time. The smaller fibroids can be tackled after the largest one or at a second sitting. This will help reduce fluid absorption.
2. Tackle the posterior fibroid first. If the anterior fibroids are resected initially, the debris of the fibroids and endometrium will settle over the posterior surface and hamper visualization.

Whether to use unipolar or bipolar systems is a personal choice. Whatever resectoscope one uses, strict fluid input and output monitoring is needed during hysteroscopic myomectomy. Bipolar systems use saline as the distension media. They cannot prevent fluid overload but only help to avoid the hyponatremic and neurologic complications of glycine.

Submucosal Fibroids

❑ Resection:
  ❖ When resecting a fibroid, limit the resection to only the fibroid without resecting the adjoining endometrial tissue. After part of the fibroid is removed, the intramural portion of the fibroid inverts into the endometrial cavity. The loop can often be used to separate the fibroid from the pseudocapsule, often called cold-loop resection, facilitating its removal and helping to identify normal myometrium and endometrium to avoid coagulation (Figs 14A to D).
  ❖ Using the cutting mode at 80–100 watts provides clean cuts through the fibroid and facilitates a rapid technique.

❖ While resecting the myoma, always start at one side and move horizontally across to the other side. Digging deeply into one area of the fibroid causes the fibroid to fold over the hysteroscope causing loss of orientation. Remove small chips so that major amount of debris gets flushed away through the outflow channel. Overdilating the cervix allows escape of fluid from the sides of the hysteroscope along with small chips of the myoma and blood thus improving visualization.

❖ Whether using monopolar or bipolar current, strictly keep fluid pressure below 100–120 mm Hg to avoid excessive absorption. Gravity based systems with the irrigation bottle perforated with multiple large holes and placed at a height of 4–5 feet above patient level are often underutilized but may be ideal in this setting since it, although providing marginally less distension, is associated with significantly lesser fluid absorption. A TURP set allows two bottles to be simultaneously connected to the resectoscope and allows change of the irrigation bottles without frequent loss of distension.

❖ Obstructed visualization due to floating tissue fragments during resection can prove difficult and may necessitate catching the loose tissue with the loop electrode, removing the hysteroscope to grab the tissue, followed by reintroduction of the scope. The chips may also be removed with a sponge-holding forceps, lithotripsy forceps or an ovum forceps. To address this problem, the Bipolar Chip E-Vac System (Richard Wolf Medical Instruments Corporation, Vernon Hills, IL) has been introduced to the market (Fig. 15). The system uses a traditional resectoscope with an automatic chip aspirator and can be used with monopolar or bipolar current. A microprocessor controlled pump pulses at an adjustable level to aspirate chips out through an operative channel in the hysteroscope while preventing fluid losses and uterine collapse.

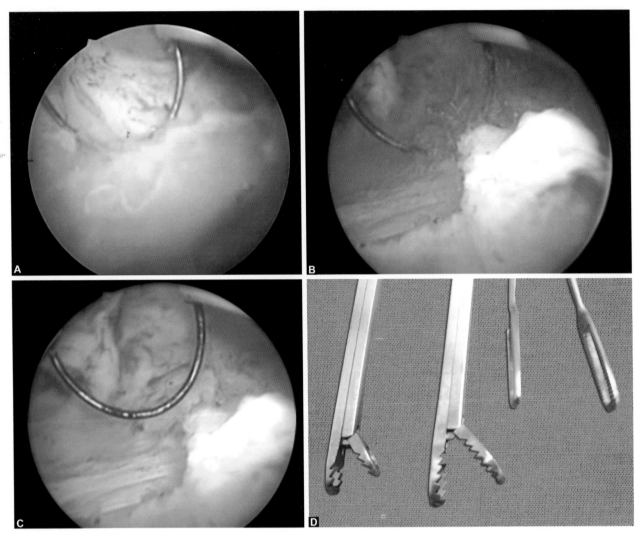

Figs 14A to D: (A) Resection of type 0 fibroid: (B) Working within pseudocapsule of fibroid; (C) Completion of resection of type 0 fibroid; (D) Instrument to remove fibroid pieces

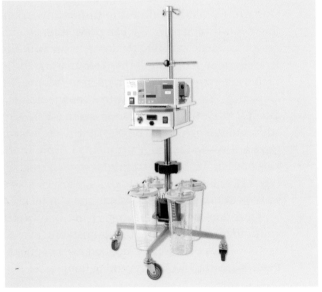

Fig. 15: Myosure tissue removal system

☐ Vaporization:
  ❖ Vaporization of a fibroid can also be performed through the use of a variety of different shaped electrodes. The chosen electrode is dragged along the surface of the myoma to directly vaporize the tissue. Perforation from prolonged use at one point can occur. However, tissue is destroyed and thus unavailable for pathologic examination (Figs 16A to C).
  ❖ The Gynecare Versapoint Bipolar Electrosurgery System (Johnson & Johnson Gateway LLC, Piscataway, NJ) provides the opportunity to use both a vaporizing electrode and resecting loop electrode with normal saline distention media for a variety of operative needs. Vaporizing electrode options include a ball or spring electrode for rapid vaporization and desiccation and a twizzle electrode for more precision.

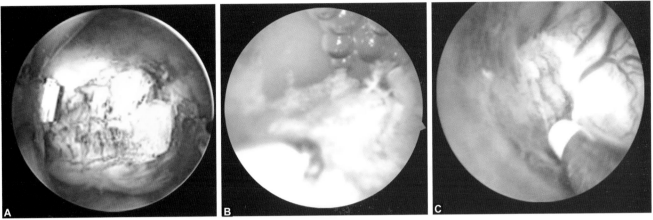

Figs 16A to C: (A) Fibroid vaporized with bipolar electrode; (B) Fibroid vaporized with bipolar spring electrode; (C) Bipolar twizzle electrode to detach fibroid

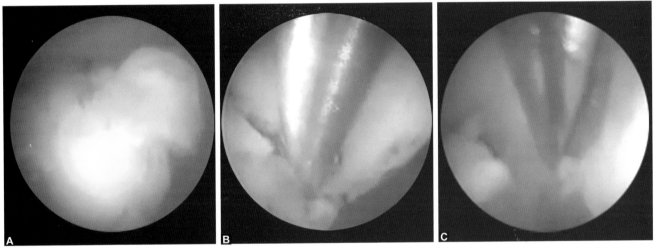

Figs 17A to C: (A) Small type 0 fibroid; (B) Hysteroscopic scissors used to cut base of fibroid; (C) Myoma completely detached from base

❖ Fibroids smaller than 2 cm can be vaporized with an Nd:YAG laser. The laser fiber is dragged over the surface of the fibroid until it is completely ablated. The tissue is not available for pathology evaluation.

❑ Excision with scissors:

❖ Small submucous myomas type 0 or I can be excised from its basal attachment with hysteroscopic scissors. It would be advisable not to detach the myoma from its attachments completely leaving a few fibrous strands undivided (Figs 17A to C). This will allow easy removal of the tethered myoma with an ovum or lithotripsy forceps. Even if the fibroid is accidentally detached completely and cannot be grasped with a forceps it will be expelled from the cavity due to uterine contractions over the subsequent few days. Administering oral methylergometrine 0.25 mg two to three times daily for a couple of days will hasten the process. A small submucous fibroid less than 1 cm in diameter can also be twisted and removed with a hysteroscopic grasper (Figs 18A to C).

Fibroids with an Intramural Component

Resection of the intramural component of type II or III fibroids is associated with the greatest risk of fluid intravasation and decreases the chance per procedure of achieving complete resection.[13] Resection of a completely intramural fibroid poses the risk of intravasation of media due to prolonged procedure time.[25]

❑ Resection:

❖ After initial excision of the intracavitary portion of the fibroid, the intramural component will typically expel into the cavity, but the volume of the remaining intramural fibroid will subsequently increase.

❖ Complete electrosurgical excision of the fibroid, including the intramural component is associated

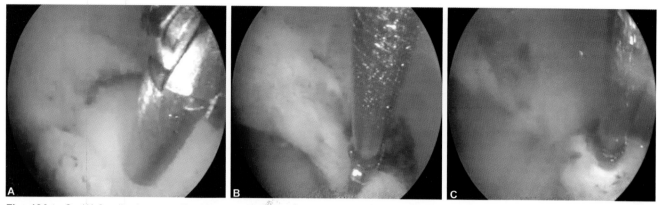

Figs 18A to C: (A) Small submucous fibroid held with grasper; (B) Fibroid twisted out of its attachment with hysteroscopic grasper; (C) Fibroid detached completely from its attachment

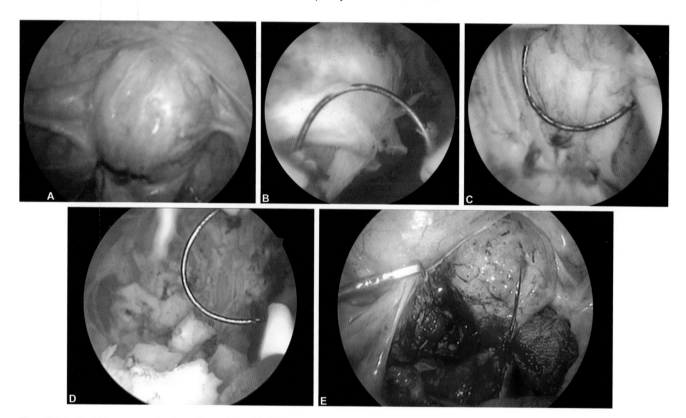

Figs 19A to E: (A) Laparoscopic view of type 2 fibroid; (B) Beginning of resection of a type 2 fibroid; (C) Retrograde dissection of fibroid working within the pseudocapsule; (D) Completion of procedure. *Note* the pink striated myometrium; (E) Laparoscopic view of uterus after resection of a type 2 fibroid

with increased risk of perforation, bleeding, thermal damage and fluid absorption (Figs 19A to E).

❖ Traditionally, the fibroid is removed in two stages. At the first procedure, as much fibroid as can be excised is removed with a Loop electrode. Repeatedly increasing and reducing the intrauterine pressure often pushes the intramural component into the cavity facilitating excision (hydrostatic massage). Concomitant administration of methylergometrine

or misoprostol induces uterine contractions and may facilitate extrusion of the intramural component. A GnRH analogue depot is administered for 1–2 doses. This will shrink the fibroid and propel the intramural component of the fibroid into the cavity turning it into a type I myoma which can be removed via a second stage hysteroscopic resection.

❖ Alternatively, the capsule of the myoma may be cut away from myometrium with a resectoscope to prevent the fibroid from sinking into the muscular layer, followed by grasping of the myoma with graspers. Rotation can then be used to pull the myoma into the intrauterine cavity.[26] This is accomplished under ultrasonographic guidance.

❏ Cold loop: The surgeon first excises the intracavitary portion of the fibroid and then uses a loop, not connected to an electrical source, for blunt dissection. The loop is used to mechanically create a plane between the fibroid and myometrium. Once the fibroid is detached from the myometrium, it can then be removed in pieces.[12]

❏ Toto enucleation: An elliptic incision is made in the endometrial mucosa covering the fibroid until the cleavage zone of the myoma and myometrium is reached. Tissue bridges between the myoma and muscle fibers are resected with electrocautery, resulting in protrusion of the fibroid into the uterine cavity. Myomectomy can then be completed by slicing.[27]

■ HYSTEROSCOPIC MORCELLATION

Hysteroscopic loop-electrode resectoscopy is a reliable method for removing submucous fibroids but problems with distension media, risks of perforation with an electrosurgical device and visual field limitation created by resected chips suggested the need to investigate alternative treatment methods. Using a modified prototype based on an orthopedic arthroscopic tissue shaver, Dr Mark Hans Emanuel of The Netherlands was able to create a first-generation device that used mechanical energy rather than electrical energy to resect uterine tissue.

In 2005, the US Food and Drug Administration (FDA) approved the TRUCLEAR hysteroscopic morcellator (Smith & Nephew, Andover, MA) as the first mechanical morcellator for intrauterine pathology. This device uses a single-use rigid metal inner tube with cutting edges that rotate and/or reciprocate within a 4-mm rigid metal outer tube. The outer tube incorporates a side-facing cutting window at its distal end. The blade assembly is secured to a reusable hand piece to which a suction tube is attached. The hand piece is also connected to a motor control unit. Suction is applied to the inner tube and tissue is then pulled into the cutting window as the inner tube rotates at 1,100 rpm. The resected tissue is then aspirated through the device into a collecting pouch for later histopathologic analysis. The entire device is introduced into the uterine cavity with a custom-designed 9-mm outer diameter, rigid, continuous-flow, 0 degree hysteroscope that requires a custom-designed high-flow Smith & Nephew fluid pump for proper functioning.[28]

In 2009, the FDA approved a second hysteroscopic morcellation device the MyoSure Tissue Removal System (Hologic, Bedford, MA). Like the first generation TRUCLEAR, the second generation MyoSure system relies on a suction-based, mechanical energy, rotating tubular cutter system to remove intrauterine tissue. However, the newer MyoSure system has a smaller 2.5-mm inner blade that rotates and reciprocates within a 3-mm outer tube at a speed as high as 6,000 rpm and presents an outer bevel rather than an inner bevel on the rotating blade edge.[18] The blade and hand piece are combined into a single-use device that is then attached to suction and a motor control unit. The device is introduced into the uterus through a 6.25-mm offset lens; custom-designed continuous flow hysteroscope that is compatible with all currently available fluid management systems (Figs 20 and 21).[29]

Newer devices for hysteroscopic mechanical morcellation such as the Bigati shaver (Karl Storz, GmBH, Germany) are being introduced into the market. Their performance vis-à-vis the first generation devices are yet to be evaluated.

Hysteroscopic Morcellation Technique

It is important to remember that the myoma must be thought of in terms of 3D rather than 2D measurements. Thus, increasing myoma diameter yields an exponential rather than linear increase in volume following the equation Volume = $\pi d^3/6$. With loop resectoscopy, the amount of tissue removed per minute will depend on how quickly the surgeon deploys each pass of the loop, how much tissue each bite with the loop resects and how quickly the tissue chips can be removed from the uterine cavity. With hysteroscopic morcellation, the amount of tissue removed per minute will only be a function of how much contact the cutting window maintains with the myoma and how quickly the device can cut tissue and aspirate it out (Figs 22A to D). Because the devices cutting speed are relatively fixed by their design characteristics, minimizing procedure time mostly depends on maintaining tissue contact between the cutting window and the pathology.

For polyps and Type I and Type II submucous myomas, hysteroscopic morcellation has been demonstrated to be both faster and easier to learn than traditional resectoscopy. The earliest published trial with a hysteroscopic morcellation device by Emanuel and colleagues showed a significant reduction in operating room time when removing polyps and Type I and Type II submucous myomas.[28] In that study, polyps were removed with a 72% reduction in operating room time with a morcellator as compared with a resectoscope (8.7 min vs 30.9 min),

	MyoSure LITE	MyoSure	MyoSure XL
Tissue recommended	Polyps ≤ 3 cm	All polyps Fibrolds ≤ 3 cm	All intrauterine pathology including large fibroisa (any fibroid where you want to experience cutting efficiency)
Scope compatibility	MyoSure, MySure XL	MyoSure, MyoSure XL	MyoSure XL
Blade material	Stalneless steel	Coated atainless steel with ultra hardness and high wear resistance	Coated stainless steel with ultra hardness and high wear resistance
Performance specification	3 cm polyp ≤ minutes	3 cm fibroid ≤ 10 minutes	5 cm fibrid ≤ 15 minutes
Tissue removal rate	7.0 g/min (polyp tissue)	1.5 g/min (fibrold tissue)	4.3 g/min (fibrid tissue)
Window size	31 mm^3	54 mm^3	98 mm^3
Blade window	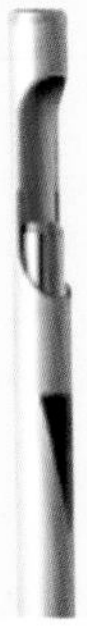	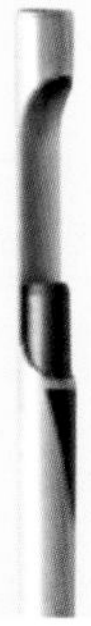	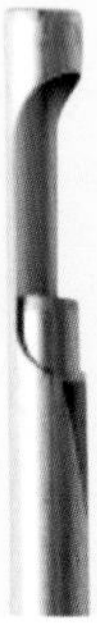

Fig. 20: Types of myosure

Comparison of device characteristics of Truclear™ Hysteroscopic Morcellator and MyspSure tissue removal system		
Morecellator characteristic	Truclear	MyoSure
Device outer diameter	4 mm	3 mm
Hysteroscope outer diameter	9 mm	6.25 mm
Pump compatibility	Smith and nephew pump	Any fluid management system
Blade rotational speed	100 rpm	6000 rpm
Blade edge	Inner bevel	Outer bevel
Maximum rate of suction	200 mm Hg	400 mm Hg

Truclear™ hysterosecopic morcellator (Smith and nephrew Andover MA)
MyoSure tissue removal system (Hologic bedford MA)

Fig. 21: Truclear hologic comparison

whereas Type 0 and Type I myomas were removed in 61% less time, respectively (16.4 min vs 42.2 min).[19] Similarly, in a 2008 trial by van Dongen and associates, 60 patients with intrauterine pathology consisting of either a polyp or a Type 0 myoma or Type I myoma smaller than 30 mm were randomized to either hysteroscopic morcellation or loop-electrode resection.[30] All the procedures were performed by residents in training under the direct guidance of an attending physician. The morcellation group demonstrated a 38% reduction in operating room (OR) time (17 min vs 10.6 min; P = 0.008) as well as a 32% reduction in distention media used (5,050 mL vs 3,413 mL; P = 0.041). Not surprisingly, the trial also demonstrated a marked reduction in the number of insertions and reinsertions of

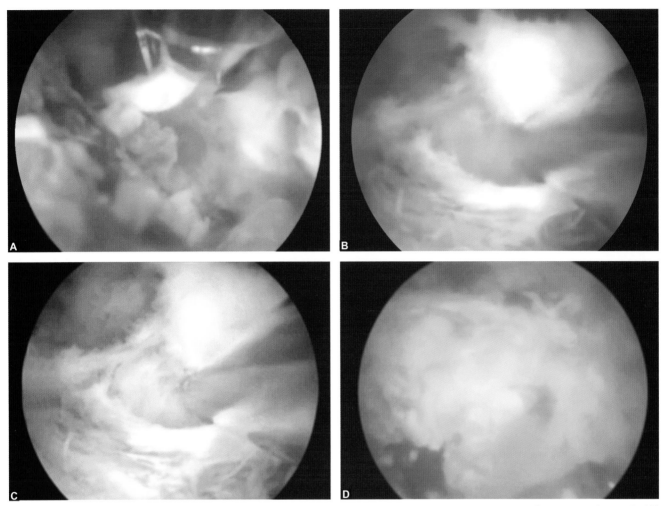

Figs 22A to D: (A) Intrauterine morcellator reciprocating blade; (B) Intrauterine morcellator lifting out a type 1 myoma from its pseudocapsule; (C) Intrauterine dissecting out a type 1 myoma from its pseudocapsule; (D) Completion of myoma morcellation. *Note* the absence of major bleeding

the hysteroscope to remove chips when the morcellator was used (number of insertions = 1) compared with the resectoscope (number of insertions = 7.2).

With the MyoSure system, Miller and coworkers reported average polyp morcellation time of 37 seconds and average myoma morcellation time of 6.4 minutes for Type 0, I and II myomas with a mean diameter of 31.7 mm.[31] These data were further validated in a recent abstract by Lukes, who reported using the MyoSure device to remove 6 myomas (average 3 cm) and 20 polyps in 13 women with a mean resection time of 84 seconds.[29] All 13 procedures were performed in an office setting using local anesthesia with average pain scores less than 1 using the Wong-Baker Faces Rating Scale (no pain = 0; worst pain = 10).

Studies have shown that both devices are capable of resecting submucous myomas 3 cm in diameter in 15 minutes or less, although the MyoSure device was consistently faster at tissue removal at every time interval despite its smaller diameter. In addition, the smaller diameter of the MyoSure hysteroscope (6.25 mm) compared

with the TRUCLEAR hysteroscope (9.0 mm) makes the MyoSure device potentially more compatible with an oral sedation/cervical block anesthesia protocol and therefore amenable to office-based treatments of polyps and Type 0 or I submucosal fibroids.[29]

HYSTEROSCOPIC RESECTION OF INTRAMURAL MYOMAS

Hysteroscopic resection of intramural myomas is a relatively new concept in gynecological endoscopy. The procedure involves localizing the intramural myoma with intraoperative ultrasound and incising the endometrium and thin layer of myometrium over the myoma with a hysteroscopic scissors or Collins knife. When the pseudocapsule of the myoma is penetrated and the fibrous attachments to the myoma divided, the myoma often protrudes into the cavity. This can be accelerated by hydrostatic massage (repeatedly increasing and decreasing intrauterine pressure by manipulating the inflow) or external bimanual massage of the uterus (Figs 23A and B). Intracervical or intramyometrial infiltration of 15-methyl PGF2 alpha, preoperative oral misoprostol (200–400 micrograms) or intramyometrial methylergometrine may aid this process. If this does not happen, a laparoscopic 5 mm myoma screw may be introduced under vision besides a diagnostic hysteroscope, the screw partially driven into the myoma (complete insertion may push the tip beyond the myoma and into the myometrium on the opposite side and interfere with delivery) and with gradual traction on the screw the myoma drawn into the endometrial cavity (Figs 24A to H). This converts the type III (ESGE-FIGO classification) into a type 0/I myoma which can be resected with a resectoscope or intrauterine morcellator.

This technique is suited for a myoma less than 5 cm and one which is placed either at the fundus or upper part of the anterior or posterior walls preferably close to the endometrium on ultrasound. The advantages of this procedure include avoidance of an intra-abdominal scar, minimum damage to the myometrium. The defect in the endometrium and myometrium immediately seals off with virtually no bleeding when the distended cavity collapses. The disadvantage of this procedure includes possibility of abandoning the procedure in case of excessive fluid absorption or perforation thus inviting the possibility of a repeat hysteroscopic procedure.

POSTOPERATIVE ADHESION PREVENTION

Prevention of postoperative adhesion formation begins with minimizing endometrial and myometrial trauma during the initial hysteroscopic procedure. The incidence of intrauterine adhesions following hysteroscopic myomectomy is 1.5% with the incidence rising to 78% following resection of multiple and opposing surface myomas (Fig. 25).[24]

A No. 8 Foley's catheter placed into the uterine cavity with the balloon inflated with 3–4 ml saline provides an adequate barrier in keeping the endometrial surfaces apart. If an intrauterine barrier is used, antibiotic prophylaxis such as doxycycline or a combination of ofloxacin with ornidazole should be considered for the duration of the stent placement.[32]

Historically, estrogen has been administered following hysteroscopic surgery to encourage endometrial regrowth across the operated surface. The estrogens used include estradiol valerate 2 mg 2–3 times daily, ethinyl estradiol 0.05 mg per day or conjugated estrogens 0.625 mg twice daily for 30 days with a progestogen administered for the last 5–10 days to induce withdrawal bleeding. Currently, the role of estrogen is being questioned.

Intrauterine use of auto-cross-linked hyaluronic acid gel has also been examined in prevention of intrauterine adhesions after hysteroscopic surgery. Administration of 10 ml of gel after adhesiolysis or hysteroscopic surgery for intrauterine lesions may be associated with a significant reduction in the development and severity of de novo adhesions.[33] Long-term reproductive outcomes are not yet available.

Cook Women's Health makes a triangular balloon catheter that may improve separation of the uterine walls at the cornua during the healing phase.

COMPLICATIONS

Major complications during and following hysteroscopy are fortunately, extremely rare. The most common

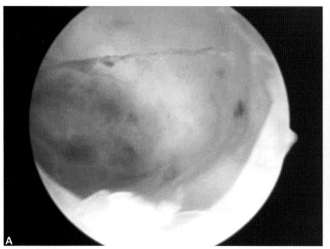
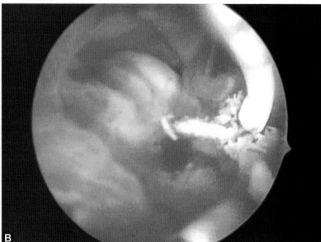

Figs 23A and B: (A) Apparently empty cavity; (B) Fibroid popping into the cavity after hydrostatic massage

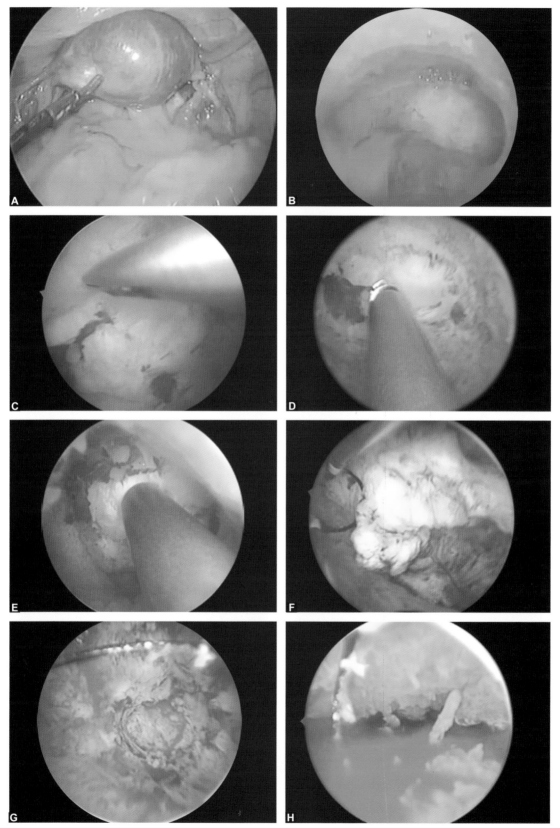

Figs 24A to H: (A) Laparoscopic view (USG showed a fundal 4 cm fibroid); (B) Normal uterine cavity; (C) Incision of fundus with hysteroscopic scissors to reach the fibroid; (D) Laparoscopic 5 mm myoma screw inserted alongside a diagnostic hysteroscopy sheath; (E) Fibroid being pulled into cavity and converted into type 0 fibroid; (F) Resection of myoma; (G) Completion of procedure; (H) *Note* how the fibroid cavity collapses on reducing intrauterine pressure

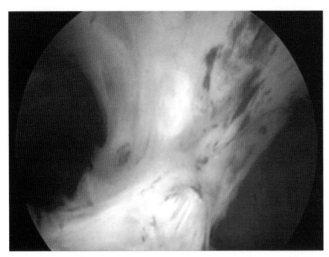

Fig. 25: Intrauterine adhesions following hysteroscopic myomectomy with incompletely resected myoma

complications are bleeding and uterine trauma. The incidence of major and minor complications during surgical hysteroscopy is 3.8%.[32]

Mechanical Complications

Perforation and cervical trauma occur in approximately 0.7–0.8% of cases and commonly occur during cervical dilatation and sometimes during resection of large type II or III fibroid (Figs 26A and B).[34] Risk factors for perforation include cervical stenosis, severe uterine anteflexion or retroflexion and distortion of the cervical canal due to lower segment fibroids.[33]

Cervical lacerations can occur from tearing of the single-toothed tenaculum from the cervix. This can be prevented by using a relatively atraumatic instrument, such as a double-toothed tenaculum, vulsellum, Allis forceps or a ringed forceps. Preoperative misoprostol reduces cervical resistance to dilatation and reduces cervical trauma. In addition, ultrasonographic guidance may help to direct dilating maneuvers. Use of the small-diameter and flexible hysteroscopes limits the need for excessive dilation.

Uterine perforations may occur during operative procedures. During resection of a fundal or cornual fibroid, care should be taken at the cornua and the lateral walls because these are the thinnest portion of the myometrium. A small midline or fundal injury with a blunt instrument does not have clinical significance if bleeding is minimal, but large rents or those caused by sharp or electrosurgical instruments may result in a need for diagnostic laparoscopy to completely evaluate the patient for bleeding or visceral injury. If a laparoscope is available, the rent should be sutured with one or two sutures of 1-0 Polyglactin 910 since this area may invite adhesion formation and may be a potential weakness in the myometrium during future pregnancies. Lateral perforations involve risk of injury to vessels and warrant an operative laparoscopy or laparotomy.

Uterine perforation with an electrosurgical instrument requires immediate exploration with a laparoscope or laparotomy. The risks of peritonitis, sepsis and death are most often associated with unrecognized and untreated thermal injuries to the viscera. The bowel should be inspected for signs of injury and a surgical consultation is mandatory.

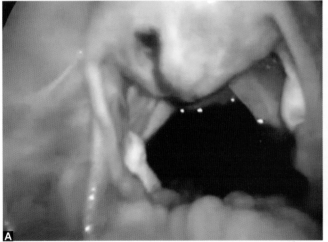
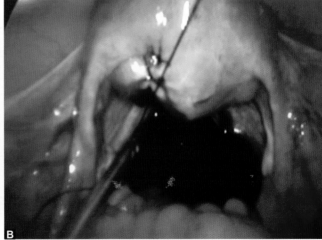

Figs 26A and B: (A) Uterine perforation during myomectomy; (B) The myomectomy may be completed using lower distention pressure after suturing the perforation

Media-related Complications

The risk of absorption of media is minimal under normal operative conditions. Risk factors for clinically significant intravasation of fluid include prolonged operative procedures, the use of large volumes of low-viscosity media, or the resection of fibroids or myometrial trauma that results in open uterine venous channels or unidentified perforations.[34] Intravasation can occur when the intrauterine pressure is greater than the patient's mean arterial pressure.[35]

Fluid overload is rare with electrolyte-containing fluids. It is treated with diuretics and restriction of intravenous fluids. On the contrary, nonelectrolyte, hypotonic media, which are nonconductive, are often used for the prolonged, complicated electrosurgical procedures. When large volumes of these solutions are absorbed, subsequent hyponatremia, hypervolemia, hypotension, pulmonary edema, cerebral edema and cardiovascular collapse can occur. For every liter of hypotonic media absorbed, the patient's serum sodium decreases by 10 mEq/L. If the patient's sodium level is less than 120 mEq/L, she is at risk for generalized cerebral edema, seizures and even death. in general, if a fluid deficit is greater than 1,500 ml or if the sodium level is less than 125 mEq/L, the procedure should be terminated. Mannitol (5%) has the safest adverse-effect profile because it can maintain a patient's osmolality despite hyponatremia, improving neurologic outcomes.[36]

If the patient's sodium osmolality is less than 125 mOsm, forced diuresis with furosemide (Lasix) 40 mg IV, fluid restriction, and administration of 3% sodium chloride at a rate to correct hyponatremia by 1.5–2.0 mOsm/L/h is required with half hourly monitoring of serum sodium levels and osmolality. Rapid correction of hyponatremia should be avoided to prevent central pontine myelinolysis. The osmolality should not be corrected above 135 mOsm.

With Dextran 70, maximal absorption should not exceed 500 ml. Dextran 70 overload does not respond to diuretic treatment because the kidneys poorly excrete Dextran 70. Plasmapheresis may be necessary.[37]

Other complications of Dextran 70 include anaphylaxis (1 in 1,500–300,000 cases), pulmonary edema and DIC. Treatment of anaphylaxis includes administration of epinephrine, hydrocortisone, and fluid and ventilatory support.[33,38]

Bleeding

Bleeding during or after surgery occurs in 0.25% of all cases.[37] GnRH analogues and paracervical or intrauterine injection of vasopressin reduce the incidence of postoperative bleeding. If bleeding persists after surgery, a 30-mL No.8 or 10 Foley catheter balloon filled with 15–30 mL of fluid can be inserted into the cavity. This balloon can be removed after 24 hours. Antibiotic prophylaxis should be given if a foreign body is placed in the uterus. Methylergometrine or misoprostol may be used to induce uterine contractions and hemostasis but their value is uncertain. Uterine artery embolization of the uterine artery or hysterectomy is the last line of management. Hysterectomy is rarely warranted.

Infection

Infection is a rare complication of hysteroscopy. Infection can be suspected on the basis of clinical symptoms (pelvic pain, fever, localized lower abdominal guarding and cervical movement tenderness and investigations (neutrophil leukocytosis, free fluid in POD on ultrasound). Postoperative infections can be treated with a combination of ceftriaxone or cefoperazone, amikacin and metronidazole. Response to therapy can be monitored with evaluation of clinical symptoms.[36,37,39]

▌TRAINING IN HYSTEROSCOPIC MYOMECTOMY

Hyteroscopic myomectomy is probably the most difficult of all hysteroscopic surgeries requiring genuine surgical skill, patience and intense monitoring during the procedure. World over there is a dearth of adequate endoscopic training due to lack of adequate number of cases in developed countries and lack of training facilities in the developing nations. In training institutions in the developed world, residents do only about 10 hysteroscopic procedures per resident per year.[40]

Endoscopic simulators are a useful method of training gynecologists in endoscopy and especially complicated procedures such as hysteroscopic myomectomy (Figs 27A to C). Studies have confirmed that hysteroscopic simulators with feedback protocols help develop surgical skills rapidly among novice hysteroscopic surgeons and also help improve surgical safety profile in already established hysteroscopic surgeons.[41]

Unfortunately, the exorbitant costs of these simulators have ensured that they are available for use only at limited training institutes across the world.

▌CONCLUSION

Hysteroscopy has revolutionized the management of uterine pathology such as submucous fibroids and

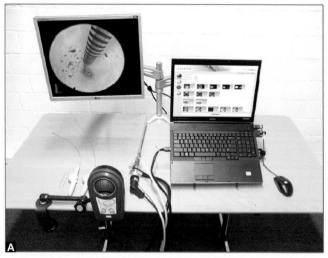

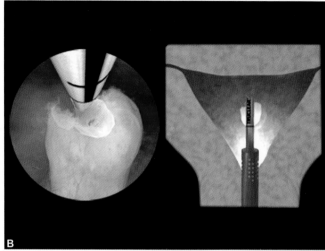

Diagnostic intervention Report
Scene: Diagnosis
show intervention movie

Visualization	Achieved	Goal
Visualized surface	69.3%	> 85%
Left tube visualized	0:09	> 0:01
Right tube visualized	0:13	> 0:01
Upper cavum visualized	0:04	> 0:01
Time out of focus	0:14	> 0:01
Ergonomics	**Achieved**	**Goal**
Intervention time	1:30	< 2:00
View horizon unstable	0:39	< 0:15
pa:h length	52.2 cm	< 50 cm
Safety	**Achieved**	**Goal**
Time coliding	0:00	< 0:01
Fluid hardling	**Achieved**	**Goal**
Distension media needed	314 ml	> 500 ml
Time view obscured	0:23	> 0:20
Time uterus collapsed	0:02	> 0:10
Number of spoil cycles	5	

Uterus surface visulization

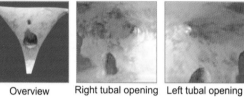

Overview Right tubal opening Left tubal opening Anterior wall

Diagnosis path

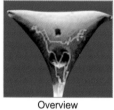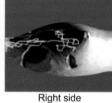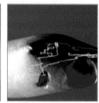

Overview Right side Left side

Figs 27A to C: (A) VR simulator; (B) Virtual reality image; (C) VR report

intramural fibroids encroaching on the uterine cavity not only in terms of their diagnosis and management but also offering a roadmap for development of other groundbreaking minimally invasive therapies such as the intrauterine morcellator.

While developing newer therapies, it is important to understand the technical aspect of complex instrumentation and the changes induced by such treatment in human physiology. This helps not only to optimize therapy but to maximize safety of surgery.

"Man has reached a stage where he evolves through his machines."

Gene Wolfe (1972)

■ REFERENCES

1. Gross KL, Morton CC. Genetics and the development of fibroids. Clin Obstet Gynecol. 2001;44(2):335-49.
2. Clevenger-Hoeft M, Syrop CH, Stovall DW, et al. Sonohysterography in premenopausal women with and without abnormal bleeding. Obstet Gynecol. 1999;94:516-20.
3. Brosens I, Deprest J, Dal Cin P, et al. Clinical significance of cytogenetic abnormalities in uterine myomas. Fertile Steril. 1998;69:232-5.
4. Brosens J, Campo R, Gordts S, et al. Submucous and outer myometrium leiomyomas are two distinct clinical entities. Fertil Steril. 2003;79:1452-4.

5. Rackow BW, Taylor HS. Submucosal uterine leiomyomas have a global effect on molecular determinants of endometrial receptivity. Fertil Steril. 2010;93:2027-34.

6. Van Dongen H, de Kroon CD, Jacobi CE, et al. Diagnostic hysteroscopy in abnormal uterine bleeding: a systematic review and meta-analysis. BJOG. 2007;114:664-75.

7. Emmanuel MH, Verdel MJC, et al. An audit of true prevalence of intrauterine pathology: the hysteroscopical findings controlled the patient selection in 1202 patients with abnormal uterine bleeding. Gynaecol Endosc. 1995;4:237-41.

8. Lasmar RB, Dias R, Barrozo PR, et al. Prevalence of hysteroscopic findings and histological diagnosis in patients with abnormal uterine bleeding. Fertil Steril. 2008;89:1803-7.

9. Stovall DW. Clinical symptomatology of uterine leiomyomas. Clin Obstet Gynecol. 2001;44(2):364-71.

10. Donnez J, Jadoul P. What are the implications of myomas on fertility? A need for a debate? Hum Reprod. 2002;17(6):1424-30.

11. Practice Committee of American. Society for Reproductive Medicine in collaboration with Society of Reproductive Surgeons. Myomas and reproductive function. Fertil Steril. 2008;90(5 Suppl):S125-30.

12. Di Spiezio Sardo A, Mazzon I, Bramante S, et al. Hysteroscopic myomectomy: a comprehensive review of surgical techniques. Hum Reprod Update. 2008;14(2):101-19.

13. Emanuel MH, Wamsteker K, Hart AA, et al. Long term results of hysteroscopic myomectomy for abnormal uterine bleeding. Obstet Gynecol. 1999;93:743-8.

14. Fernandez H, Sefrioui O, Virelizier C, et al. Hysteroscopic resection of submucosal myomas in patients with infertility. Human Reproduction. 2001;16:1489-92.

15. Pritts EA, Parker WH, Olive DL. Fibroids and infertility: an updated systematic review of the evidence. Fertil Steril. 2009;91:1215-23.

16. Klatsky PC, Tran ND, Caughey AB, et al. Fibroids and reproductive outcomes: a systematic review from conception to delivery. Am J Obstet Gynecol. 2008;198:357-66.

17. Hunt RE, Siegler AM. Uterine tumors. In: Hunt RE, Siegler AM (Eds). Hysterosalpingography: Techniques and Interpretation. Year Book Medical Publishers Inc.; 1990. pp. 65-84.

18. Merchant SA, Sarvagod TV. Normal pelvic anatomy and endosonographic scanning techniques. Ind J Med Ultrasound. 1994;11:1-7.

19. Cicinelli E, Romano F, Anastasio PS, et al. Transabdominal sonohysterography, transvaginal sonography, and hysteroscopy in the evaluation of submucous myomas. Obstet Gynecol. 1995;85:42-7.

20. Shimizu B, Fukuda K, Yomura W, et al. Transvaginal hysterosonography for differential diagnosis between submucous and intramural myoma. Gynecol Obstet Invest. 1993;35:236-9.

21. Bradley LD, Falcone T, Magen AB. Radiographic imaging techniques for the diagnosis of abnormal uterine bleeding. Obstet Gynecol Clin N Am. 2000;27(2):245-76.

22. Weinraub Z, Herman A. Three dimensional hysterosonography. In: Merz E (Ed). 3-D Ultrasound in Obstetrics and Gynecology. Philadelphia: Lippincott Williams and Wilkins; 1998. pp. 57-64.

23. Parent B, Guedj H, Barbot J, et al. Uterine leiomyomas. In: Parent B, Guedj H, Barbot J, Nodarian P (Eds). Panoramic Hysteroscopy. Baltimore: Williams and Wilkins; 1987. pp. 39-46.

24. American Association of Gynecologic Laparoscopists (AAGL): Advancing Minimally Invasive Gynecology Worldwide. AAGL Practice Report: Practice guidelines for the diagnosis and management of submucous leiomyomas. J Min Invasive Gynecol. 2012;19:152-71.

25. Vercellini P, Zaina B, Yaylayan L, et al. Hysteroscopic myomectomy: long-term effects on menstrual pattern and fertility. Obstet Gynecol. 1999;94(3):341-7.

26. Lin B, Akiba Y, Iwata Y. One-step hysteroscopic removal of sinking submucous myoma in two infertile patients. Fertil Steril. 2000;74(5):1035-8.

27. Litta P, Cosmi E, Sacco G, et al. Hysteroscopic permanent tubal sterilization using a nitinol-dacron intratubal device without anaesthesia in the outpatient setting: procedure feasibility and effectiveness. Hum Reprod. 2005;20(12):3419-22.

28. Emanuel MH, Wamsteker K. The intra uterine morcellator: a new hysteroscopic operating technique to remove intrauterine polyps and myomas. J Min Invasive Gynecol. 2005;12:62-6.

29. Lukes AS. MyoSure tissue removal system-comparative sedation study in an office setting. J Min Invasive gynecol. 2007;17(6):S67.

30. Van Dongen H, Emanuel MH, Wolterbeek R, et al. Hysteroscopic morcellator for removal of intrauterine polyps and myomas: a randomized controlled pilot study among residents in training. J Min Invasive Gynecol. 2008;15:466-71.

31. Miller C, Glazerman L, et al. Clinical evaluation of a new hysteroscopic morcellator-retrospective case review. J Med. 2009;2:163-6.

32. March CM. Hysteroscopy. J Reprod Med. 1992;37(4):293-311.

33. Bosteels J, Weyers S, Mol BW, et al. Anti-adhesion barrier gels following operative hysteroscopy for treating female infertility: a systematic review and meta-analysis. Gynecol Surg. 2014;11:113-27.

34. Jansen FW, Vredevoogd CB, van Ulzen K, et al. Complications of hysteroscopy: a prospective, multicenter study. Obstet Gynecol. 2000;96(2):266-70.

35. Morrison DM. Management of hysteroscopic surgery complications. AORN J. 1999;69(1):194-7, 199-209; quiz 210, 213-5, 21.

36. Cooper JM, Brady RM. Late complications of operative hysteroscopy. Obstet Gynecol Clin North Am. 2000;27(2):367-74.

37. Borten M, Seibert CP, Taymor ML. Recurrent anaphylactic reaction to intraperitoneal dextran 75 used for prevention of postsurgical adhesions. Obstet Gynecol. 1983;61(6): 755-7.

38. Jedeikin R, Olsfanger D, Kessler I. Disseminated intravascular coagulopathy and adult respiratory distress syndrome: life-threatening complications of hysteroscopy. Am J Obstet Gynecol. 1990;162(1):44-5.

39. Gimpelson RJ. Hysteroscopic treatment of the patient with intracavitary pathology (myomectomy/polypectomy). Obstet Gynecol Clin North Am. 2000;27(2):327-37.

40. Miller CE. Training in minimally invasive surgery—you say you want a revolution. J Min Invasive Gynecol. 2009;16(2):113-20.

41. Janse JA, Ruben S, et al. Hysteroscopic sterilization using a virtual reality simulator: assessment of learning curve. J Min Invasive Gynecol. 2013;20:775-82.

CHAPTER 25

Complications in Hysteroscopic Surgery— Prevention and Management

Vivek Salunke, Shinjini Pande

■ INTRODUCTION

It would not be an understatement to say that hysteroscopy—both diagnostic and operative—has evolved in modern gynecology not as an alternative method of diagnosis and surgery, but as a philosophy and science which has changed the whole dimension of surgical approach, management and patient care.

In this era of evidence-based medicine, what could be more than direct visualization of pathology and also its treatment in most cases.

The ability to perform surgery within the intracavitary space is minimally invasive in the true sense.

As the spectrum of operative hysteroscopy is expanding concern about the early recognition and management of complications associated and risks involved must be highlighted upon. As a growing number of physicians endeavor to perform more advanced hysteroscopic surgeries the significance of complications also rises. Keen vigilance, high index of suspicion and good operative skills are an integral part of operative hysteroscopy which will minimize risks in surgery and ensure good outcome.

To start with, there is an exaggerated fear of complications associated with hysteroscopy.

American Association of Gynecologic Laparoscopists (AAGL) surveyed its members in 1993 and found a complication rate of only 2% for operative hysteroscopy.[1] The risk with diagnostic procedures is very low and is more with operative procedures. (Complication rate quoted in various studies varies from 0.95% to 3% of cases).[2-4] Similarly, a large multicentric trial of 13,600 procedures in Netherland found a higher complication with operative procedures (0.95%) than diagnostic procedures (0.13%).[3]

Complications cannot be avoided completely and may occur even when a procedure is done correctly by an experienced surgeon. However, they are more likely if techniques and equipment used are improper.

The rate of major complications i.e., *perforation, hemorrhage, fluid overload, bowel/urogenital injury comprises less than 1% of cases.*

Despite the encouraging figures the sad fact is that only 30% gynecologists perform operative hysteroscopic procedures.

Broadly any complication could be due to—
❑ Lack of informed consent or counseling
❑ Improper surgical techniques or lack of skill
❑ Improper use of equipment and instruments
❑ Incorrectly chosen patients
   ❖ Poor surgical candidates who may go into fluid overload easily due to preexisting cardiac diseases etc.
   ❖ Patients having conditions like acute pelvic inflammatory disease (PID), genital tract malignancy, pregnancy, acutely stenotic cervical os
❑ Lack of trained staff who are not familiar with equipment or procedure.

■ PREOPERATIVE PRECAUTIONS

The general complication rate can be made to decrease by following a few simple protocols:
❑ Taking proper consent
❑ Adequate counseling of patients, for instance some patients may assume that amenorrhea achieved would be complete after endometrial ablation though in

practicality this might not be so. In some instances more than one hysteroscopic procedure may be required and patient might not be relieved with single procedure, e.g. large myoma, Asherman's syndrome

❑ Proper training of surgeon and also the staff especially those who maintain fluid monitoring system
❑ Using good equipment
❑ "Time out" before every operation is very useful in briefing everyone in the operation theater (OT) about the surgery and may be valuable in preventing errors.

CLASSIFICATION OF COMPLICATIONS

❑ Entry-related mechanical causes
  ❖ Entry-related trauma/perforation
  ❖ Failed Entry
❑ Method-related complications
  ❖ Technique related
    – Perforation
    – Intraoperative hemorrhage
    – Vasovagal attacks
    – Gas embolism
  ❖ Media-related complications
  ❖ Electromechanical burns
❑ Delayed postoperative complications
  ❖ Infections
  ❖ Endometrial cancer
  ❖ Iatrogenic adenomyosis
  ❖ Hematometra
  ❖ Postendometrial ablation tubal ligation syndrome
  ❖ Pregnancy-related concerns.

ENTRY-RELATED MECHANICAL CAUSES

Entry-related Trauma and Perforation

Cervical Laceration

This may occur at times and cause cumbersome bleeding. In such cases suture the cervix. Occasionally a touch of ball electrode at low power on coagulation mode can cause hemostasis.

Entry-related Perforations

These are generally caused by dilators or the hysteroscope itself when undue force is applied in the wrong direction. The management of these will be dealt in conjunction with technique-related perforations mentioned later.

It is important to remember that about 50% of perforations are made during entry.

Failed Entry (Flow chart 1)

Its causes are:
❑ Stenotic os, nulliparous cervix
❑ Menopausal flushed cervix
❑ Previous surgeries—cervical biopsy, cone biopsy, cryosurgeries
❑ Acute anteflexion or retroflexion
❑ Use of gonadotropin-releasing hormone (GnRH) agonists.

Acute Flexion Problems

These may be solved by giving good traction by vulsellum on the anterior lip of cervix in cases of acute anterior flexion or on posterior lip in retroflexion.

Also, compensatory hand movements, taking the guidance from the opening of the os as seen on the screen will help the surgeon to enter in the right direction.

Cervical Stenosis

❑ Some studies advocate the use of laminaria tents in the evening before surgery. But these may also cause false passages.[5]
❑ Alternatively cervical ripening drugs like Misoprostol either orally or vaginally can be used. Dosage is 200 mg vaginally or 400 mg orally before 8–12 hours before surgery.
❑ Intracervical injection of vasopressin 4 IU in 100 mL of normal saline (NS) is diluted and injected at 4 and 8 O'clock positions. This decreases the force needed to dilate markedly. Note: Half sized dilators should be used for smoother dilatation.
❑ Ed's solution: This causes very effective and smooth dilatation of the cervix. This is prepared by mixing 5 IU of vasopressin (one-fourth of an ampoule) with 30 mL of 1% lignocaine. Inject about 6–10 mL at 4 and 8 O'clock positions. In the author's own experience this works very effectively in dilating markedly stenotic cervical os also. Apart from easing out dilatation, it also reduces media absorption to about one-third and also causes lesser intraoperative bleeding.
❑ Ultrasonography (USG) guidance: In difficult cases USG guidance may be taken.
❑ Laparoscopic guidance: If concurrent laparoscopy is to be done, laparoscopic guidance may be helpful.

Flow chart 1: Troubleshooting difficult dilation

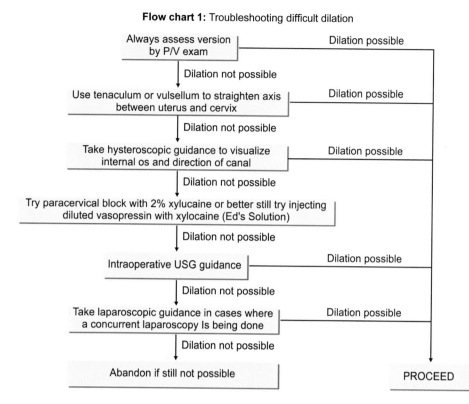

Always assess version by P/V exam → Dilation possible

Dilation not possible

Use tenaculum or vulsellum to straighten axis between uterus and cervix → Dilation possible

Dilation not possible

Take hysteroscopic guidance to visualize internal os and direction of canal → Dilation possible

Dilation not possible

Try paracervical block with 2% xylucaine or better still try injecting diluted vasopressin with xylocaine (Ed's Solution)

Dilation not possible

Intraoperative USG guidance → Dilation possible

Dilation possible

Take laparoscopic guidance in cases where a concurrent laparoscopy Is being done → Dilation possible

Dilation not possible

Abandon if still not possible

PROCEED

■ METHOD-RELATED COMPLICATIONS

Technique-Related Complications

Perforations (Figs 1 and 2)

In an AAGL survey[1] the rate of perforation was 14/1,000 cases. It was even more when procedures which required cuts to be made on lateral walls were done and also when fundal/lateral wall adhesions were released (2–3/100 cases).

Intraoperative perforations may be cold perforations as with cold scissors or with the hysteroscope itself or may be due to active energy source being used. And these may cause thermal energy-related damage.

Procedure-related risk of perforation: A multicentric study report[3] reported the following:

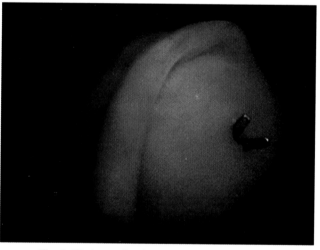

Fig. 1: Uterine perforation by hysteroscopic scissors

Procedure	Percentage (%)
Adhesiolysis	4.48
Transcervical resection of the endometrium (TCRE)	0.8
Myomectomy	0.75
Polyp removal	0.38

Analysis of other studies has also identified adhesiolysis as the one procedure which carries the highest risk that is 12 times as compared to polyp removal. Adhesiolysis has a statistically significant rate of complications as compared

to other procedures. Also noteworthy is the fact that many patients in the series received GnRH analogs so the uterine size was in postmenopausal range.

Risk factors associated with perforation (Figs 3A to E):
- ❏ Postmenopausal status
- ❏ Nulliparous status
- ❏ Postpartum status
- ❏ Small sized uterus due to other causes
  - ❖ Chronic anovulation
  - ❖ Pretreatment with GnRH agonists
  - ❖ History of uterine artery embolization

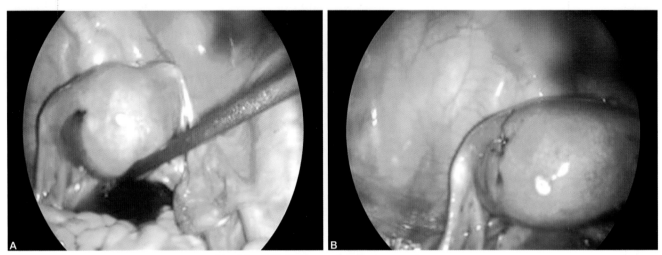

Figs 2A and B: Uterine perforation by resectoscope

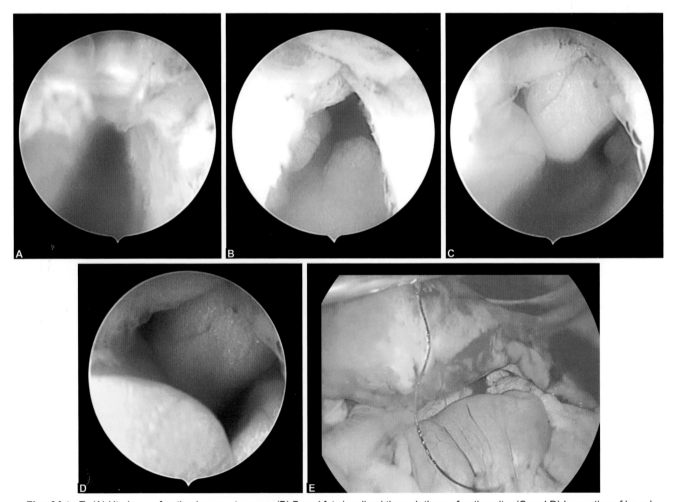

Figs 3A to E: (A) Uterine perforation by resectoscope; (B) Bowel fat visualized through the perforation site; (C and D) Inspection of bowel being done with the hysteroscope through the primary perforation site; (E) Laparoscopic evaluation and repair

❑ Surgery on the uterus
  ❖ Previous lower segment Cesarean section (LSCS)
  ❖ Previous myomectomy
  ❖ Previous cone biopsy
❑ Pelvic Koch's disease
❑ Endometrial cancer (friable uterus)
❑ Acutely retroverted uterus
❑ Operator related (undue force).

False passage: This is created in the cervical canal when scope enters in the wrong way (Fig. 4) or it may be created during hysteroscopic adhesiolysis when dissection of the adhesions is in the wrong plane and an intramyometrial space is created; this false passage might actually distend with pressure of the fluid and further fool the surgeon (Figs 5A and B).

So always suspect false passage if you see crisis cross muscle fibers with no evidence of ostia.

Always abandon the surgery and repost the patient after 2–3 months as the false passage can cause significant amount of glycine to get absorbed because the false space created in between the myometrial muscle walls has lot of vascularity (Flow chart 1).

Often the force required to dilate the internal os so that the 27 Fr resectoscope passes is quite significant. In such circumstances using the Ed's solution and also using the forward column of fluid pressure to slowly distend and dilate the os will help.

Repeat surgeries: In a series of analysis it has been found that repeat hysteroscopic surgeries are more risky than primary procedures. In a study of endometrial ablation it was found that risk of major complication during second surgery was much more (9.3% vs. 2.0%).[6]

Tackling the perforation: Cold perforations caused by scissors (Fig. 1) or dilators can be managed conservatively in most cases. However, when the perforation has happened with thermal energy then rigorous step to step management approach should be undertaken (Figs 2 and 3). The first step is to call for immediate laparoscopic inspection of the entire abdomen. While the arrangements for the laparoscopy are made, it is always worthwhile distending the pelvis through the perforation site with normal saline and gently inspecting the local area with the hysteroscope itself which is navigated through the perforated site into the abdominal cavity. Further management depends on the laparoscopic findings. Even if no positive findings are found, it is always wise to advise the patient to observe for any signs and symptoms of perforation, to monitor her temperature twice daily and report in the event of any abnormality (Flow chart 2).

Caution: Thermal injury at times may present as late as 2 weeks after surgery.

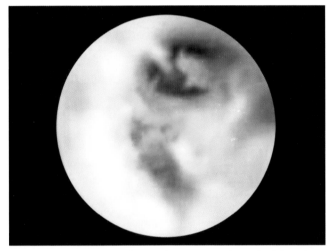

Fig. 4: False passage in the cervix seen posterior to the internal os

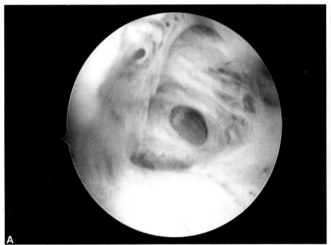
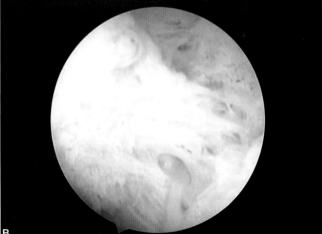

Figs 5A and B: False passage: Notice the crisscross myometrial fibers and the bleeding vessel (shown with an arrow) indicating wrong plane

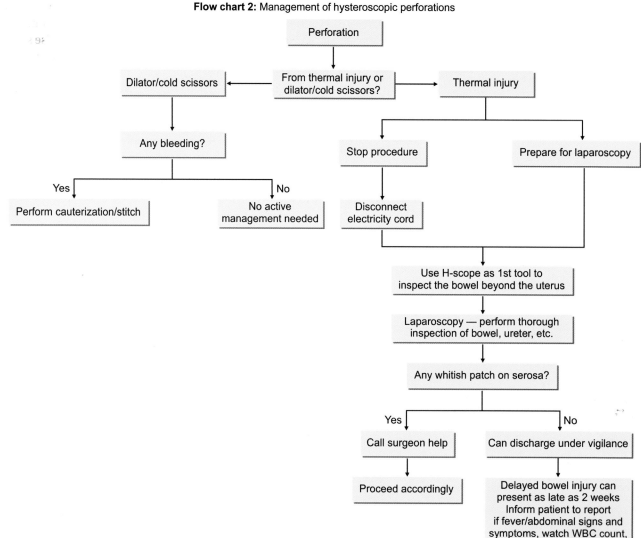

Flow chart 2: Management of hysteroscopic perforations

Intraoperative Hemorrhage

This is the second most common complication (Fig. 6) and at times may be severe. Mostly it happens in procedures like myomectomies and ablations. Significant bleeding is seen rarely if a vessel is lacerated or in procedures where myometrial layers are disrupted. In different series 0.5–1.9% of cases required interventions to stop bleeding.

Management strategies:

❑ Balloon tamponade method: A Foley's catheter No. 12 or 14 (30 cc capacity of balloon) is inserted into the cavity and injected with 10–20 mL according to uterine size. This is left in situ and removed after 8–10 hours if there is no bleeding. If 20 mL of saline has been used we generally reduce it to 10 mL after about an hour when

bleeding has settled to avoid endometrial pressure necrosis.

❑ Uterine packing: In this about half an inch roller gauze which is previously dipped in a solution of normal saline containing vasopressin (20 IU of vasopressin mixed with 60 mL of NS) is used to pack the uterus using an artery forceps.

❑ Using vaporizing electrode: This method can be effectively used if a solitary large pulsatile vessel is noted intraoperatively. Touch the vaporizing tip to actively bleeding spot keeping the coagulation mode on at about 60–80 Watt but not more than that.

Caution: Sometimes near the cornual areas myometrium may be very thin especially if resectoscope has been used near this area and perforation with intra-abdominal burns can happen while coagulating these areas.

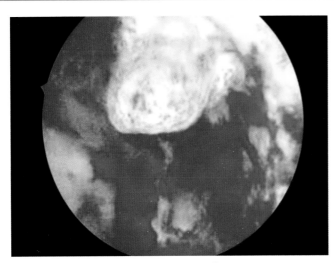

Fig. 6: Intracavitary bleeding seen in resectoscopy

Media-related Complications

This is a major problem while using resectoscope and glycine as media.

Overall incidence of dilutional hyponatremia is 0.2% as seen by AAGL survey in 1993.[7]

It is known that monopolar current is not compatible with electrolytic solutions. Thus, operative hysteroscopy requires media like 1.5% glycine, 3% sorbitol or mannitol. All these may be associated with dilutional hyponatremia, overload and hypo-osmolality.

The advent of bipolar energy using resectoscopes has relieved this problem to a great extent as these use NS as media. The deficit of media allowed is quite high to almost 2 L before overload sets in.

However, with judicious use monopolar resectoscopes are a good option as the technique is time tried, fast and effective for large pathology. Also, in experienced hands studies have found the same results in terms of complications associated with media use when bipolar and monopolar methods are compared.

Who is at risk: It is noted that it is actually the premenopausal young female with a good intrinsic estrogenic load who is at maximum risk of glycine associated complications. This is because the estrogen (E) and progesterone (P) both act to inhibit the Na-K-ATPase pump in the brain. This pump protects against cerebral edema. So when glycine related dilutional hyponatremia sets in, the brain swells as it tries to become isosmotic with vascular system. This can cause severe brain damage and even permanent neurological damage and death. This is less often the case with men and postmenopausal women although dilutional hyponatremia may develop in them too.

Protocols and vigilance drill in OT to avoid media-related complications: High degree of vigilance not only from the surgeon but the entire team is effective in performing safe surgery without media complications. We take the following measures to ensure the same:

❑ *Outflow inflow tracking:* An accountability of the entire fluid input and output should be strictly adhered to. There is no scope for "assuming" losses by fluid in wet drapes or spilt on the floor. State-of-the-art monitoring of fluid can be done by electronic inflow outflow systems (Fig. 7). However if this is not available, even then meticulous monitoring of outflow is possible by collecting entire fluid in suction bottle and good plastic pouch like drapes (Fig. 8) which are easily available nowadays.

❑ *Understanding the pressure mathematics of operative hysteroscopy (Flow chart 3):* The secret of avoiding media-related problems is to minimize the absorption.

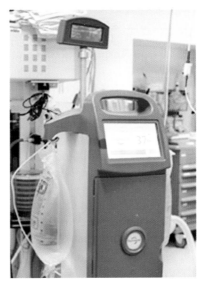

Fig. 7: Electronic fluid monitoring system in operative hysteroscopy

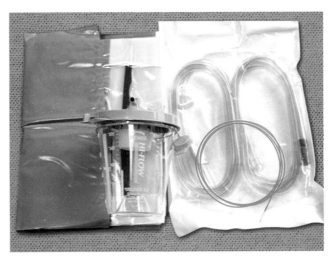

Fig. 8: Draping set for operative hysteroscopy

Flow chart 3: Drill to avoid media complications

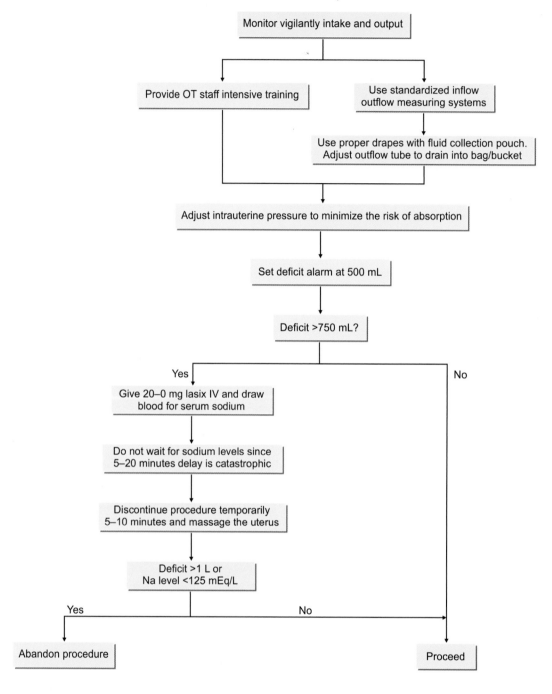

This can be achieved by operating in and around the mean arterial pressure (MAP). But in practicality this is difficult to maintain as hysteroscopy is not a closed system and fluid from the uterine cavity leaks out at many points. This causes difficulty in maintaining a particular set operating pressure.

The leaky points from where fluid escapes are:
❖ Tubal ostia
❖ Patulous cervix

❖ Absorption from vascular myometrial bed (large pathology like large myomas can cause more absorption).

Although the electronic ENDOMAT® units do tell us the pressure at which we are operating but the exact intrauterine pressure might be different. Thus, a good practical tip is to adjust the pressure levels of ENDOMAT® unit seeing the MAP and also adjust the outflow such that minimal bleeding is seen in the operating field ensuring that the intrauterine pressure is lower than the MAP because we are actually seeing the blood being pumped in by the patient's vascular system.

❑ Use of dilute vasopressin as described—Ed's solution
❑ Seal all bleeders at the time with coagulation current to minimize bleeding and hence absorption
❑ Some surgeons recommend giving preoperative GnRH-a, leuprolide for 2 months prior to surgery will shrink the size of the myomas but the author personally does not favor this approach as these agents may cause shrinkage of myometrium more than the myoma rendering operative hysteroscopy, i.e. dilatation and resection more difficult. However, for very large myomas more than 4–5 cm, it is worth giving these agents
❑ If possible, we operate under locoregional anesthesia spinal or epidural anesthesia as patient's sensorium can be judged continuously. Confusion and irritability are the early signs of hyponatremia
❑ Always a preoperative electrolytes level is sent before starting surgery
❑ During surgery the first alarm is set at 500 mL of deficit and second at 750 mL of deficit. At this time 20–40 mg of Lasix* may be given and serum Na level is again calculated
❑ Make massaging movements on the uterus to cause contractions of the blood vessels
❑ Stop surgery preferably at deficit of 1.2 L, never proceed if deficit has reached 1.5 L
❑ While using bipolar devices a false sense of security should be avoided as deficit of about 2 L of fluid may lead to overload related problems.

VASOVAGAL REACTION/SYNCOPE

Usually seen with inadequate anesthesia or while performing cervical dilatation during office procedures. This entity is rare and at times may be severe. Usually it is accompanied by a nausea, dizziness, pallor or sweating.

Treatment is supportive like:
❑ Stopping the surgery
❑ Leg raising/Trendelenburg position
❑ Fluid administration
❑ Atropine if reaction is severe.

Note: Instillation of local anesthetic agent into the cervical canal may not reduce pain but decreases the incidence of vasovagal reaction [Level A evidence Royal College of Obstetricians and Gynaecologists (RCOG) guidelines].

GAS EMBOLISM

This is a potentially serious complication which can turn into a real emergency as it can be lethal.

The difference between gas and air embolism differs in the composition of gases.

In gas embolism the embolus is composed of electrosurgical vapors or carbon dioxide (CO_2) which is used as media while in air embolism it is due to the improper purging of tubings or entry of air from insertion or reinsertion of scope causing *pistoning* effect of air into cervical and uterine veins.

CO_2 is a soluble gas so embolism reverts back fast but in contrast air embolism is likely to be lethal.

In a survey[8] which was conducted to analyze seven cases of air embolism it was noted that:
❑ 5 patients underwent hysteroscopy for abnormal uterine bleeding
❑ 2 patients had intrauterine septae and synechiae
❑ 5 out of 7 patients were in Trendelenburg position (head low) while operating
❑ 3 out of 7 had difficult dilatation of cervix.

In each of these cases first sign was noted by anesthetist like sudden decrease in end tidal CO_2, bradycardia, decrease in oxygen saturation and precordial mill wheel murmur (classic sign of air in the heart).

Thus looking into these a fairly clear consensus evolves:
❑ Position of patient's heart and vena cava should never be below the level of uterus. This is often seen as surgeon requests for head low to be able to put speculum easily and see the cervix well. This facilitates the air entry into the large veins. So never perform hysteroscopy in head low position
❑ Avoid dilatation of the cervix with force and creation of false passage. These are an invitation ground for air to enter into abnormally exposed vessels
❑ Expose the cervix and vagina to minimal room air. Do not introduce and take out the scope very frequently. Also keep the last dilator in place in the cervical canal till the resectoscope is fully ready to go in
❑ The intracervical injection of vasopressin especially when operating large pathology helps to block gas from entering circulation.

Management: Standard Protocol

❑ Stop procedure and call help
❑ Increase inspiratory oxygen
❑ Give Durant's position (left lateral decubitus position)

❏ Hemodynamic support like large NS bolus, dobutamine, norepinephrine, etc.
❏ If able and appropriate conditions exist, start hyperbaric oxygen plus central venous catheter, aspiration of air from right atrium may be attempted
❏ If needed, continue with cardiopulmonary resuscitation (CPR) protocol.

ELECTROSURGICAL COMPLICATIONS

Most electrosurgical complications are similar to those in laparoscopy.
❏ Perforation of uterus with active electrode—already dealt with
❏ Current diversion to outer sheath
❏ Vilos et al. have reported current diversion to outer sheath due to insulation failures in cases of endometrial ablations. To avoid this, inspect carefully and ensure intact insulation.[9,10] Thermal injury can be due to overheating of the returning plate. Use of second dispersive pad to dissipate the heat can be done to avoid this
❏ Capacitive coupling may also divert current. This effect can happen due to the inherent sheath within sheath design of the resectoscope and can happen especially when high voltage coagulation current is used. So restrict the use to maximum of 60–80 watt. The best way to avoid damage is to use:
  ❖ Short bursts of current, and
  ❖ Place a damp mop from the posterior vagina over the introitus and perineal region.

POSTOPERATIVE AND LATE COMPLICATIONS

These may be:
❏ Infections
❏ Endometrial cancer
❏ Iatrogenic adenomyosis
❏ Hematometra
❏ Postendometrial ablation tubal ligation syndrome
❏ Pregnancy-related concerns.

Infection

Most series report an incidence rate of 0.2%. Rate of 0.3–2% is reported in the form of endometritis, PID, pyometra, etc. These are most common after resection of submucous myomas. Prophylactic antibiotics, e.g. a single dose of IV ceftizoxime 1 g 30–60 minutes before surgery and doxycycline 100 mg BD for 7 days is generally given to reduce the infection.

Endometrial Cancer

This is an area of concern as it has been found that many females who have been evaluated for peri- and post-menopausal bleeding have a risk of dissemination of endometrial cells into the peritoneal cavity. Endometrial sampling should be done before patients are put for endometrial ablations to prevent wrong treatment. Performing office hysteroscopy with biopsy under low pressure is a good option to diagnose early endometrial cancer.

There is a fear of burying endometrial glands deeper into myometrial layers during ablation and this, in theory, can implant an early cancer in deeper layers. If a patient comes with a bleeding after ablation then such a woman should be again evaluated with office hysteroscopy and endometrial sampling. In fact, a study by Cooper[11] et al. suggests that females with high risk for endometrial cancer and abnormal uterine bleeding which is not relieved by hormonal therapy should undergo hysterectomy rather than ablation.

Note: If atypia is present on biopsy report, there is no role of hysteroscopic ablation and hysterectomy becomes mandatory.

Iatrogenic Adenomyosis

This happens possibly due to two mechanisms:
1. During ablation islands of incompletely resected endometrium may be left behind. Scarring over this tissue causes these endometrial glands to get embedded into deep myometrium.
2. Viable endometrial glandular cells may reach deeper layers of the myometrium via opened up blood vessels and get implanted there. This may be avoided by using the roller ball after the cutting loop so that there is deeper and more uniform spread of energy. This ensures that no viable endometrium is left behind.

Hematometra

Hematometra can be formed if after any operative procedure there is formation of adhesions at the level of internal os or lower uterine segment. This prevents egress of blood through os.

This is more so if during an ablation procedure the endocervical endometrium gets ablated. Treatment is to repeat hysteroscopy and perform adhesiolysis and drain the hematometra.

Postendometrial Ablation Tubal Ligation Syndrome

This is a peculiar condition that develops typically in females who have history of tubal ligation and later underwent ablation due to abnormal uterine bleeding. When such women undergo ablation if the cornual areas are improperly resected leaving behind viable endometrium then this cornual area bleeds cyclically leading to hematometra localized in the cornual region and proximal part of the tubal stump. This causes discomfort and pain.

Prevention

Performing cornual ablation with care and using the roller ball in inaccessible areas can prevent this.

Treatment

❑ Hysterectomy
❑ Bilateral salpingectomy
❑ Repeat resection at cornu.

Pregnancy-related Issues

❑ Pregnancy after ablation has a complicated outcome. Incidence is 0.2–1.6%. Patient must always be told that ablation does not prevent pregnancy. In those patients who choose to continue pregnancy, outcome is very poor with a high chance of intrauterine growth restriction (IUGR), placenta accreta, and preterm labor.
❑ Uterine ruptures after myoma or septum resection and lateral metroplasty have been reported. In an analysis of such cases it was found that an intraoperative perforation which happened during procedure greatly increased the chance of uterine rupture during pregnancy. Lateral metroplasty is a myometrial scarring procedure. Such cases should be very judiciously chosen and posted for elective cesarean section with continuous obstetric monitoring.

■ CONCLUSION

Complications are more frequent when devices are misused and safety margins are neglected. Prevention of complication starts by raising awareness of the risks and precautions. About half of all complications are due to entry-related injuries. Adoption of standard protocols and techniques regarding the insertion of hysteroscope and technical improvement in instruments and also proper skill acquisition by surgeons will reduce complications on their own.

■ REFERENCES

1. Hulka JF, Peterson HA, Philips JM, Surrey MW. Operative by hysteroscopy: American Association of Gynecologic Laparoscopists 1993 Member Survey. J Am Assoc Gynecol. 1995;2:131-2.
2. Shveiky D, Rojansky N, Revel A, Benshushan A, Laufer N, Shushan A. Complications of hysteroscopic surgery "Beyond the learning curve". J Minim Invasive Gynecol. 2007;14(2):218-22.
3. Jansen FW, Vrederoogd CB, van Ulzen K, Hermans J, Trimbos JB, Trimbos-Kemper TC. Complications of hysteroscopy: a prospective multicentric study. Obstet Gynecol. 2006;96(2):266-70.
4. Propst AM, Liberman RF, Harlow BL, Ginsberg ES. Complications of hysteroscopic surgery: predicting patients at risk. Obstet Gynecol. 2000;96(4):57-70.
5. Ostrzenski A. Resectoscopic cervical trauma minimized by Laminaria digitata insertion preoperatively. Int J Fertil. 1994;39;111-3.
6. Mac Lean Fraser E, Peneva D, Vilos GA. Perioperative complication rates of primary and repeat endometrial ablations. J Am Obstet Gynecol. 1983;147:869-72.
7. Loffer FD. Complications of hysteroscopy—their cause, prevention and correction. J Am Assoc Gynecol Laparosc. 1995;3(1):11-26.
8. Corson SL, Brooks PG, Soderstrom RM. Gynecologic endoscopic gas embolism. Fertil Steril. 1996;65(3):529-33.
9. Vilos GA, Brown S, Graham G, McCulloch S, Borg P. Genital tract electrical burns during hysteroscopic endometrial ablation, report of 13 cases in United States of Canada. J Am Assoc Gynecol Laparosc. 2000;7:141-7.
10. Munro MG. Factors affecting capacitative current diversion with a resectoscope: an in vitro study. J Am Assoc Gynec Laparosc. 2003;10:450-60.
11. Cooper JM, Brady RM. Late complications of operative hysteroscopy. Obstet Gynecol Clin North Am. 2000;27:367-74.

Index